HEALTH AND HEALTH CARE

2010

THE FORECAST, THE CHALLENGE

SECOND EDITION

CONTRIBUTORS

Authors: Roy Amara, Karen Bodenhorn, Mary Cain, Rick Carlson, Janet Chambers, Diana Cypress, Hank Dempsey, Rod Falcon, Roberto Garces, Jaycee Garrett, Danielle Gasper, Katherine Haynes Sanstad, Matthew Holt, Susannah Kirsch, Nandini Kuehn, Heather Kuiper, Elaina Kyrouz, Robert Mittman, Ellen Morrison, Ian Morrison, Geoffrey Nilsen, Marina Pascali, Andrew Robertson, Denise Runde, Jane Sarasohn-Kahn, Greg Schmid, Charlie Wilson, Kathy Yu

Editors: Charles Grosel, Melinda Hamilton, Julie Koyano, Susan Eastwood

Art Director: Janet Chambers

Graphic Designers: Adrianna Aranda, Robin Bogott, Diana Cypress, Jeanné Haffner, Melinda Hamilton

HEALTH AND HEALTH CARE

2010

THE FORECAST, THE CHALLENGE

SECOND EDITION

Prepared by

The Institute for the Future

Support for this publication was provided by

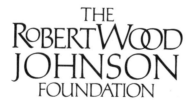

THE
ROBERT WOOD
JOHNSON
FOUNDATION

Princeton, NJ

January 2003

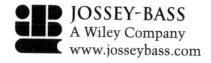

JOSSEY-BASS
A Wiley Company
www.josseybass.com

Published by Jossey-Bass
A Wiley Imprint
989 Market Street, San Francisco, CA 94103-1741   www.josseybass.com

Jossey-Bass books and products are available through most bookstores. To contact Jossey-Bass directly call our Customer Care Department within the U.S. at 800-956-7739, outside the U.S. at 317-572-3986 or fax 317-572-4002.

Jossey-Bass also publishes its books in a variety of electronic formats. Some content that appears in print may not be available in electronic books.

Library of Congress Cataloging-in-Publication Data

Health and health care 2010 : the forecast, the challenge / [contributors, Roy Amara . . . [et al.]]
     p. cm.
  "To recognize the 25th anniversary of its founding, The Robert Wood Johnson Foundation asked the Institute for the Future (IFTF) to forecast the future of health and and health care in America . . ."—Introduction.
  Includes bibliographical references and index.
  ISBN 0-7879-5974-x
    1. Medical care—United States—Forecasting. 2. Public Health—United States—Forecasting. I. Amara, Roy. II. Robert Wood Johnson Foundation. III Institute for the Future.

SECOND EDITION
PB Printing 10 9 8 7 6 5 4 3 2 1

HEALTH AND HEALTH CARE 2010

Contents

FIGURES

TABLES

SIDEBARS

ABBREVIATIONS AND ACRONYMS

AAMC	American Association of Medical Colleges
AAPCC	adjusted average per capita costs
AARP	American Association of Retired Persons
AFDC	Aid to Families with Dependent Children
AHA	American Hospital Association
AIDS	acquired immunodeficiency syndrome
AMA	American Medical Association
AMC	academic medical center
CBO	Congressional Budget Office
CDC	Centers for Disease Control and Prevention
COGME	Council on Graduate Medical Education
CPR	computer-based patient record
CPS	Current Population Survey
CT	computed tomography
DRG	diagnosis-related group
DSH	disproportionate share hospital
EBRI	Employee Benefits Research Institute
EMR	electronic medical record
ETS	environmental tobacco smoke
FDA	Food and Drug Administration
FFS	fee for service
FTE	full-time equivalent
GDP	gross domestic product
GME	graduate medical education
HCFA	Health Care Financing Administration
HEDIS	health plan employer data and information set
HIPAA	Health Insurance Portability and Accountability Act
HIV	human immunodeficiency virus
HMO	health maintenance organization
HPV	human papilloma virus
IMGs	international medical graduates
IOM	Institute of Medicine

IPA	independent practice association
IVR	interactive voice response
LPN	licensed practical nurses
MRI	magnetic resonance imaging
MRN	magnetic resonance neurography
MSA	medical savings account
MSO	management services organization
MTBE	methlytertiary butyl ether
NAFTA	North American Free Trade Agreement
NCQA	National Committee on Quality Assurance
NHE	National Health Expenditure
NHIS	National Health Insurance Survey
NP	nurse practitioner
OTC	over the counter
PA	physician's assistant
PC	personal computer
PET	positron emission tomography
POS	point of service
PPM	physician practice management
PPO	preferred provider organization
PPS	prospective payment system
PSN	provider service network
RN	registered nurse
SAMHSA	Substance Abuse and Mental Health Services Association
SES	socioeconomic status
SIDS	sudden infant death syndrome
SNF	skilled nursing facility
SV40	simian virus 40
WHO	World Health Organization

HEALTH AND HEALTH CARE 2010

Introduction

To recognize the 25th anniversary of its founding, in 1997 The Robert Wood Johnson Foundation asked the Institute for the Future (IFTF) to forecast the future of health and health care in America for the period between 2000 and the year 2010. This is the Second Edition of that Forecast, revised and updated to reflect the changes that have occurred since our initial work in 1997–1998. As we originally stated, the purpose of this forecast is to provide the reader with a description of critical factors that will influence health and health care in the first decade of the 21st century.

In this book, we have singled out the trends most likely to influence the course of Americans' health and the state of the American health care delivery system in the next decade. The drivers of this system are relatively stable and predictable from now to 2005. Beyond 2005, and through to 2010 and beyond, the future of health and health care is much more volatile.

To cope with the uncertainties that exist in these later years, IFTF has created three different scenarios that describe emerging visions of health care in this country. They are titled Stormy Weather, The Long and Winding Road, and The Sunny Side of the Street, and they are

described in the first chapter of this report and depicted in the map that is bound to the inside of the back cover. We hope that the findings of this study will be of value to community service organizations, hospitals, providers, payers, and researchers in the long-term planning processes that support their own visions of the future.

This forecast is organized in the following way:

- *Health and Health Care Forecast*
  This first chapter provides an overview of the important issues covered in greater detail throughout the forecast. It functions as an executive summary of the topics that are covered in greater detail in the subsequent chapters.

- *Demographic Trends and the Burden of Disease*
  In 2010, the American population will be older and more ethnically and racially diverse. The burden of disease is shifting toward chronic illnesses that stem from our behaviors. This chapter draws attention to the importance of these shifts.

- *Health Care's Demand Side*
  The growth rate of American health care costs steadily increased from

1960 through the early 1990s, then slowed dramatically. This chapter reviews the historical factors that drove these changes and forecasts the health care cost increases in both the public and private sectors over the next 10 years.

■ *Health Insurance*
Changes in the health insurance system and in the numbers of the uninsured are discussed in this chapter. The growth of Medicare and Medicaid, as well as new versions of managed care products, are projected through the year 2010.

■ *Managed Care*
During the 1990's, managed care became the dominant health care insurance and delivery system, covering more than 60 percent of publicly and privately insured lives. It was instrumental in controlling national health care expenditures during that decade, and promised to deliver comprehensive, coordinated health care. Despite a recent backlash from physicians, consumers, and the media, managed care will persist as a mechanism to control costs and coordinate the delivery of care. This section outlines three scenarios that depict the evolution of managed care over the next decade.

■ *Health Care Providers*
There will be continued change in the way health care is organized and delivered over the next 10 to 15 years. The surplus of hospital beds will contribute to a buyer's market, and a new role for intermediaries will emerge.

This chapter examines in depth the battle that will evolve in the medical management arena.

■ *Health Care Workforce*
There has been little real change in the way physicians practice medicine since the invention of the telephone. Although physicians are still the central figures in American health care, the current oversupply of doctors and the emergence of new health care provider roles may create changes in the health care delivery system over the next decade. The supply and demand of these providers are projected through 2010.

■ *Medical Technologies*
New medical technologies have been one of the key driving forces in both the cost and the organization of 20th-century health care. This chapter reviews eight new medical technologies that will affect the provision of patient care in the next 10 years and examines both their potential positive effects and the barriers that may stand in the way of their adoption.

■ *Information Technologies*
The health care industry has lagged behind other industries in implementing information technologies that streamline business and clinical processes. We forecast that changes in information technology as applied to health care will be a prime catalyst of change in the future.

■ *Health Care Consumers*
As a new, educated generation of informed consumers begins to use

more health services, it is demanding more information, choice, and control than ever before. These empowered consumers have the capacity to change dramatically the culture of health care. In addition, the press of health care cost containment may lead to a three-tiered system of access to care that seriously disenfranchises people who do not have insurance.

■ *Public Health Services*
Modern public health is practiced in an environment of increasing globalism and resource scarcity. New developments in technology, public health strategy, and public-private partnerships will shape future successes and failures in public health. This chapter examines and forecasts the future of public health services, including organizational and environmental health issues.

■ *Mental Health*
The incidence and prevalence of mental illness in our society and the effects that reverberate through our economy and culture are daunting. This chapter explores the issues that surround the provision of mental health services, and forecasts the future of new approaches, emphasizing community-based programs.

■ *Children's Health*
Children are the backbone of our future. The integrity of their health, especially in terms of prevention of disease and the establishment of healthy behaviors, is paramount to a flourishing and productive society. This chapter describes the challenges facing child

health today, and forecasts the progress we will make during the next ten years in creating an environment in which to raise healthy children.

■ *Health and Health Care of America's Seniors*
As the Baby Boom cohort of the population ages, there will be an increased demand for medical services and a greater interest in adopting healthy lifestyles as a way to age gracefully. Increased demands on the Medicare Program to finance the health care of people over 65 years will put significant pressure on the health care delivery system. These new demands may well outstrip our ability to provide services. This chapter analyzes the effect that the change in demographics and consumer behaviors will have on care for our aging population.

■ *Chronic Care in America*
The numbers of chronically ill people in America will grow significantly in the next decade, as our aging population lives longer and confronts the illnesses inherent in growing older. We estimate the growth in patients with chronic diseases, and forecast the new services and technologies that will be available to them.

■ *Disease Managemen*
The U.S. health care system originally was created to treat patients with acute conditions. Today, the leading diseases that cause death and disability are no longer acute, but rather chronic illnesses. By 2010, 40 percent of Americans will have a chronic illness, and caring for them will cost up

to $600 billion each year. Disease management is quickly becoming the key strategy for easing the health and economic burdens of chronic disease. This chapter provides a description of the evolution of disease management into the 21st century, with implications for key players in the health care system.

- *Health Behaviors*
  Our health behaviors, namely smoking, poor dietary habits, lack of exercise, alcohol abuse, the use of illicit drugs, and violence, influence up to 50 percent of our health status. Although we do not anticipate radical improvements in these health behaviors in the coming decade, the emphasis that managed care has placed on prevention will help us begin to decrease these harmful behaviors. In addition, community-based programs that change or restrict the environment will also be very important.

- *Expanded Perspective on Health*
  A definition of health must have equal applicability to everyone: to the fully well, to people who are unwell because of disease or illness that is treatable or curable, and to that growing segment of the population with genetic or acquired impairment, such as people with chronic disease or disability. Over the next decade, our view of health will be expanded to encompass mental, social, and spiritual well being.

WILD CARDS

Wild cards are events that have less than a 10 percent chance of occurring, but will have a tremendous impact on society and business if they do occur. The point of wild cards is not to predict an outcome but to expand our peripheral vision regarding the total range of possibilities that exist; to offer a larger context within which to consider mainstream forecasts; and to prepare for surprises in the event that wildcards do come to pass.

ABOUT THE INSTITUTE FOR THE FUTURE

Located in Menlo Park, California, IFTF is an independent, nonprofit research firm that specializes in long-term forecasting. Founded in 1968, IFTF has become a leader in applied research for nonprofit organizations, corporations, industries, and governments. IFTF has a cross-disciplinary professional staff that works internationally, analyzing health, technology, and broad public policy, forecasting potential scenarios for the future, and identifying markets for new products and next-generation technologies.

IFTF's Health Team is in its 17th year of providing health care data tracking and forecasting based both on primary and secondary research data. Our research projects focus on emerging trends in the organization, financing, and delivery of health care services, technologies, and products, with an emphasis on public policy changes as well as on the impact of private sector markets. The Health Team evaluates the forces that both drive and resist innovation and forecasts not only the direction but also the pace of change in the health and health care environments.

ACKNOWLEDGMENTS

The idea for this study originated with Ruby Hearn, Ph.D., and Steven Schroeder, M.D., of The Robert Wood Johnson Foundation. They believed that there would be value in developing the forecast as a long-range strategic planning tool for health organizations. Along with Dr. Hearn and Dr. Schroeder, Frank Karel, Ann Searight, Maureen Cozine, Connie Pechura, Ph.D., Beth Stevens, Ph.D., Nancy Kaufman, Ph.D., and Jeanne Weber provided consistent oversight and cogent direction to the project, helping all of us to focus, refine, and improve the final product. Lois Shevlin and Phyllis Kane were invaluable in guiding us through the planning and development processes. We are indebted to them and are extremely grateful for their support and guidance throughout this project.

The IFTF staff could not have completed the research necessary to formulate this forecast without the help of many colleagues, experts, and friends. Among those who were instrumental in identifying and refining issues and trends with us, we would like to thank particularly the following people:

Nancy Adler, Ph.D.; Adrianna Aranda; Morris Barer, Ph.D.; John Berthko; Katherine Binns; Bob Blendon, ScD; Robin Bogott; Janet Chambers; Rick Carlson; Toby Cole, M.D.; Rena Convissor; John Danaher, M.D.; Karen Davis, Ph.D.; Joe DeLuca; Paolo del Vecchio;Al Dembe; Susan Edgman-Levitan; Amy Einshorn; Carroll Estes, Ph.D.; Robert Evans, Ph.D..; Brian Finch, Ph.D.; Barbara Fuller; Brianna Gass; Suzanne Gelber Ph.D.; Michael Goldberg; Howard H. Goldman, M.D. Ph.D.; Michael Goze; Peter Grant, Jessie Gruman, Ph.D.; David Gustafson, Ph.D.; Melinda Hamilton; David Hansen; Kathy Harty; David Hayes-Bautista, Ph.D.; David Hemenway, Ph.D.; Rona Hu, M.D.; Patrick Jeffries; Don Kemper; Bill Kerr; Quita Kirk; Nandini Kuehn, Ph.D., Paula Lack; Kim Lawrence; Julia Lear, Ph.D.; Bob Leitman; Jeff Lemieux; Katherine Levit; Karen Linkins, Ph.D.; Marty Lynch; Ron Manderscheid, Ph.D.; Alexandra Matveyeva; Molly Mettler; Arnie Milstein, M.D.; Al Mulley, M.D.; Al Martin, M.D.; Gordon Moore, M.D.; H. Richard Nesson, M.D.; Robert Newcomer, Ph.D.; Mark Petrakis; David Reuben, M.D.; Dorothy Rice, Ph.D.; James Robinson, Ph.D.; Richard Rockefeller, M.D.; John Rother; Joan Rummelsburg; Pamela Russell; Bill Scanlon; Andrew Scharlach, Ph.D.; Monica Seghers; Cary Sennet, M.D.; J. J. Singh; Mark Smith, M.D.; Elliott Sternberg, M.D.; Felicia Stewart, M.D.; Jon Stewart; Humphrey Taylor; Sally Tom; Joan Trauner, Ph.D.; and Leonard Zegans, M.D..

Their thoughtfulness, insightful comments, and generous contributions of time and energy added significantly to our own knowledge and to the robustness of the forecast.

Special thanks go to Jean Hagan, Julie Koyano, Sue Reynolds and Susan Eastwood for their sensational editorial work and patience, and to Jon Peck for his guidance in publishing this work.

Andy Pasternack, our publisher at Jossey-Bass, achieved early sainthood for his continuing patience and support during this process.

This forecast was submitted to the Foundation as a report to RWJF and is solely the responsibility of the Institute for the Future and its afffiliates.

With thanks,

Wendy Everett
Director

Roy Amara

Mary Cain

Rick Carlson

Janet Chambers

Diana Cypress

Hank Dempsey

Rod Falcon

Jaycee Garrett

Danielle Gasper

Katherine Haynes Sanstad

Matthew Holt

Susannah Kirsch

Nandini Kuehn

Heather Kuiper

Elaina Kyrouz

Robert Mittman

Ellen Morrison

Ian Morrison

Geoffrey Nilsen

Marina Pascali

Andrew Robertson

Denise Runde

Jane Sarasohn-Kahn

Greg Schmid

Charlie Wilson

Kathy Yu

*Institute for the Future
Menlo Park, California*

Karen Bodenhorn

Roberto Garces

California Center for Health Improvement

HEALTH AND HEALTH CARE

2010

THE FORECAST, THE CHALLENGE

SECOND EDITION

CHAPTER 1

Health and Health Care Forecast

Executive Summary

Fifteen years ago, the key issues in the American health care system were classic: containing *costs* while improving *access* to care for people and maintaining *quality* of services. Then the rapid cost increases of the late 1980s, combined with the recession of the early 1990s, added a new issue to the list: ensuring *security of benefits*.

unholy △

After the political dust of the 1992–1994 debate about health reform settled, several structural shifts in the system became apparent. Managed care—designed to contain costs—went from being an aberration to being the mainstream method of providing health insurance. Several new issues came to the forefront of health policy: monitoring the activities of managed care plans, organizing health care providers, and evaluating the quality of care delivered to patients. Although the recent strong economy and job market has increased the security of health benefits for some people, the issue of how to pay for care for a growing number of uninsured Americans remains with us.

None of these issues will be completely resolved in the next few years. Instead, a new group of issues will join them. They include organizing insurers and intermediaries, along with providers; incorporating consumers into health care decision making; determining responsibility for medical management; and improving the health behaviors of the American people. These will be the health battlegrounds of the next decade.

This chapter provides an overview of our 10-year forecast of health and health care. We describe the path from now until 2005 in terms of the future legislative and regulatory contexts; changes in the demographics and attitudes of patients, populations, and consumers; the concerns of payers about health care costs; the organization of health plans and insurers; the structure of hospitals, provider organizations, and the public health system; the role of medical information technologies; and the forthcoming shifts in care processes and medical management. Beyond 2005, our forecast splits into three scenarios—one optimistic about the impact of changes on the health of the population, one pessimistic about the ability of American society to provide coverage and access to care, and one in which incrementalism reigns supreme.

LEGISLATION

Legislative activity will be set against a background of incremental legislative reform. The failure of the health reform effort from 1992 to 1994 dulled the appetite of most politicians for significant health regulation. In addition, there is almost no support for large-scale social programs targeting the poor or the uninsured. Major government reform is therefore unlikely. Strong support for the current Medicare and Social Security systems means that change in the benefits of these systems will be slow. There will be few initiatives to design new government programs beyond the limited programs enacted in the past few years—insurance portability and children's coverage. Neither of these two initiatives will have a significant impact on the overall number of uninsured or the general health insurance market.

Government legislation in two significant areas will have some impact on the mainstream health care system.

First, there will be legislative outcomes as a result of a backlash against managed care. While there are few clearly articulated alternatives to market-based health care in the United States, there is considerable support for legislation to curb what are seen as health plan abuses. Given that these regulations will require little money from public coffers, we can expect more regulation of health plan activity, including disclosure rules, mandates for clinical protocols such as the 48-hour hospital stay for maternity patients, and medical records privacy laws. Although the effect of such regulations on the overall market may be slight, there will be significant effects on plan and provider operations.

Second, Medicare may look very different than it did in the early 1990s, when its financial future became uncertain. Many Medicare recipients will not be in the traditional fee-for-service (FFS) program but instead will be in health maintenance organizations (HMOs), preferred provider organizations (PPOs), or some other organized health plan arrangement. Cost controls enacted in the 1997 Balanced Budget Act will have changed the way providers deal with Medicare patients, in particular placing the reimbursement for outpatient, home health, and skilled nursing facilities (SNFs) on a prospective payment system. It's plausible that the baseline will be sufficiently different that "incremental" legislation in the future could make a big change in the nature of the program. But Medicare remains the second most popular program among the most powerful demographic group in America—the elderly—and politicians have learned to tamper with it at their peril.

Consequently, our forecast for legislation is one of continued incremental program change directed primarily at providers and with little direct effect on beneficiaries. The real challenge—changing Medicare so that it can afford to cover the vast number of baby boomers retiring after 2010—will not be dealt with until later in the decade.

DEMOGRAPHICS: PATIENTS, POPULATIONS, AND NEW CONSUMERS

In the next decade, Americans will be getting older and living longer. By 2010 the average life expectancy will be up to

Figure 1-1. Increasing diversity of the United States population

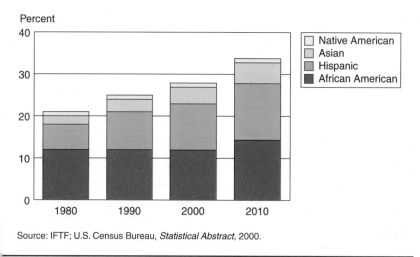

Source: IFTF; U.S. Census Bureau, *Statistical Abstract*, 2000.

Figure 1-2. The real story of diversity in 2010 is regional.

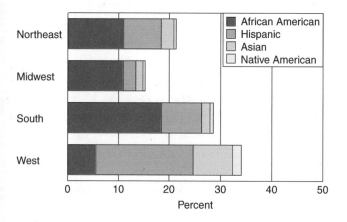

Source: IFTF; U.S. Census Bureau, *Statistical Abstract*, 2000.

Tiers of Coverage

Empowered Consumers:	38 percent
Worried Consumers:	34 percent
Excluded Consumers:	28 percent

86 years of age for a woman and 76 years for a man. In addition, there will be more than 100,000 people over the age of 100 in the year 2010. However, the first baby boomers will not turn 65 until 2010, so although the population is aging, it's aging quite slowly.

[margin note: major gap]

America will soon be a more ethnically diverse nation (see Figures 1-1 and 1-2). Currently 74 percent of the population is white, but that will decrease to about 64 percent by the year 2010. Asians will make up 5 percent, and African Americans 13 percent. In the more densely populated western states, approximately 15 percent of the population will be Hispanic.

The population will also be better educated in 2005: 55 percent of the population age 25 years and older will have the equivalent of one year of college (see Figure 1-3). Income disparity— a critical factor in determining health— will increase slightly. In the year 2005, 50 percent of the population will have a family income of $53,000 or more in constant 1998 dollars, and the distribution will be slightly more equal.

Access to care will remain "tiered" and that tiering will become much more extreme. The top tier, the "empowered consumers," have considerable discretionary income, are well educated, and use technology (including the Internet) to get information about their health. These new consumers increasingly will engage in shared decision making with their physicians.

Chapter 1: Health and Health Care Forecast   3

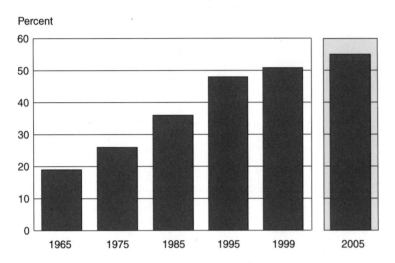

Figure 1-3. A growing number of adults in the United States have attended college. (Percentage of people age 25 years and older who have attended college)

Percent

Source: U.S. Census Bureau, *Statistical Abstract*, 2000.

discuss/define "tiers"

The second tier is made up of the "worried consumers." These are consumers who have access to some health insurance but have little or no choice of health plans. This tier includes those whose employers only offer one type of coverage and those who may be temporarily employed and face an even less secure health insurance outlook. This "worried" group also includes early retirees and others who do not have the same access to discretionary income as the empowered consumers.

The third tier is composed of the "excluded consumers." In this group are the uninsured, people on Medicaid, and others who don't have access to market-based health insurance. Throughout our forecast, these three groups are affected in varying ways by different aspects of the health care system.

PAYERS AND HEALTH CARE COSTS

The health care system has been dominated by cost concerns for the better part of 30 years, but that domination will wane during the next decade. From 1965 to 1991—from the inception of Medicare and Medicaid through the recession that precipitated the health care reform debate of 1992–1994—health care grew from 5 percent of the gross domestic product (GDP) to more than 13 percent. It is now at about 14 percent of GDP, with virtually all the reduction in cost growth coming from savings in the private sector.

We forecast a moderate but consistent increase in the cost of health care between now and 2005. Health care will grow as a share of the economy,[1] albeit more slowly than in the 1960s, 1970s, and 1980s. By 2005, the health care sector will account for about 15 percent of GDP. Employers in the private sector will see the short-lived cost decreases of the mid-1990s fade away.[2] They'll see nominal cost increases of 3 to 6 percent per year. Despite the best efforts of Congress to reduce spending in the Medicare system, public programs will continue to grow between 6 and 9 percent per year.

Between now and 2005, business and government will put several strategies in place to repress large cost increases. These strategies tend to assuage the symptoms rather than to attack the cause of the increases. The strategies include reducing insurance coverage, passing on the costs of health care premiums to beneficiaries, and increasing the restrictions on access to care via financial disincentives for utilization.

Figure 1-4. Americans move into HMOs.

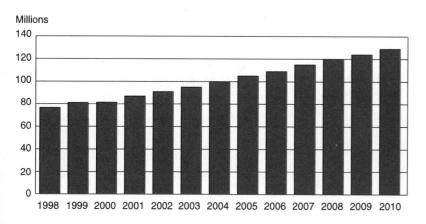

Source: Group Health Administration of America, Interstudy, American Association of Health Plans.

The health insurance market will evolve into a mix of different health plan models, many of which will spend the next several years in a constant flurry of reorganization and mergers. Four dominant "intermediary" models will emerge by 2005: the case manager, the provider partner, the high-end FFS broker, and the safety-net funder. As a result, in 2007 close to 50 percent of the population will be in health plans for which cost containment is a key issue.

Despite all the pressures toward increasing costs in the system, these new strategies will be successful enough to keep costs from exploding again as they did from 1960 to 1990.

HEALTH PLANS AND INSURERS

The biggest change in the health insurance market over the past 10 years has been the fast growth of HMO enrollment. In 1998, more than 76 million Americans were enrolled in HMOs, and a majority were in some kind of a managed care plan. By 2005, HMOs will capture the majority of the commercial market and more than 25 percent of the Medicare market. Sixty percent of Medicaid recipients will be in some form of HMO by the year 2010.[3]

Among this plethora of new products, it will be increasingly difficult to distinguish one health plan from another. They'll all offer similar—and often the same—providers and pay those providers through a mixture of discounted FFS and capitation (a flat fee per patient). By 2005, more than 100 million people will be in these "HMO descendants." (See Figure 1-4.)

HOSPITALS AND PHYSICIANS

As the demand side evolves, changes in the ways providers are organized will occur in the context of significant provider oversupply (see Figure 1-5). There are approximately 630,000 physicians in the United States and another 170,000 in the medical school pipeline. There are nearly three new physicians for every one doctor who retires. Moreover, the numbers of nurse practitioners (NPs), physician's assistants (PAs), and other non-MD clinicians will increase rapidly over the next decade. Physicians are moving into group practices, yet it will be 2005 before most office-based physicians are in groups, and most of those will be in groups of six or fewer.

On the hospital side, occupancy percentage rates have fallen from the low 80s to the low 60s in the past decade, but neither beds nor hospitals have closed at a

excess supply

Figure 1-5. In excess: Physician supply and estimated requirement (including residents and interns)

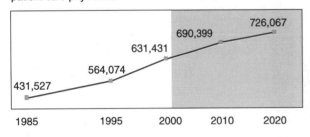

Total supply of nonfederal
patient-care physicians

431,527   564,074   631,431   690,399   726,067

1985   1995   2000   2010   2020

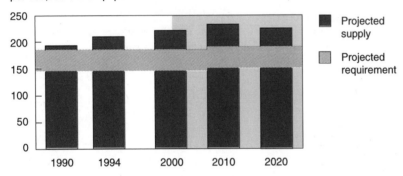

Nonfederal patient-care physicians
per 100,000 civilian population

250
200
150
100
50
0

1990   1994   2000   2010   2020

■ Projected supply
■ Projected requirement

Source: IFTF; Bureau of Health Professions, American Medical Association, Council on Graduate Medical Education.

interventions of health plans that have driven much activity out of the inpatient setting will continue, but at a relatively slower pace.

MEDICAL AND INFORMATION TECHNOLOGIES

Technological change is accelerating in two areas that will affect health care dramatically: medical and information technologies. Medical technology has been one of the major drivers of the health care system since the introduction of effective pharmacological agents in the early part of this century. Its impact will continue in the next decade. However, health care has not made significant use of the advances in information technology that have transformed most other industries. That situation will not continue for much longer as the boundaries between information and medical technologies begin to blur.

MEDICAL TECHNOLOGIES

The health care system has quickly adopted new medical technologies, both devices and pharmaceuticals. Despite increased interest in cost-benefit assessment techniques, the pace of introducing new technologies is unlikely to slow, and there will be a significant increase in the number of new technologies available in the coming decade. Some of the most interesting new technologies include:

■ *Rational drug design.* The use of computers to design drugs that target a particular receptor.

■ *Advances in imaging.* The use of new imaging technologies—such as

rate that's close to the drop in demand. Set against this background of institutional inertia, no dominant model will emerge to replace the large teaching hospital and smaller community hospital models that provided medical care from the 1930s to the early 1990s.

There will be some hospital closings and bed reductions, but hospitals will continue to be difficult to shut down. From a total of just over 850,000 beds in 1997, we anticipate a further reduction of 130,000 beds by 2005.[4] The advances in medical technology and the aggressive

# of hospital beds?

Chapter 1: Health and Health Care Forecast

electron-beam computed tomography (CT), harmonic ultrasound, high-resolution positron emission tomography (PET), and functional magnetic resonance imaging (MRI)—to look at the form and function of organs that were once examined only in surgery.

■ *Minimally invasive surgery.* The use of miniaturized devices, digitized imaging, and vascular catheters in neurosurgery, cardiology, and interventional radiology.

■ *Genetic mapping and testing.* The identification and testing of genes and genetic interactions that cause disease.

■ *Gene therapy.* The use of site-specific genes to treat a variety of inherited or acquired diseases.

■ *Vaccines.* The use of vaccines to bolster immune systems, target tumors, or immunize against viruses, and of delivery methods including oral and nasal sprays to simplify the vaccination processes.

■ *Artificial blood.* The use of recombinant hemoglobin, using *E. coli,* to create a blood substitute.

■ *Xenotransplantation.* The transplantation of tissues and organs from animals into humans, primarily bone marrow and solid organs.

INFORMATION TECHNOLOGIES

The information and communications revolution will move into the health care system in the next 5 to 10 years. We forecast that four main areas will be affected by new information technologies and that

together they'll be the drivers behind new clinical care processes. They are:

■ *Automation of basic business processes.* The transaction standards mandated in the 1996 Health Insurance Portability and Accountability Act (HIPAA) legislation are beginning to move plans and providers toward automation of the submission and adjudication of claims, determination of patient eligibility, coordination of benefits, and authorizations of referrals.

■ *Clinical information interfaces.* The creation of an electronic medical record (EMR) has stumbled because of resistance from providers, even while many of the basic building blocks are being put into place. Over the next decade, the availability of computers, sophisticated decision support systems, and voice recognition will create interfaces that are clinician-friendly. A combination of low equipment prices, younger, computer-savvy clinicians, and the move of physicians into groups will cause a slow but certain adoption of computerized medical records in the years after 2005.

■ *Data analysis.* In the next few years, administrative and claims data sets will be extensively "mined" to gain a better understanding of a population's future illnesses and an improved ability to risk-adjust payments to health plans and providers. After 2005, there will be more data available directly from clinical records. There will be close to real-time online analytical processing of information about patient and provider outcomes, and that information will be used in all aspects of health care.

- *Telehealth.* A combination of computer-supported case management, remote telemetry via sensors, and better-informed patients will create new ways of delivering health care. Chronically ill patients will be monitored remotely by using a variety of sensor devices, such as video cameras, blood pressure monitors, blood glucose readers, and smart pill boxes. Sensors will be linked to computer systems that enable the provider to catch adverse events almost before they happen. The vast increase in information about health that the Internet, interactive TV, and other communications media bring into the home will also affect the health care system. Patients will use these media for disease-specific research, psychosocial support groups, self-care, and shared decision making.

We forecast that the impact of medical technologies on the health care system will continue to be significant, although the true gains from using information technology and computerizing clinical care processes will not be seen until after 2005.

CARE PROCESSES AND MEDICAL MANAGEMENT

Medical management—the active management of the care of patients and populations—is currently applied sporadically, if at all. There are two main issues in the future of medical management. The first is the debate over which care processes are used. Many groups are developing guidelines and practice protocols, but none has agreed how, where, or when to use them. The second is the need to reduce variations in practice, thereby reducing costs and improving clinical outcomes. Since an individual clinician is less able to judge adherence to protocols than is a manager reviewing records of an entire organization, decisions about medical management will continue to shift away from the prerogative of the independent physician. Instead, internal managers in provider organizations and external managers working for intermediaries and plans will assume increasing authority in managing physicians' behavior and patients' compliance. Because medical management will depend on information systems to monitor and track both processes and outcomes, we forecast that putting these medical management processes in place will take closer to 15 years than 5 years.

In the interim, disease and demand management programs for the well population—advice nurses working with patients using the telephone and the Internet—will be commonplace. The advent of disease management programs and the adoption of clinical guidelines will have a significant impact on medical practice and patient management by 2005 and a sporadic but discernible effect on practice variation a few years later. However, the struggle between intermediaries and providers and among different provider organizations over who controls patients' and physicians' behavior will not be resolved by 2010.

PUBLIC HEALTH

Over the past 30 years the public health system has operated under pressures of resource scarcity, limits in leadership, and organizational fragmentation. As the public health system assumed the role of safety-net medical provider, the economic burden upon it became almost unbearable. Public health also suffered an identity crisis as the public confused public health with indigent medical care, further diminishing support for a population-based health infrastructure. At the same time, new health challenges emerged, such as HIV/AIDS and environmental contamination, that required strong leadership and an integration of population-based approaches into public health.

Overarching global forces will determine the context in which public health functions in the future. By the end of this decade the currently inchoate social vision reshaping government will have fully emerged and will determine the players and resources in future public health leadership and action. Furthermore, global economies and populations will drive increases in health risks, and by the next decade, national public health concerns will be embedded in a global context of threats and opportunities. Cost-effective technological advances, while mitigated by ethical debate, will enhance screening, surveillance, and environmental health. Finally, public health will increasingly employ "ecological" strategies that simultaneously address multiple human and structural determinants of health and health behavior.

During most of the next decade, public health will continue to be underfunded and marginalized, and efforts to address these underlying problems will be largely incremental. Breaches in public health prevention systems will become increasingly evident, but the system will not totally collapse because support for public health will increase enough to maintain at least a minimal system. The rise of the new consumer will also increase support for public health measures.

Over the next decade, national public health policy will be generally piecemeal, but dynamic state-level actions will generate enough momentum to reignite federal comprehensive health care reform debate. Community coalitions that assure access to basic personal and public health services will become more common. Managed care will continue to dominate, but will be augmented by the integration of population and personal health, public and private patient bases, and a variety of reimbursement strategies. The full potency, limitations, and consequences of public health litigation, à la tobacco, also will be evident in the next decade.

The future of public health service delivery will be shared among the local public health agencies, the community's private health care providers and organizations, and community-based organizations and leaders. The science of epidemiology will continue to be one of public health's most useful guides and will extend beyond biomedical applications to evaluate innovative and comprehensive public health prevention strategies.

Tobacco use will continue its steady decline, but at a very slow pace. In some geographic regions, use may remain at the current plateau. Community-based actions and local legislation will remain effective tactics in curbing tobacco use in public places. A persistent influx of youth smokers will require constant vigilance,

Forecast Through 2005

Health Care Spending Growth:	2 percent per year above nominal GDP growth
Health Care Spending:	15 percent of GDP, $6,424 per capita
Uninsurance Rate:	44 million uninsured, 15 percent of population

especially as smoking interacts with alcohol and illicit drug use. Abuse of these substances, in the absence of significant augmentation of treatment and prevention programs, will continue to fluctuate at high but not record-breaking levels. Barring a massive economic recession, firearm injuries related to violence will continue their decline, which began in the mid-1990s, with slower declines in nonviolent firearm injury gaining momentum as an array of interventions take effect. Although levels of infectious disease in the early 21st century will not approximate those of the early 20th century, (re)emerging infections, drug resistance, resurgence in risky behaviors, threats of bioterrorism, and the interaction of infec-

What Level of Health Care Spending Growth Is Sustainable in the Long Run?

A sea change in health care spending took place in the early 1990s. The annual growth rate dropped from 11 percent—a rate that had been sustained since the 1960s—to 6.75 percent. A combination of forces converged to lower spending growth: strong price pressure from employer coalitions and other large purchasers; a low point in the health insurance underwriting cycle; and providers' and suppliers' keeping their prices in check during the health reform debate and its aftermath. A key question for the next 10 years is this: Do we sustain the 1990s pattern of low growth rates in spending or do we return to the historical, 30-year pattern of higher growth? Scenario One reflects the 30-year pattern of spending growth. Scenarios Two and Three reflect the more recent pattern of spending growth.

tious and chronic disease will keep infectious diseases on the public health attention list. Finally, the by-products of our modern society will gain markedly increased attention in the next decade as food safety and air and water quality reach critical points. The crucible for environmental health action will be child health and safety actions and standards.

THREE SCENARIOS

Our forecast is relatively certain and stable through the year 2005. Beyond 2005, we have created three scenarios to describe how the health care landscape might evolve.

SCENARIO ONE: STORMY WEATHER

In the Stormy Weather scenario, pressures from rising costs, dissatisfied providers and patients, marked inequality of access to care, greedy profit takers, and repeated health care scandals accumulate through the year 2005. None of the fundamental problems of cost, quality, or access are addressed in a meaningful way. Between 2005 and 2010, the barometer drops, winds converge, and stormy weather erupts. The primary driving forces in this scenario include:

- Managed care programs that fail to deliver on their promises to contain costs or to improve quality. Instead, they default to more hassling of providers and gaming of utilization management systems.

- Consumers and providers who react to the adversarial climate with a strong, unified backlash to managed care. They succeed in getting legislation

Scenario One Indicators

Health Care Spending Growth:	2.5 percent per year above nominal GDP growth
Health Care Spending:	19 percent of GDP, $10,200 per capita
Uninsurance Rate:	65 million uninsured, 22 percent of population

passed that further erodes the effectiveness of managed care by intervening in a variety of clinical and structural decisions, such as regulation of lengths of stay for various procedures, staffing ratios, and any-willing-provider laws.

■ Health plans that engage in substantial adverse selection and cream-skimming of beneficiaries as Medicare moves toward managed care and a wider range of choices for its beneficiaries. Medicare risk plans manage to get the bulk of low-cost, healthy beneficiaries, leaving the sick, costly people to the conventional indemnity plan. Each attempt at risk adjustment is met with strategies that boost overall Medicare spending.

■ Provider oligopolies, including large group practices, physician practice management firms, national single-specialty groups, and large hospital chains, that are able to sustain high prices in an environment that demands open provider networks. They threaten to leave the networks of plans that don't pay well and the plans blink first.

■ Large employers that continue to offer insurance as a benefit of employment in the face of a tight labor market and are unable to demand substantial price

breaks from health plans. Many small employers, meanwhile, drop insurance benefits altogether, substantially increasing the number of uninsured.

■ The march of new medical technologies, which continues unabated. Consumers, prompted both by pharmaceutical companies' direct-to-consumer advertising and by "gee-whiz" articles in the popular press, demand access to the latest, greatest, and most expensive drugs and medical technologies. Beleaguered health plans concede the point and lose control over cost and quality.

■ Costly medical technologies for extending life that are not restricted, as no social consensus develops to limit spending on health care near the end of life.

■ Information technologies, once thought to be the way to efficiency, consistency, and higher-quality care, that prove to be costly and ineffective. Plans and providers find that their investments in the late 1990s and early 2000s don't pay off, but seeing no better way, they continue to invest after 2005.

■ The public health system, which will be in tatters, with local public health departments retreating from service provision and only minimally fulfilling mandated functions, and no compensatory response from the private sector.

Scenario One plays out with a range of difficult consequences. Health care spending, by 2010, constitutes almost one-fifth of gross domestic spending. Even with expenditures at that level, more than one in five Americans remains uninsured. A majority worry about losing their health benefits. Insecurity of benefits is widespread as many people are just one job change away from being without health insurance. Even those who retain insurance are a lot less happy as their out-of-pocket costs rise.

The health system exhibits radical tiering, with much poorer access to care for the uninsured and people on Medicaid. Medicaid itself puts enormous strain on states, as the state programs are faced with medical costs that overwhelm recession-depleted state budgets. A number of major public hospitals are forced to close their doors. Although their closing helps bring the supply of hospital beds into closer relation to the demand, it also strands many people who have nowhere else to go. The Medicare program finds itself unprepared to absorb the baby boomers, who begin to become eligible in 2010. By the end of the forecast period, health reform is again on the public policy agenda.

SCENARIO TWO: THE LONG AND WINDING ROAD

In Scenario Two, The Long and Winding Road, incrementalism reigns. The successive attempts at revising a portion of the health care system work sufficiently well that tinkering continues well past 2005. As costs get pushed down in one place, they pop up in another, but the system is able to respond rapidly and keep costs in balance. The primary driving forces for this scenario include:

- Employers who continue to pay close attention to health care costs and their

benefit structures. They keep substantial price pressure on health plans, limiting increases on the commercial side to 3 to 4 percent per year. They also shift cost and risk to employees by moving increasingly from a defined benefit plan to a defined contribution program. As beneficiaries' out-of-pocket costs increase, utilization of health care services drops off in response.

- Health plans that, in turn, increase pressure on providers. They convince employers that they can only control utilization in a more closed network, so the expansive networks of the late 1990s disappear. In their place are more tightly controlled networks that exert both clinical control and strong price pressure on providers.

- Providers who—stung by the high cost and organizational difficulty of forming large units and integrating care—adopt few of the innovations of the leading-edge provider groups. Instead, they engage in sustained, and largely unsuccessful, resistance to being "hassled" by insurers.

- The cost-containment provisions of the 1998 federal budget, which rein in both Medicare and Medicaid spending. The provisions stick. That bill sets the standard for budget bills for the first 10 years of this century.

- The public health system, which will engage in the dynamic competition with the private sector in service delivery.

The period of 2005 through 2010 is one of turbulent, disorganized change. The health care landscape changes as much in

Scenario Two Indicators

Health Care Spending Growth:	1 to 2 percent per year above nominal GDP growth
Health Care Spending:	16 percent of GDP, $8,600 per capita
Uninsurance Rate:	47 million uninsured, 16 percent of population

those 5 years as it did in the period from 1993 to 1998.

In Scenario Two, costs grow only a little faster than nominal GDP growth, reaching 16 percent of GDP by 2010. Federal and commercial cost containment work well enough to make insurance coverage affordable for most employers. About one in six Americans (47 million) is uninsured.

The health care system remains tiered, with about 20 percent of Americans in the bottom tier of public coverage and uninsurance, 60 percent in managed care plans that substantially restrict their choice of providers and limit providers' autonomy, and 20 percent in high-end, indemnity-type programs.

The bottom tier safety-net providers face tighter conditions, with cuts in disproportionate share hospital (DSH) funding, an end to cost-based reimbursement for outpatient clinics, and tight state and local budgets. But they manage to muddle through as usual by patching together a range of disparate funding sources.

Care delivery is still fragmented, as national players remain relatively rare and small. The majority of physicians now practice in groups of three or more,

but most of those are in three- to six-doctor groups. These groups are not large enough to accept global capitation safely, align with a hospital, or influence their physicians' practice patterns radically.

Comprehensive health reform does not enter the public policy debate, as incremental changes each year reassure elected officials that they are "doing something about health care."

SCENARIO THREE: THE SUNNY SIDE OF THE STREET

In the Sunny Side of the Street scenario, all the hard work and investment from now until 2005 pays off after 2005 in the form of a sustainable, efficient health care system. Competition helps drive excess capacity out of the system. We learn what does and does not work in medicine, and especially how to get providers and patients to work effectively together. Health plans and providers put in place information and management systems that can take the health care system through the next 2 decades. The driving forces for this scenario include:

- Competition at all levels of the health care system, but especially among providers, which helps drive costs down. Young physicians enter the market with lower income expectations and more of an employee mentality than their predecessors.

- The wave of consolidation of the late 1990s, which continues through the early 2000s. Efficient health care organizations, which can assimilate the best practices from their constituent parts, emerge. Consolidation also

Chapter 1: Health and Health Care Forecast

Scenario Three Indicators

Health Care Spending Growth:	1 percent per year above nominal GDP growth
Health Care Spending:	15 percent of GDP, $8,100 per capita
Uninsurance Rate:	30 million uninsured, 10 percent of population

serves to drive some excess capacity, especially of hospital beds although not necessarily hospitals themselves, out of the system.

■ The provider service networks (PSNs) that form to contract with Medicare. PSNs find that they have efficient administrative structures. They begin to contract directly with employers in certain parts of the country. Medicare encourages further growth in its risk contracting as it develops effective risk-adjustment methods that make risk contracting cost-neutral for the program.

■ Innovative payment approaches that are developed throughout the health care system. Prospective payment for outpatient services is put in place first by Medicare, then by commercial health plans.

■ Health care information systems, which make significant progress beyond their current administrative functions. Clinical information systems are put in place that successfully improve care processes and outcomes. The EMR sees the light of day.

■ Developments in medical technology that focus both on improving outcomes and on reducing costs. Regulators favor technologies that can demonstrate their cost-effectiveness as well as their safety and efficacy with more rapid approvals. Health plans and providers, through their improved information systems, develop the capacity to make trade-offs among therapies according to their cost-effectiveness.

■ The public health sector, which will embrace public-private community partnerships, where service delivery occurs in the private sector and government focuses on assessment, development, and assurance.

In Scenario Three, cost growth is also just 1 percent above the nominal growth of GDP. By 2010, it reaches 15 percent of GDP. These moderate cost increases make health insurance more affordable. People experience more security of benefits, leaving an uninsurance rate of 10 percent (30 million people).

The good news is that the basics are in place—health systems are equipped to minimize unnecessary variation in practices, they operate efficiently, they can track what they're doing. The time spent cultivating a well-organized health system pays off in the long run. The bad news is that we still have 30 million people who are uninsured.

Medicare and private plans begin thinking about the long term. They put in place incentives to reward population management in addition to individual patient care. They also provide incentives for a longer-term focus on today's health care decisions. The system appears well equipped to take on the wave of baby boomers who will begin to be eligible for Medicare starting in 2010.

ENDNOTES

[1] We forecast that, until 2010, real economic growth will remain at 2.5 percent, with general inflation in the economy averaging 3 percent. Health care cost growth at 5.5 percent will mean no change in the share of GDP going to health care. Faster growth of health care costs will mean that health care will grow as a share of GDP.

[2] Overall private sector cost increases averaged 4.8 percent from 1991 to 1995, but many large employers extracted actual premium decreases from health plans in a string of "famous victories" between 1993 and 1997.

[3] These 60 percent will account for only 30 percent of the costs of the program, as the blind, disabled, and dual-eligible elderly will still consume most of the resources.

[4] This doesn't tell the whole story as beds are often allocated to SNFs, 23-hour beds, or long-term care without moving from the same facility, but this projection is based on the official American Hospital Association (AHA) data for inpatient beds.

CHAPTER 2

Demographic Trends and the Burden of Disease

Increasing Diversity

Demographic shifts will shape the future. An increasing number of debates and discussions are surfacing around the social, economic, and health implications of demographic and social change. All of these concerns present new challenges for public policy, government, business, and the health care industry. Several critical issues and trends deserve attention—the aging baby boomers, the increasing ethnic and racial diversity, the growing disparity between the richest and the poorest households, and the future burden of disease.

This chapter examines each of these issues and sets the broad demographic context for examining the future of health and health care in America.

THE UNITED STATES POPULATION IS GROWING OLDER AND LIVING LONGER

The United States population is growing older, a demographic trend that will have far-reaching effects as the baby boom generation—those Americans born between 1946 and 1964—ages (see Figure 2-1). People 65 years of age and older are the

fastest-growing segment of the population. Their numbers will increase from 35 million in 1999 to 40 million in 2010 (see Figure 2-2). This "age wave" will have a transformational impact across many institutions, levels of government, and segments of society. The health care industry should begin planning now—well before 2010—to respond adequately to the needs of an older American population. The average life expectancy has increased by more than 30 years in the last century and will be 81 for women and 76 for men who are 65 in the year 2010 (see Figure 2-3).

The health care industry will certainly feel the effects of this demographic change in the next decade. Baby boomers have transformed many institutions and aspects of society along their life cycle—including the workplace, financial institutions, and government. As baby boomers interact with the health care system, their expectations and preferences will also transform these institutions as the health care industry adapts to accommodate baby boomers' demands and numbers. They will access the system not only for themselves but also for their parents and children. Boomers' involvement

Figure 2-1. The changing age structure of the population (number of people per age group, in millions)

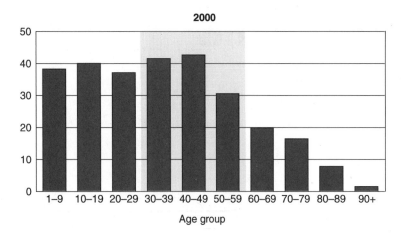

2000

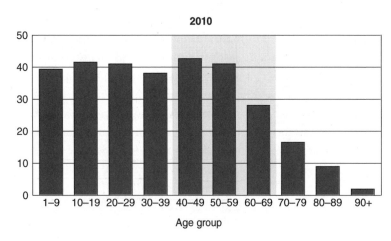

2010

Source: U.S. Census Bureau.

Figure 2-2. The coming surge in the population of age 65 years and older

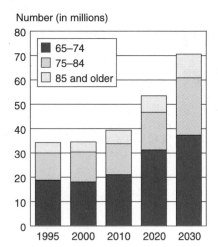

Source: IFTF; U.S. Census Bureau.

in their own care will be distinctly different from that of past generations of older Americans. They will accelerate the movement and awareness of self-care and wellness and will irreversibly alter the traditional doctor–patient relationship.

However, the full impact of the aging population will not be felt until well after 2010, when baby boomers reach retirement age. Many baby boomers will enjoy better health and longer lives due in part to advances in health and medical technologies. With increasing longevity, boomers will lead more active and productive lives rather than simply retiring in old age, illustrating just one of the many social changes associated with this demographic shift. Not until 2030, when the youngest baby boomer has

Chapter 2: Demographic Trends and the Burden of Disease

Figure 2-3. Life expectancy at age 65 increased throughout the 20th century in the United States and this increase is projected to continue.

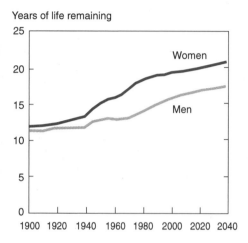

Source: Economic Report of the President, February 1999.

Figure 2-4. Increasing diversity of the United States population

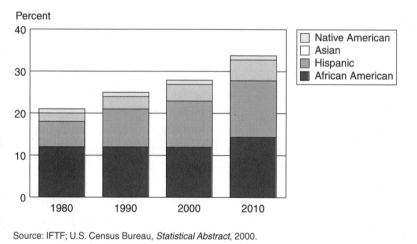

Source: IFTF; U.S. Census Bureau, *Statistical Abstract*, 2000.

reached the age of 65 and the entire baby boom's health care is subsidized by Medicare, will the nation's health and welfare system feel the true social and economic impact of this large age cohort. This trend signals the urgent need to resolve the problems of financing and delivering health care, social services, and long-term care for the population, as well as managing the health and health behaviors of this group.

THE FACE OF AMERICA CONTINUES TO CHANGE—DIVERSITY IS INCREASING

The United States is growing increasingly diverse. Although the population remains largely white non-Hispanic (69 percent), the Hispanic, African American, Asian, and Native American populations are all growing faster than the population as a whole—a trend driven by both higher immigration and higher birthrates among these groups. By 2010, minority ethnic and racial groups will account for 34 percent of the population, up from 22 percent in 1980. Yet the absolute number of ethnic and racial minorities will remain small and will continue to account for less than 50 percent of the population until well after 2050 (see Figure 2-4).

However, national data do not tell the full story—the real story of diversity is regional.

Hispanic, African American, Asian, and Native American populations are not evenly distributed across the United States, making the issue of diversity more pronounced in certain regions than in others. Although the degree of diversity is increasing throughout the United States, the highest concentration of ethnic and racial minorities is found in the West, followed by the South, the Northeast, and the Midwest—a pattern that will continue (see Figure 2-5). In 2010, the concentration of African Americans will be highest in the South. The West will continue to be the most diverse multiethnic and multiracial region of the United States with the largest concentration of Hispanic, Asian, and Native American populations.

In addition to examining this issue at the regional level, it is important to look at specific states and metropolitan areas—a level where demographic profiles have more strategic meaning to health care providers. California, Illinois, New York, Florida, and Texas are all states where the issues of diversity are being confronted now. For example, in

California, the Hispanic, Asian, African American, and Native American populations already account for 53.3 percent of the population and no one ethnic or racial group (including whites) is in the majority (see Figure 2-6). In cities such as Los Angeles, where 45 percent of the population is Hispanic, clinical providers are already facing the challenges of delivering care to a diverse population.

The increasing diversity of the population will place new demands on the health care industry. As the patient profile shows increasing proportions of Hispanic, African American, Asian, and Native American patients, the demand will become more pronounced for services that are culturally appropriate, beyond simple language competency. The concept of culturally appropriate services includes awareness of the complex issues related to the underdiagnosis of certain conditions and diseases among minority groups, the effects of lifestyle and cultural differences on health status, the implications of the diverse genetic endowment of the population, and the impact of patterns of assimilation on health status.

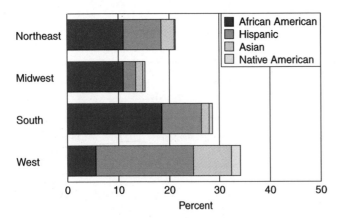

Figure 2-5. The real story of diversity in 2010 is regional.

Source: IFTF; U.S. Census Bureau, *Statistical Abstract*, 2000.

HOUSEHOLD INCOME IS INCREASING, BUT THE GAP BETWEEN THE EXTREMES IS WIDENING

Another key demographic shift is the growing number of households with high incomes. This trend is particularly important to consider in examining the future of both health and health care because income is related to both health

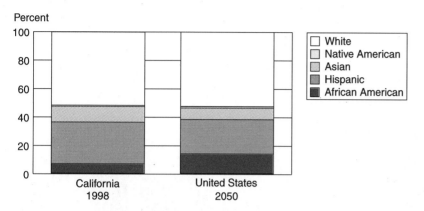

Figure 2-6. California is ahead of the nation.

Source: IFTF; State of California, Department of Finance; U.S. Census Bureau.

By 2010, the number of households with an income of $50,000 or more will reach 48 million, or 52 percent of all households—a number that is driven by the large number of baby boomers who will be well into their peak earning years.

However, the pattern of income distribution reveals a second, more disturbing trend: a widening of the gap between the richest 25 percent and the poorest 25 percent of the population (see Figure 2-7). The prosperity of the 1980s and 1990s has moved many middle-class households into higher income tiers. By 2010, this pattern will be even more pronounced. Research has also shown that when income disparity among the population widens, the overall health status of the population worsens.[2] This projected income disparity will have negative consequences on the nation's overall health status and will remain a significant social and health issue well into the future.

status and access to health care services. Although various demographic characteristics are correlated with differences in health status, none is more highly correlated than income.

The boom in the United States economy in the late 1990s resulted in extraordinarily low unemployment rates, low inflation, high productivity, and a generally favorable economic outlook. This economic growth (2.5 percent in real terms) moved many people into higher household income brackets. Households with higher incomes have higher levels of discretionary income and have better health status and access to care.

An examination of income distribution in the United States from 1970 to 2010 shows two significant trends emerging. First, the average per capita income in America will increase in real dollars. The good news is that higher income is associated with improved health status.[1]

THE SHIFTING BURDEN OF DISEASE: CHRONIC DISEASES, MENTAL ILLNESS, AND LIFESTYLE BEHAVIORS

In reviewing disease prevalence and causes of death over the past century, it is impossible to ignore the significant decrease in, and even eradication of, many infectious diseases. Vaccines, antibiotics, and biotechnological advances have curbed the communicable diseases of the 20th century. Simultaneously, there has been an increase in the incidence of chronic diseases, such as cancer and cardiovascular disease. One reason for this increase is the greater

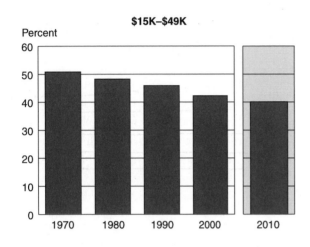

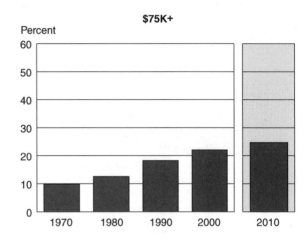

Source: IFTF; U.S. Census Bureau, *Money Income in the United States*, 1999.

life expectancy enjoyed by many Americans. Many chronic illnesses, such as cardiovascular disease, generally strike people in their later years. Increases in life expectancy and in the proportion of elderly people are accompanied by an increased prevalence of chronic diseases. Although new medical innovations promise to make a dent in the prevalence of some noncommunicable, chronic diseases in the 21st century, between 1990 and 2020 the absolute number of deaths in the United States from noncommunicable disease will increase by 77 percent, from 28.1 million to 49.7 million.[3]

An important shift in the burden of disease in the future is related to the huge impact of chronic disease around the world. The World Health Organization (WHO) defines "burden of disease" as a combination of untimely death and disability.[4] The WHO Global Burden of Disease Study attempts to assess

comprehensively current mortality and disability rates from diseases, injuries, and risk factors and to project them out to 2020. To assess the relative impact of different diseases, the study uses "1 year of healthy life lost" as a unit of measurement with which to compare disability and death from each disease. This approach reveals that the burden of a condition such as depression, alcohol dependence, or schizophrenia has been seriously underestimated by traditional approaches that take into account only deaths and not disabilities.

The overall effect of heart disease in terms of both death and disability rates will continue to be greater than that of any other illness. When looking only at mortality rates, cancer will continue to rank second. What is surprising in the current forecast is that—taking into account the extent to which an illness causes both death and disability—

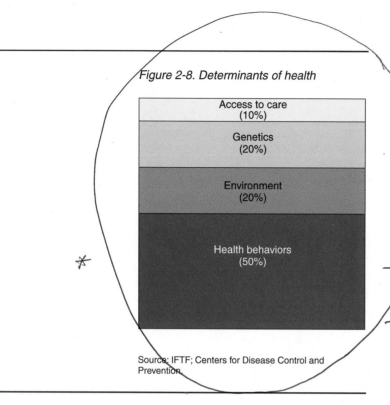

Figure 2-8. Determinants of health

| Access to care (10%) |
| Genetics (20%) |
| Environment (20%) |
| Health behaviors (50%) |

Source: IFTF; Centers for Disease Control and Prevention.

mental illness, especially unipolar major depression, will have a larger impact than cancer by the year 2010.

The burden of disease is also shifting from diseases caused by infectious organisms to disorders with behavioral causes, such as illnesses related to smoking and to alcohol abuse. It is estimated that lifestyle behaviors alone contribute to 50 percent of an individual's health status (see Figure 2-8). The biomedical model of health care, which focuses on a single causative agent for an illness and is concerned primarily with curing, is necessary but not sufficient. Much more needs to be done to create and implement effective health management and disease prevention programs. Our culture's current focus on wellness is encouraging but is primarily a phenomenon in the wealthier, more educated cohorts of society—which tend to have a better health status anyway.

ENDNOTES

[1] Adler, N. *Black Report*. Report of the Working Group on Inequalities in Health. London: DHSS, 1980.

[2] Wilkinson, R. G. Income distribution and life expectancy. *British Medical Journal* 1992; 304:165–168.

[3] Unless otherwise noted, the information presented here is from 2000 United States Census data.

[4] *The Global Burden of Disease*. Murray, C.J.L, and Lopez, A. D. (eds.). Cambridge, MA: Harvard University Press, 1996.

Chapter 2: Demographic Trends and the Burden of Disease

CHAPTER 3

Health Care's Demand Side

Changing Trends in Growth Rates 1960–2010

From 1960 to 1990, American health care saw steady cost increases in excess of the growth of the rest of the economy: health care's share of GDP went from 5 percent in 1960 to 12 percent in 1990, as shown in Figure 3-1. But after annual growth averaging more than 11 percent per year between 1960 and 1990 (3 percent above the nominal growth of the economy), annual growth in health care costs fell to 5.8 percent between 1992 and 1995 and fell each year after that until 1999. For the first time in decades, health care costs were stable as a share of GDP.[1]

To understand the components of health care cost growth, we need to know where the money comes from. The United States has had a balanced public-private health care financing system since the introduction of Medicaid and Medicare in 1965. Spending is fairly evenly split between government and the private sector, including out-of-pocket costs and insurance premiums paid by individuals. Any growth in overall health care costs will be a function of the growth in private costs, paid by both employers and individuals, and public costs.

Figure 3-1. Total health care expenditures as a percentage of GDP, 1960–1999

Percent of GDP

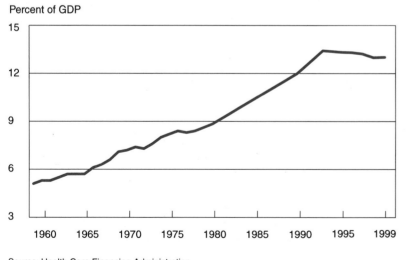

Source: Health Care Financing Administration.

HISTORICAL TRENDS
THE PRIVATE SECTOR

So far it's the private sector that has experienced the greatest reversal in cost growth. From 1960 to 1990, private sector costs grew an average of 10.6 percent a year. From 1991 to 1995—in a period viewed by some as the triumph of market-based managed care and by others as the ultimate nadir of cost shifting from employers to consumers and government—private-sector health care costs fell below the growth rates of the rest of the economy, averaging under 5 percent per year[2] (see Figure 3-2). Many employers saw an actual *decrease* in their health care expenditures. How was

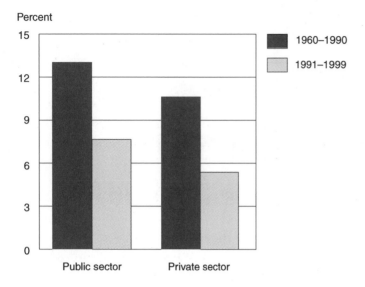

Figure 3-2. *Average annual growth rate of health care costs by sector*

Percent

Legend:
- 1960–1990
- 1991–1999

(Bars: Public sector, Private sector)

Source: Health Care Financing Administration.

this achieved? First, employers passed more costs on to employees by demanding greater contributions in premiums and forcing higher copays and deductibles. Second, employers reduced the number of people for whom they provided insurance. But most of these cost decreases resulted from lower payments to health plans. In particular, HMOs and PPOs have actively intervened with care providers to lower costs and have become the staple form of insurance plan used by most employers, rather than the more traditional indemnity products.

THE PUBLIC SECTOR

From 1960 to 1990, public spending on health care grew at an annual average rate of 13.3 percent, about 3 percent more than in the private sector. But most of that difference related to the 1960s and 1970s when Medicare and Medicaid were expanding fast. In fact, the experience of the 1990s is in contrast to that of the early 1980s, when costs in the private sector grew faster than in the

public sector. In the 1990s, the private sector saw cost growth slow to below 5 percent, whereas the public sector had average cost growths of over 9 percent from 1990 to 1995. The difference between the two widened to nearly 5 percent at that time, indicating that a greater share of health care spending was going to the public sector, and that public sector cost growth was a greater concern for the future.

While there are several reasons for this fast growth in public sector costs, a casual observer would notice that neither of the major public programs—Medicare and Medicaid—was as quick to follow the private sector's lead in adopting HMOs or PPOs. Medicare's basic infrastructure supports an FFS cost-reimbursement system for virtually all types of services apart from hospital inpatient care, which was changed to a per-episode prospective payment system in 1983. This may partially explain why public program cost increases did not tail off as they did in the private sector. Even if these were not the causative factors, they encapsulated two underlying legacies of Medicare and Medicaid—a typical FFS payment system and the peripherality of managed care—each of which will see dramatic changes during the next decade.

THE ISSUES: WHAT DRIVES COST INCREASES?

Several factors are responsible for the slowing growth in health care costs in the early 1990s. They includ the

Chapter 3: Health Care's Demand Side

movement toward HMOs and PPOs, a reluctance to raise prices during the health care reform debate, and a technological shift away from hospitalization. The question is whether these trends will continue through 2010.

In general we believe they will continue because the experiences and drives of consumers purchasing health care have changed since the mid-1990s. Some of these purchase factors include:

- *A more conservative Congress* passed a budget bill aimed in part at cutting back Medicare expenditures and delegating Medicaid decisions to the states. Managed care options will expand, quickly and involuntarily for people in Medicaid and more slowly (because of market factors) for those in Medicare. Other entitlements such as Social Security are coming under consideration for future cuts in a political era when a balanced-budget mentality appears dominant, even if subdued by pressures from industry lobbies.

- *Private (and some public sector) employers* have successfully maneuvered a majority of their workforce into managed care products. They've also either prodded health plans (intermediaries) into more aggressive cost-containment efforts with providers or have increasingly purchased coverage from plans that have taken that stance. Now that employers know they can influence costs, they are not likely to loosen that control.

- *Consumers* experienced a steady decrease in their share of national health care spending from 1960 to 1990, even though health care costs increased as a share of household spending. But with a combination of fewer employers offering insurance and, of those who do, more demanding premium contributions and increased deductibles and copays, consumers are picking up more of the financial slack. They are likely to be more cost conscious in the future.

- *Providers are more "sophisticated."* While higher health care costs ultimately translate into higher provider incomes, in recent years payers have clearly communicated their demands for cost containment. In this equation, specific providers may be rewarded for reducing costs—despite the myriad pressures to increase health care spending—and all providers are aware of that pressure.

Although these factors indicate that a slowing of the underlying growth in health care costs has taken place, several traditional factors ensure that cost inflation will not die easily. For instance:

- The vast majority of providers are paid on some type of *FFS basis*. FFS medicine stimulates increased use of services in contrast to capitation, the most extreme form of managed care payment. Although pure FFS medicine is in decline, most forms of provider payment still encourage more utilization of services rather than less.

- New, and usually more expensive, *drugs and medical technologies* are

The Economy Is the Crucial Denominator

Because health expenditures react slowly to cost-cutting measures, the amount government and employers spend on health care goes up much faster than the rest of the economy in times of recession. This rise has a noticeable impact on both the share of GDP and the share of public sector revenues and private sector profits. Figure 3-3 shows that health care costs grew continually from 1985 to 2000, but the economy was less predictable. The difference in real health care spending growth and the growth in real GDP was greatest during recessions and least during economic booms. Historically, health care costs are regarded as a problem during and immediately after recessions while on average they increase only a little faster than economic growth.

Figure 3-3. Health care cost increases get noticed during recessions. (Real changes in national health expenditure [NHE] as compared to real changes in GDP over time)

Percent

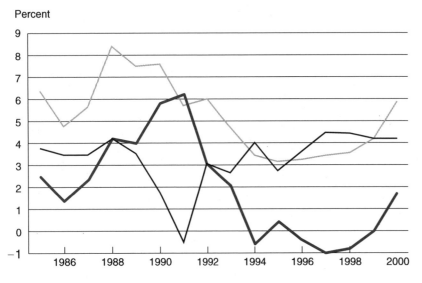

— Change in GDP, in constant 1996 dollars
--- Real change in NHE
— Difference between NHE and GDP

Source: Health Care Financing Administration, Office of the Actuary, National Health Statistics Group.
Note: Current dollars deflated by the Gross Domestic Product (GDP) chain-type price index.

becoming available all the time. Use of these drugs and technologies tends to spread quickly whether or not they are cost-effective. Even with cost-shifting to the employee via multiple-tiered pharmacy benefit programs, new drugs in the pipeline will be in great demand. This will especially be true for the field of pharmaco-genomics, when both consumer demand and quality of care issues will help pharmaceutical companies to thrive.

- *The growing labor force*, as evidenced by the number of both high-cost employees (e.g., physicians) and low-cost employees in the health care industry, increased at an average annual rate of 3.78 percent between 1980 and 1998. That's 2.73 percent more than the rate of population growth, yet overall wage rates have remained roughly constant. So as more resources go to health care employment, it appears that the supply-driven demand demonstrated during the 1970s is still in evidence.[3]

MARKET DYNAMICS

In the United States, the basic trend of real growth in the gross domestic product (GDP) over any extended period is about 2.5 to 3 percent per year. This growth rate has held true over the past hundred years with only a few exceptions—for example, during the Great Depression in the 1930s, when the GDP declined at a rate of 13 percent, and during the World War II recovery, when GDP growth soared to 18 percent.

The 1990s produced one of the longest expansionary periods for the U.S.

economy in the past hundred years—nine years of expansion that compares favorably to the nine years of expansion during the Vietnam War and the eight years during the 1980s. In the last four years of the decade, annual GDP growth hovered at about 4 percent and unemployment dropped to 3.9 percent, the lowest level since 1970. Strong growth and low unemployment meant that employers competed fiercely for workers to fuel increasing productivity. When health insurance premiums began to rise precipitously, employers were only too willing to cover the bulk of the increases in order to retain their workers.

The third quarter of 2000 brought an end to that nine-year expansion. Though the year 2000 ended with a 4.1 percent annual growth in GDP, that annual rate masked the dramatic drop in growth from a second-quarter high of 5.7 percent to a third-quarter low of 1.3 percent.

Figure 3-4. Future spending projections
(Health care expenditures as a share of GDP)

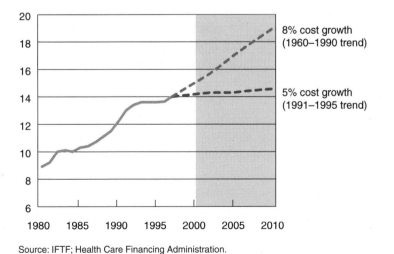

Source: IFTF; Health Care Financing Administration.

The Bureau of Economic Analysis pegs GDP growth at 0.2 percent for the second quarter of 2001. As GDP growth declines, unemployment inches up, and consumer confidence wilts, many economists see the beginning of a recession (defined either as two consecutive quarters of declining GDP or as the downward movement of employment, industrial production, real income, and sales[4]).

THE FORECAST: REAL COST GROWTH AT 1 PERCENT

The underlying question is whether the future will look more like the private sector's experience in the 1990s—health care cost growth in line with economic growth—or the public sector's experience of cost growth at a higher level. The first possibility continues the trend from 1990 to 1995. The second takes us back to the high cost-growth rates of the previous 30 years. Figure 3-4 shows the share of GDP that would end up being consumed by health care under each scenario.

There are good reasons to believe that the dramatic growth rate of the period between 1960 and 1990 is a thing of the past. But there are still sufficient factors to warrant suspicion that the experience of the private sector—a reduction in health cost rates below overall economic growth—in the early 1990s is unlikely to be replicated in the next decade.

Overall, we forecast that health care expenditures between 2002 and 2010 are likely to grow at 6.5 percent annually—roughly equivalent to just under

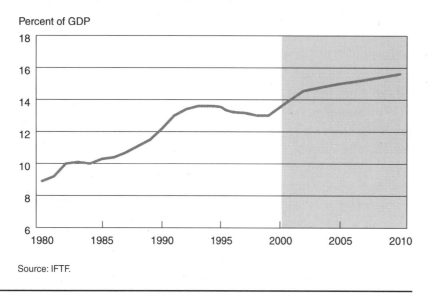

Figure 3-5. Projection of future health care spending
(Health care expenditures as a share of GDP)

Percent of GDP

Source: IFTF.

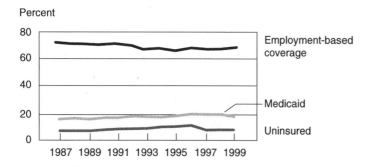

Figure 3-6. Percent of American adults, ages 18–64, with employment-
based health benefits or Medicaid, and without health insurance, 1987–1999

Percent

Source: Fronstin, P. *Employment-Based Health Benefits: Trends and Outlook*. EBRI Issue Brief
No. 233. Washington, DC: Employee Benefit Research Institute, May 2001.

1 percent more than GDP growth. If
this forecast is correct, then health care,
which currently consumes 14.3 percent
of GDP, will reach 15.7 percent in 2010
(see Figure 3-5). Within that steady
growth, the gap between rates of cost
growth in the private and public sectors
will narrow.

Why will the gap narrow? So far, much
of the private sector's gains have come at
the expense of consumers, the public sector, and providers. For instance, there are
relatively fewer people insured by their
own or their family's employers now
than there were in the late 1980s—
73.3 percent in 1999, compared with
76.1 percent in 1987 (see Figure 3-6).
The increase in the number of working
uninsured and the fact that most
employers are demanding greater contributions toward insurance costs mean
that more pressure is put on safety-net
providers, such as public hospitals and
inner-city academic medical centers
(AMCs). Consequently, the financial
health of these institutions has suffered
and the amount of compensation the
government has paid out in disproportionate share payments (DSH) made to
hospitals that deliver a higher than average amount of uncompensated care
reflects this impact (see Figure 3-7).
Similarly, the Medicaid expansion of the
late 1980s added about 10 million people to the program at a time when fewer
people were receiving coverage from
employers.

In addition, the mainstream Medicare
and Medicaid programs have either experienced cost shifting from private insurers or simply haven't shared as greatly in
the productivity improvements that
providers, especially hospitals, have
experienced over the past few years.

We don't believe that this discrepancy
between cost growth in the public and
private sectors can continue at the 5 percent differential seen in the 1990s. It
appears that the gains made in the private sector at the public sector's expense

Chapter 3: Health Care's Demand Side

Figure 3-7. DSH spending exploded in the early 1990s. It is projected to increase 1 percent annually between 1998 and 2010.

Billions of dollars

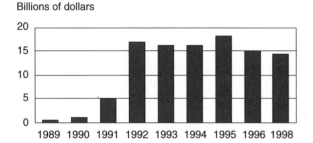

Source: U.S. General Accounting Office, The Urban Institute, Health Care Financing Administration.

were mostly a one-time gain, and the gap is now starting to narrow.

Evidence of such a reversal is accumulating. Private insurance premiums increased between 3 percent and 11 percent in 2001, due mostly to poor margins among health plans and to increased utilization of pharmaceuticals and physician services. Meanwhile, the Medicare and Medicaid cost increases in excess of 10 percent seen during the early 1990s slowed to 8 percent and less than 5 percent, respectively, in 1996 and 1997. The 1997 balanced-budget legislation attempt to put an overall cap on the growth of Medicare costs at 6 percent for the period from 1998 to 2002 caused a precipitous drop in Medicare cost increases, to 0.1 percent in 1998 and 1.0 percent in 1999. This reduction in Medicare spending may put more pressure on providers, who in turn will try to transfer their costs to the private sector.

We forecast that private sector cost growth will move closer to the 3 to 6 percent range over the next 10 years,

and public sector cost increases will end up in the 6 to 9 percent range. Hence, our forecast of overall costs averages 6.5 percent per year.

Why will costs stay at that level rather than go much higher? In the private sector, employers and other payers now understand that they don't simply have to accept large cost increases year after year. Meanwhile, recent Medicare legislation appears to be the most comprehensive attempt yet to implement cost containment across the entire program. Previous efforts simply squeezed one part of the Medicare cost balloon and let it bulge out elsewhere.[5]

Nonetheless, given the greater pressures on the Medicare and Medicaid programs and the traditional ability of providers to take advantage of the comparative inflexibility of these programs, we project that—although cost growth will slow—the government's share of all health care expenditures will increase rapidly. The government's share of spending on health, *excluding* the government as employer, will increase from around 46.75 percent today to as much as 47.5 percent in 2002, when the current Medicare budget plan expires, and to as much as 52 percent by 2010.[6]

Consumers will be the other major source of increased spending because they will be paying more for health care. Currently, out-of-pocket costs (direct spending on medical services) are $202.5 billion a year, or about 15.4 percent of total health care expenditures. In addition, individuals pay $126.4 billion in private insurance premiums, either for their primary insurance, as a contribution to what their employer provides, or for Medigap coverage.[7] Combined, these costs account for 25 percent of total health care spending.

Because of the reduction in scope of benefits, increased consumer demand for over-the-counter (OTC) medical products and complementary services such as chiropractic care, and the higher growth rate of both individual and group insurance premiums, we forecast that this share of total spending will rise to as much as 28 percent by 2003. After that, growth in the public sector will absorb some of the increase and it will fall back to 26.5 percent by 2010. But in the next decade, health care will rise as a share of overall consumer spending.

In 2010, employers will be paying a smaller share of overall costs and government and consumers will be paying a greater proportion (see Figure 3-8).

THE SIGNIFICANCE OF OUR COST FORECAST FOR THE REST OF OUR 10-YEAR OUTLOOK

We broadly agree with forecasts suggesting that the health care cost problem is not going to go away. The nominal rate of health care cost growth for the period 2000 to 2010 will be about 6.4 percent, or 1 percent over GDP, as opposed to 3 percent over GDP for the period 1960 to 1990. But we believe (with some temerity) that this relatively slower cost growth may not be the dominant issue for the next 10 years. The period up to 2010 is likely to be a cost-containment hiatus given the impact of the soon-to-retire baby boomers in the years between 2010 and 2030.

WILD CARDS

Wild cards are events that have less than a 10 percent likelihood of occurring, but should they occur they would have a significant impact. Which wild cards could derail this forecast for information-driven cost control in managed care?

- Market forces and risk selection sink Medicare savings: Health plans will withdraw from Medicare managed care programs because it will be such an unprofitable system. Medicare managed care will end up with medical savings accounts (MSAs), PSNs, and HMOs cream-skimming on a noticeable scale.

- Cost-reduction strategies in fast-growing parts of Medicare such as SNFs or home health and outpatient services either don't work or are

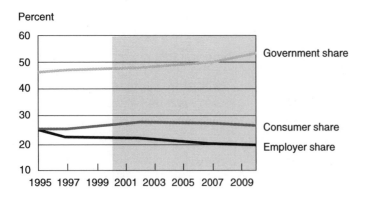

Figure 3-8. Share of costs borne by government, employers, and consumers

Source: IFTF; Health Care Financing Administration.

counterproductive because they create fast-growing exceptions. Those rapidly growing programs are joined by other new programs like telemedicine, which are equally expensive.

- Cost shifting to providers and public payers causes a collapse of the safety net, forcing large influxes of federal funding to several inner-city areas.

- The 2001–2002 recession is deeper than anticipated, requiring more services for the indigent and hence a greater share of government revenue and GDP for health care while taxes and other revenues decline.

- The weapons are taken out of the hands of managed care. A combina-

tion of legal and regulatory restrictions on health plans, such as more "any-willing-provider" laws, and bans on capitation and utilization review tilt negotiating power back toward providers.

- A provider surplus, plus aggressive HMOs, plus Medicare's actually sticking to 6 percent cost increases and Medicaid's getting tougher, keep costs below our forecast and below 4.5 percent. As a consequence, health care shrinks as a share of GDP.

- The technology revolution increases the rate of economic growth. Health care costs shrink as a share of GDP because GDP grows so quickly.

ENDNOTES

[1] Since the mid-1980s, the economy has generally grown at an annual rate of 5.5 percent in nominal terms (2.5 percent real growth and 3 percent inflation). Thus, for health costs to maintain their share of GDP they would have to grow at an average annual rate of 5.5 percent in nominal terms.

[2] That is, less than 5.5 percent, the average growth of the economy in nominal terms (not adjusted for inflation).

[3] Fuchs, V. R., and Kramer, M. J. Determinants of expenditure for physicians services. In Fuchs, V. R. *The Health Economy*. Cambridge, MA: Harvard University Press, 1986.

[4] Ranking, K. Recession defined. The Dismal Scientist, May 3, 2001. www.dismal.com.

[5] Medicaid too appears to be growing more slowly. However, the recent falls in Medicaid cost growth (i.e., to below 4 percent) came during an economic expansion. Because Medicaid costs grow fastest during recessions, we forecast Medicaid growth to remain at about 8 percent.

[6] This does not include the government's spending as an employer. We consider that spending as private health insurance (as does the Health Care Financing Administration [HCFA] in some versions of the national health expenditure [NHE]) and believe that it will increase at the rate of private spending. In 1995, government spending on insurance for federal, state, and local government employees amounted to roughly $58 billion of the $242 billion spent by employers on private health insurance in 1995. If this were to be counted as part of government health expenditures, it would mean that the government accounted for 52 percent of health expenditures in 1995.

[7] This does not include $16 billion paid as premiums by individuals for Part B of Medicare, which is included in our Medicare numbers.

CHAPTER 4

Health Insurance

The Three-Tiered Model

The American health insurance system developed out of a need for hospitals and physicians to make their product affordable to ordinary people. Health insurance first became a reality for Americans in the 1930s with the creation of specialized health insurance companies—the Blue Cross and Blue Shield plans. The system was given a boost when health insurance became an employment benefit during and after World War II, and when Medicare (for the elderly) and Medicaid (for the poor) were created in 1965. It was this indemnity-based system of mixed public and private insurance sources that constituted the mainstream of American health care until the early 1980s. Only in some regions, notably in the West, were any substantial number of people enrolled in the prepaid health plans that were later called health maintenance organizations (HMOs).

During the 1970s and 1980s, a series of legislative and court decisions fostered the growth of selective contracting. Selective contracting allowed insurance plans, which came to be known as preferred provider organizations (PPOs) and HMOs, to contract with networks of providers. The plans could arrange the contracts at a predetermined price and reimburse providers for their services in a number of different ways, still including (but not limited to) a traditional fee-for-service (FFS) model. Generally, the Medicare and Medicaid programs were not included in these arrangements.

By the early 1990s, the cost advantages that HMOs and PPOs afforded employers were great enough that most large employers, such as the California Public Employees Retirement System (CalPERS), moved their employees to this type of insurance arrangement. This caused a rapid growth in the numbers of people enrolled in HMOs and PPOs, and later in hybrid models like point-of-service (POS) programs. By 1995, most companies had moved their workers away from indemnity plans, and by 2000 more than 80 million people were enrolled in HMO plans (see Figures 4-1 and 4-2).

SCOPE OF EMPLOYMENT-BASED COVERAGE

Moving employees into managed care plans was not employers' only response to rising health care costs. They also offered insurance to fewer employees. There has been a long-term erosion of coverage that has been modestly ameliorated by gains in the past several years. The Employee Benefit Research Institute (EBRI) estimates that 73.3 percent of workers, ages 18 to 64, had employment-based health

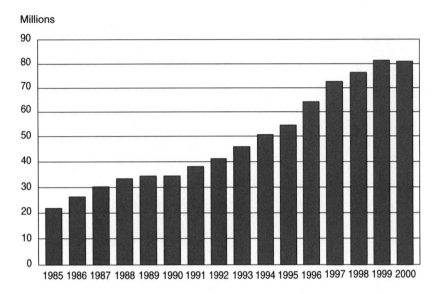

Figure 4-1. HMO membership takes off in the 1990s.
(Number of HMO enrollees in millions)

Source: Group Health Administration of America, Interstudy, American Association of Health Plans.

Figure 4-2. Health plan enrollment for covered workers,
selected years 1996–2001

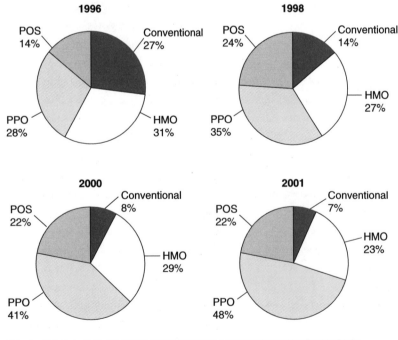

Source: Gabel, J., et al. Job-Based Health Insurance in 2001: Inflation Hits Double Digits, Managed Care Retreats. *Health Affairs* (September/October) 2001; 20(5): 180–186.

insurance in 1999, compared to 76.1 percent in 1987. The majority, 55.6 percent, received benefits from their own employer, while 17.7 percent got them through a family member's employer. This marks a slight gain in employer-sponsored benefits in the second half of the 1990s (see Figure 4-3).

RETIREE BENEFITS ARE GETTING WORSE

Although there has been some good news regarding health insurance for the active workforce, retiree benefits are in free fall. Employers have changed retiree health benefits because of rising costs—the costs of retiree benefits were rising faster than those of the active workforce—and because of a 1992 change in accounting procedures that required employers to record unfunded retiree benefits as liabilities on their financial statements. As a result, the share of firms with 500-plus employees that offer health benefits to early retirees fell from 46 percent in 1993 to 31 percent in 2000. For Medicare-eligible retirees, the share fell from 40 percent to 24 percent over the same period. There is no end in sight to this trend.[1] Thus, the health benefits cost-containment efforts already have begun. Employers moved to cut health care costs in a way that did not affect their core businesses.

THE UNINSURED

What has changed over the past few years is the number of people who are uninsured. This number rose during the 1980s and most of the 1990s. By 1998, 16 percent of nonelderly Americans were uninsured, compared to 14.8 percent in 1987.

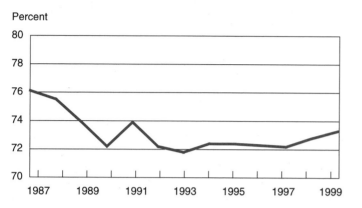

Figure 4-3. Employment-based insurance (Percentage of workers aged 18 to 64 with employment-based health insurance)

Source: Little, J. S. *New England Economic Review*, 1995.

However, by 1999, the booming economy helped decrease the ranks of the uninsured to 14.3 percent of nonelderly Americans and the actual number of uninsured from 44 million to 39.3 million.[2]

The uninsured are not necessarily those you might expect—the poor and the unemployed. Indeed, in 1999 35.4 million of the 39 million uninsured Americans were members of families in which the head of household worked.[3] More than 24 million working adults—employees and self-employed—were uninsured in 1999. Workers most likely to be among the uninsured were young white men, without a college diploma, who worked full-time in the retail or wholesale trades for wages of less than $20,000. Although white men formed the majority of uninsured workers, Hispanic men were disproportionately likely to be among the working uninsured.

One in four self-employed workers is also likely to be uninsured. In contrast to typical uninsured workers, self-employed

workers are more likely to have college and graduate school education, their income is higher, they are slightly older, and they are more likely to be skilled. Self-employed workers number around 8.5 million. If the number of uninsured among them grows, they may combine forces with small-business owners who struggle to offer benefits and to create skilled and vocal advocacy for health care reforms to which politicians may begin to respond.

THE ISSUES: HOW WILL PEOPLE RECEIVE HEALTH INSURANCE?

Both the source of health insurance funding and the type of insurance coverage people receive have great influence on the health care system. Some of the factors determining how people receive health insurance between now and 2010 are predictable. These include the source of funding: employee-funded health insurance will remain the mainstream, and most people will have their insurance paid for by the same source it comes from now.

An assessment of the sources of health insurance for Americans (see Figure 4-4) shows that in 1999 approximately 174 million Americans (62 percent) received private health insurance from their employer or purchased it themselves. Of the remainder, 40 million (10 percent) were in the Medicaid program, 39 million (14 percent) were in Medicare, and about 42 million (16 percent) had no health insurance and relied on self-pay, county and local programs, or charity.[4]

Chapter 4: Health Insurance

Employer-Sponsored Health Insurance and the Economy

Employer-sponsored health insurance is particularly vulnerable to recession. As business profits and stock market valuations fall, companies are under severe pressure to improve cash flow or reduce costs.

Lowering the costs of health benefits is the primary way to fight rising costs in general because the costs of health benefits are not only the biggest chunk of indirect costs but are also rising the fastest. Already the magnitude of the difference between the growth of health premiums and growth in other economic measures is striking. Premiums are growing at more than three times the rate of overall inflation, greater than twice the rate of increase in workers' earnings, and more than twice the rate of medical inflation. At a rate of 4.7 percent, medical inflation is just slightly higher than growth in GDP, but premiums are growing two-and-a-half times as fast. This is a red flag for employers facing an economic recession.

Tight Labor Markets Limit Employers' Options

Though employers experienced 5 years of accelerating premium growth in the late 1990s, there was little explicit cost shifting to the covered employees.[5] Between 1996 and 2000, both employees' monthly contribution to premiums and percent of premium paid fell significantly for single coverage.[6] (The dollar amount rose and percentage stayed steady for family coverage.) Because the economy was booming and unemployment was dropping to its lowest point in 30 years, employers used health benefits to compete for labor (see Figure 4-5).

The economic downturn of 2001–2002 pushed unemployment toward 5 percent. If unemployment continues to grow, employers will have a larger labor pool to draw on and more latitude for shaving health benefits costs. The first line of attack is likely to be altering existing benefits structures, changing waiting periods and eligibility requirements, and shifting more costs to employees.

Sources of insurance will remain fairly stable. For the next 5 years, we know who the Medicare population will be; any future policy changes related to eligibility will not kick in until late in the next decade. In the near future, employment-based insurance will remain the predominant form of insurance for most people under 65. There will be a continuing group of Medicaid recipients and uninsured, but their numbers cannot be known for certain. The major categories of Medicare, Medicaid, uninsured, and private health insurance will remain the core sources of coverage, or lack thereof.

However, the question is not only from which source do people receive health insurance—we must also ask what form that insurance takes. During the past few years, most people with employer-based insurance have moved from indemnity plans into a variety of more complex models, including several types of open-panel HMOs and PPOs. The shift from indemnity to PPO and HMO models will continue, with the shift accelerating in the public programs.

Contrary to popular opinion, the growth in PPOs and HMOs was not primarily due to an increase in the number of enrollees of traditional staff- and group-model health plans, such as Kaiser Permanente or Harvard Pilgrim Health Plan. Instead, most of the growth came from independent practice association–based (IPA) HMOs that developed new contracting arrangements with community providers (see Figure 4-6). In other words, the delivery system used by the new intermediaries was the same one that Blue Cross, Blue Shield, and traditional indemnity systems had been using all along.

In the mid-1990s, more Medicare and Medicaid recipients enrolled in HMOs. Some state governments forced Medicaid recipients to join HMOs, and for a while it became more attractive for private-sector health plans to recruit senior citizens into specialized HMOs. This "Medicare risk contracting" was a complicated arrangement for health plans. Beginning

Figure 4-4. Sources of health insurance for Americans over time

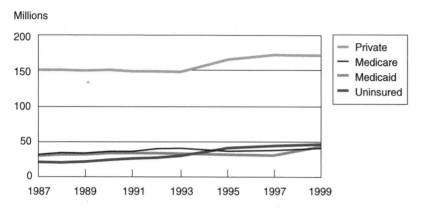

Source: IFTF, using data from Health Care Financing Administration, Employee Benefits Research Institute, and Current Population Survey.

Figure 4-5. Strong economy, low unemployment made employers stomach premium growth.

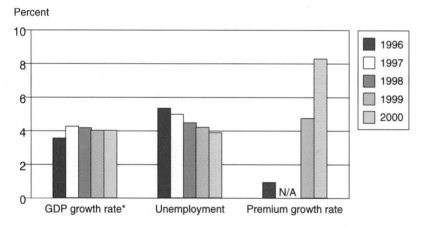

*GDP growth based on chained 1996 dollars.

Source: IFTF, based on data from U.S. Census Bureau Statistical Abstracts, Bureau of Labor Statistics, and Kaiser Family Foundation/Health Research and Educational Trust.

a reimbursement policy that encouraged the recruitment of seniors in high-cost markets such as Los Angeles, Miami, and New York City. Membership of Medicare recipients in risk-contracting HMOs grew from 4 percent at the end of 1989 to 6 percent at the end of 1994, to 13 percent at the beginning of 1998. It then declined to 7.2 percent in 2001, reflecting the health plans' reluctance to continue coverage for this population.

Two major issues, then, have influenced our forecast for health insurance. One is the *source* of insurance. The major sources of health insurance will remain fairly constant through 2010, although the relative proportions will change slightly.

The other is the *type* of insurance. Although we estimate the numbers enrolled in the classically defined products—indemnity, PPO, and HMO—the distinction among different types of HMOs, PPOs, POSs, and all the rest of the players in the alphabet soup is becoming irrelevant. Continued innovation in the benefit plans' contractual arrangements will rapidly erode the distinction among the classic gatekeeper HMOs, PPOs, POSs, and other models of managed care.

THE FORECAST: SOURCE OF INSURANCE —WHERE ARE THE PEOPLE? . . .

PRIVATE INSURANCE

The downward trend in the number of people with employment-based insurance and the upward trend in the numbers

in 1998–1999, health plans began dropping their Medicare risk programs in regions that were unprofitable. For each member enrolled, HMOs were paid 95 percent of the average costs of a Medicare recipient in that particular county—

Figure 4-6. It's been the IPAs that have grown fastest. (HMO enrollment growth split by IPA and network models versus group and staff models)

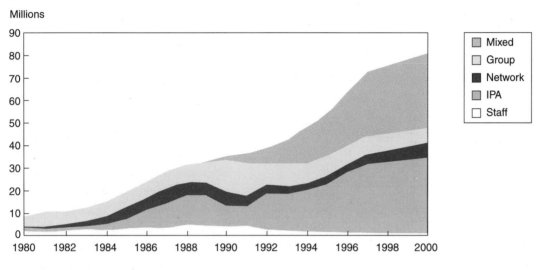

Millions

Source: IFTF, using data from Interstudy.

Figure 4-7. Future sources of health insurance for Americans

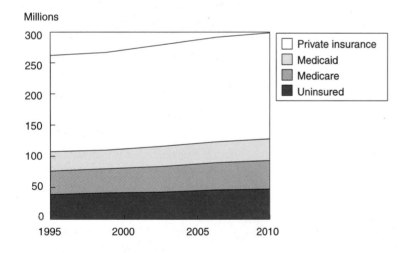

Millions

Source: IFTF, based on data and projections from Health Care Financing Administration, Urban Institute, Lewin Inc., and Congressional Budget Office.

population, at 1 percent every 5 years, from about 59 percent in 1997 to about 56 percent in 2010 (see Figure 4-7). Due to overall population growth, their total number will increase by about 13 million.

MEDICARE

Meanwhile, the population insured through Medicare will increase at a slightly faster rate than the rate of over-all population growth, increasing from just under 38 million (14.2 percent of the population) currently to 45 million in 2007 (15.5 percent) and 49 million in 2010 (16.8 percent). While the numbers of the elderly will increase, the fastest-growing segment of the Medicare population is now the disabled, which is growing at 6 percent annually. Considering that no eligibility changes were made in 1997, a policy that is unlikely

with Medicaid will remain constant over the next 10 years. The number receiving health insurance from employers will decrease, *as a proportion of the overall*

What's Behind Medicaid's Growth?

The Medicaid program has grown in both size and complexity since its inception in 1965.[7] The program now accounts for about 15 percent of all health care spending ($202 billion in 2000) and provides four major types of coverage:

1. acute medical insurance coverage

2. coverage for the disabled, including residential care for the long-term mentally disabled

3. long-term care for the poor elderly (those who have "spent down" to poverty level and need nursing home care)

4. state Medicaid programs paying the Medicare Part B insurance premiums for poor elderly and disabled (known as dual eligibles)

Sixty-five percent of people enrolled in Medicaid are in the first category, and 65 percent of the money is spent on the 35 percent in the last three categories. As that spending tends to fall outside of the traditional acute care model, it is difficult to include in managed care programs.

A series of legislated eligibility expansions in the late 1980s, followed by the 1990–1992 recession, increased the number of people covered by Medicaid from 23 million in 1987 to 36 million in 1996. Currently, about 28 million people use Medicaid as their primary source of health insurance (our model counts the dual eligibles in the Medicare numbers). Federal legislation in 1996 gave states far more freedom to alter Medicaid plans, both in terms of implementing new benefit arrangements and in changing eligibility levels. Meanwhile several states, notably Tennessee, had already moved their Medicaid population into managed care programs.[8] Most other states have announced an intention to do the same, and we forecast that about 60 percent of Medicaid recipients will be in managed care plans by 2005, although they will account for only 35 percent of spending.

The 1997 Balanced Budget Act also gave the states funding to increase the number of children covered by health insurance. States may use these funds to increase Medicaid eligibility levels for children or they may create separate child health programs.

old, owing to the baby boom after World War II, will not begin until 2010 and will continue until 2040.

MEDICAID

There are now about 28 million Americans (10.3 percent of the population) who use Medicaid as their primary source of health insurance. That number does not include the nearly 6 million people who are eligible for both Medicaid and Medicare. It also does not include an estimated 6 million additional people who are eligible for the Medicaid program but are not enrolled in it—we classify these people among the uninsured. The rate of growth of the Medicaid population depends on both federal and state government policies and the economy, and it is notoriously difficult to forecast. However, we do not forecast a substantial expansion in Medicaid eligibility other than for some children covered under the 1997 Balanced Budget Act.

We estimate that the number served by Medicaid will grow from 28 million to 34 million by 2010.[9] Several factors could inflate this forecast, including a faster uptake of children into Medicaid or a severe recession that would cause an expansion in the ranks of the poor. However, states now freed from federal mandates could tighten eligibility requirements, which would reduce the number of people served.

THE UNINSURED

The uninsured will still constitute a sizable proportion of Americans, but our core forecast is that they will continue to

to change during the next several years, we think that Medicare will continue to cover people over 65 years of age, at least until 2010. There are now 36 million Americans over 65 and there will be 40 million in 2010. The significant growth in the population over 65 years

be about 15 percent of the population. Although counting the number of uninsured is problematic, their number appears to be increasing at about 750,000 people per year. Because health insurance costs dropped in the late 1990s, we project that this number will fall over the next 5 years, although the recession may keep the average growth at 750,000.

There will also be a modest impact on Medicaid as between 1.5 and 2 million children receive coverage over the next 5 years through the Children's Health Insurance Program (CHIP) provision of the 1997 Balanced Budget Act (10 million of the 42 million currently uninsured are under 18 years of age).

We forecast that by 2002 the numbers of uninsured will increase from the current 43 million to around 44 million. After 2002, the average rate of increase will decline, partly because of the shifting age structure in the population. Lack of insurance is most common among people of age 18 to 34 years, and most of the baby boomers will be age 40 to 60 years by the next decade. Overall, we estimate that the rate of growth in the uninsured will be close to an additional 500,000 per year through 2010. We estimate that, in 2007, 16 percent of Americans (46.4 million) will be uninsured, a percentage that will rise to 16.1 percent or 47.9 million in 2010.

The important factor in these projections is the *proportion* of the population that is uninsured at any one time. About 21 million of the 42 million uninsured will be uninsured for a year or more. Twice that number will be uninsured at some time over a 2-year period.

. . . AND WHAT TYPE OF INSURANCE WILL THEY HAVE?

While the distinctions among indemnity, PPO, and HMO are breaking down, the people moving into managed care have been counted in the increase in HMO membership, and that's how managed care enrollment will be forecast in the near future. Figure 4-8 shows the change in type of insurance coverage held by the insured over the next decade.

Among people with private insurance HMO membership grew at about 7 percent each year during the 1990s. We expect that rate to drop to 5 percent from 2002 to 2007, and to 4 percent after 2007. Indemnity programs are increasingly turning into PPOs, and PPO membership increased to about 60 million by 2002. But by 2010 the number will decline to below 50 million as PPO members begin to move into HMOs. However, the distinctions among these products will be hard to discern by then and we will call them "HMO descendants" (see Figure 4-9).

Two key issues will be of concern to insurers in 2010:

- What the components of the benefits package will be, in terms of the insured's obligations such as coinsurance, deductibles, and copayments.

- The way in which insurance plans pay the providers.

The first issue, benefits packages and the insured's obligations, will reflect the underlying tiering that is developing among consumers in the population as a

*Figure 4-8. The future is much more of the present.
(Type of insurance coverage for the insured)*

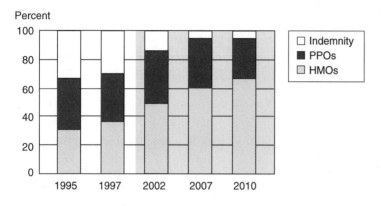

Source: IFTF.

*Figure 4-9. HMO descendants move from mainstream to majority.
(Number of Americans in HMOs, by source of insurance)*

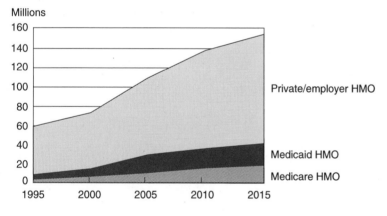

Source: IFTF.

on the employment status and wealth of the participants:

- *Carriage trade indemnity or PPO, including traditional Medicare:* These will remain traditional programs with high deductibles and coinsurance, copayments, and free choice of providers.

- *HMO descendants:* Most Americans will have excellent benefits in terms of low or no deductibles, and low copayments (the current HMO standard) if they stay within the provider network and work through their plans' referral processes. The option to self-refer to other providers will be covered in general, but at a lower percentage of reimbursement with higher copayments and most likely higher coinsurance.

- *The low tier:* This tier will include most Medicaid enrollees, who face a more restrictive set of provider choices but with better access to them than they've experienced in the traditional program. The providers for this group will be dealing with most of the uninsured. There will also be continued but limited efforts to help uninsured individuals and small groups buy into these low-tier plans.

To see how these factors will translate into reimbursement and affect the provider system, see the "Reimbursement Models: Between Finance and Delivery" section in Chapter 6.

whole (see Chapter 11). We look at the second question, provider reimbursement, in Chapter 6.

TIERING WILL INCREASE

Three types of insurance models (see Figure 4-10) are likely to develop based

WILD CARDS

- A severe, protracted recession increases the number of uninsured and Medicaid eligibles by 75 percent each.

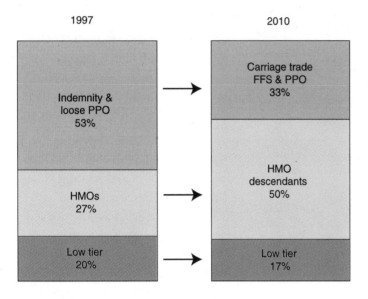

Figure 4-10. Tiers 'R' Us . . . and will be.

1997

| Indemnity & loose PPO 53% |
| HMOs 27% |
| Low tier 20% |

2010

| Carriage trade FFS & PPO 33% |
| HMO descendants 50% |
| Low tier 17% |

Source: IFTF.

- Universal health insurance legislation is enacted, reducing the number of uninsured to nearly zero.

- Health insurance premiums become a taxable benefit; employers stop providing coverage and abandon the market as purchasers.

- MSAs, vouchers for Medicare, and other individual-based buying become significant forces, changing the group nature of the insurance market.

- HMO enrollment growth in either Medicare or the commercial market slows substantially or even declines due to legislative, market, or other pressures.

- A national health insurance system is adopted; private-sector insurance is eliminated.

ENDNOTES

[1] Hewitt Associates. *Health promotion/managed health provided by major U.S. employers in 2000.* Lincolnshire, IL: Hewitt Associates, 2001.

[2] National Center for Policy Analysis. Fewer uninsured than previously estimated. *Daily Policy Digest*, *Health Issues*, August 9, 2001.

[3] Fronstin, P. *Sources of health insurance and characteristics of the uninsured.* EBRI Issue Brief No. 228. Washington, DC: Employee Benefit Research Institute, December 2000.

[4] About 20 million (7 percent) buy health insurance themselves.

[5] William M. Mercer, 15th Annual Mercer/Foster Higgins National Survey of Employer-Sponsored Health Plans, 2000.

[6] Kaiser Family Foundation/Health Research and Educational Trust, Employer Health Benefits Survey, 2001.

[7] The expansion in Medicaid eligibility in the late 1980s, which increased the population covered from about 19 million to closer to 30 million, kept the number of uninsured lower than it would otherwise have been.

Few of those new Medicaid recipients had previously been uninsured—in fact most of them had been insured by an employer—but this expansion of Medicaid eligibility did make a one-time impact on the underlying trend of uninsurance.

[8] Until the 1996 legislation, it was necessary for states to receive a waiver from the federal government to make substantial changes in their Medicaid programs. Several waivers were granted, including one that allowed Tennessee to introduce the TennCare managed care program for Medicaid recipients and the uninsured.

[9] There is some controversy over forecasting Medicaid enrollment. The Congressional Budget Office (CBO) estimates annual Medicaid growth of 2.7 percent. The Urban Institute reworked the CBO number in 1997 and established, to our satisfaction, that CBO had overestimated the growth in the core Medicaid populations of Aid to Families with Dependent Children (AFDC) mothers and children and disabled people. They projected a 1.6 percent annual growth rate, which we've used here.

CHAPTER 5

Managed Care

Experiments in Reinvention

Twenty years ago, "managed care" was nearly synonymous with the term health-maintenance organization (HMO). Today, managed care includes the continuum from staff- and group-model HMOs, through network-model HMOs, to preferred provider organizations (PPOs). PPOs are the dominant form of managed care, holding 48 percent, versus HMOs' 23 percent, of the employment-based insurance market.[1]

THE ISSUES: MANAGED CARE IS OUT OF BALANCE

After successfully restraining premiums and health care inflation in the early to mid 1990s, managed care has ceased to deliver promised savings and many question its ability to deliver quality care. Both health care costs and premiums are rising at ever increasing rates. Consumers and providers alike are expressing concern about the quality of care.[2,3] In a struggle for survival, health care institutions—together with physicians seeking to regain control over clinical decision making—are rejecting both low reimbursement rates and restrictive practice management. Consumers want ready access to providers and choices among doctors and treatments.[4] As providers and consumers have made their case about

damage wrought by the restrictions of traditional managed care, health plans, the courts, regulators, and employers have responded. The established managed care techniques for controlling costs, for administration and utilization review, and for restricting patients to set physician networks and denying service have fallen prey to lawsuits, regulation, and bad press. At the same time, health care faces immutable cost drivers. Managed care may not be at a breaking point, but the current situation is unsustainable.

MAKING UP FOR LOST TIME: PRICES SOARED

Between 1994 and 1998, health plans scrambled to respond to purchasers' demands for cost containment and to gain market share by dramatically suppressing the growth of premiums. To do this, they used a familiar set of management tools to control costs.

- *Capitation and shared-risk arrangements* place providers at risk for some or all components of care at a predetermined fixed price.

- *Utilization review and restriction of services* use a centralized process of either prospectively or retrospectively reviewing and approving payment for medical procedures.

Chapter 5: Managed Care   47

- *Bargaining down payment rates* to providers simply attempts to set an advantageous rate for payers.

With these tools, managed care plans did, in fact, deliver what they promised to health care purchasers: the growth of premiums slowed. While inflation of medical costs dropped to 4.6 percent in 1996, the growth of premiums plummeted to 0.8 percent per year—one-quarter of the overall inflation rate (see Figure 5-1). Managed care kept premiums artificially low by restricting access to care, cutting staff, and reducing professional fees. But plans and providers failed to attack the underlying problems, including poor information systems, weak administrative support to identify and track costs, and lack of discipline among providers. Thus managed care did little to cut the underlying costs of delivering health care. Public and private purchasers were much happier with lower premiums, but physicians, health systems, and consumers were not.

PREMIUMS WERE UNSUSTAINABLE

As medical costs continued to rise, albeit more slowly, plans, providers, and hospital systems could not sustain the discounted prices. HMOs experienced 4 years of net losses from 1995 to 1999.[5] Parsimonious reimbursement wreaked financial havoc on providers. In California, where managed care realized the greatest penetration and the lowest premiums, the California Medical Association found that 113 out of 300 medical groups failed or quit between 1996 and 1999.[6] The industry saw a precipitous rise and fall of physicians' practice-management companies that could neither manage nor squeeze profits out of medical groups.[7] The value of privately owned hospitals fell by 33 percent between January 1999 and January 2000.[8] The financial markets began to reappraise health care.

Evidence that established managed care techniques are crumbling is abundant.

- Many Independent Practice Associations (IPAs) and medical groups in heavily capitated areas have struggled to find the capabilities to manage effectively under capitation, and many have failed.[9,10]

- Highly publicized cases have caused plans like United Healthcare and Aetna to back away from utilization review. New laws enabling consumers to sue HMOs for denial of service are chilling enthusiasm for this form of medical management.

- Health plans in the public managed care market rebelled, pulling out of the Medicare market in response to

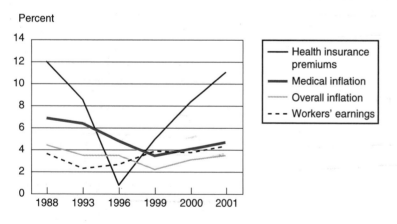

Figure 5-1. Inflation rates diverge.

Percent

Health insurance premiums
Medical inflation
Overall inflation
Workers' earnings

Source: Kaiser Family Foundation/Health Research and Educational Trust, Employer Benefits Survey, 2001.

the low reimbursement rates introduced by the Balanced Budget Amendment of 1997.

- Consolidation among providers made them much less likely to accept low payments in order to be included in a managed care network.

ENTER THE EMPOWERED CONSUMER

To make matters worse, managed care faced the increasingly demanding "New Consumer" of health care. With disposable income, computers, and at least a year of college education, these New Consumers want choices, access, control, and information[11]. Managed care's efforts to reduce utilization and costs by limit-

ing access ran afoul of the New Consumer's demand for choice. Consumers were more satisfied with loose managed care than strict managed care.[12] As a result, PPO enrollment grew from 28 percent to 48 percent of insured workers between 1996 and 2001 (see Figure 5-2).

REGULATORS RESPONDED TO ANTI–MANAGED CARE SENTIMENT

As clinicians and consumers bridled at managed care's restrictions on access to care and on providers' decision-making prerogatives, regulators responded. Building on sweeping federal legislation, including the HMO act of 1973, the Employee Retirement Income Security Act (ERISA) of 1974, the Consolidated Omnibus Budget Reconciliation Act of 1985 (COBRA), the Health Insurance Portability and Accountability Act of 1996 (HIPAA), and the Balanced Budget Amendment of 1997, regulators passed laws to protect patients' rights to access and treatment and to ensure that medical decision making is squarely in the hands of qualified clinicians. The effect has been to make managed care organizations more wary of denying care.[13]

DRIVERS

Five drivers of change will force managed care to invent new tools to manage care and control costs—or to fail.

- Relentlessly **rising health care premiums and costs** that compel purchasers to push for cost containment

- Dissemination of new **information technology (IT)** that allows for

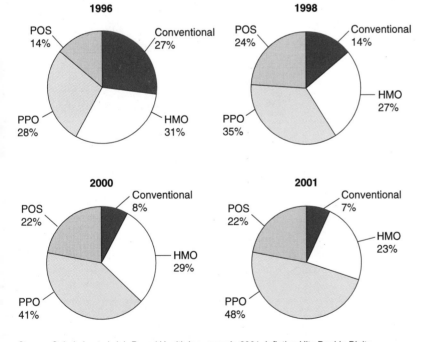

Figure 5-2. Enrollment in PPOs grows.
(Health plan enrollment for covered workers, selected years 1996–2001)

Source: Gabel, J., et al. Job-Based Health Insurance in 2001: Inflation Hits Double Digits, Managed Care Retreats. *Health Affairs* (September/October) 2001; 20(5):180–186.

improved clinical and administrative oversight

- The **New Consumers** of health care, who demand choice, information, and control over their health care

- **Increased regulation** of managed care plans and of access to patients' medical data

- **Innovation** in business models to coordinate the financing and delivery of health care

RISING HEALTH CARE PREMIUMS AND COSTS DRIVE A PUSH FOR COST CONTAINMENT

Despite its initial success at cutting health care costs, managed care has lost its fiscal way. The easily won savings have been realized. An aging population, advancements in medical technology, and the rising cost of pharmaceuticals are intractable forces driving health care expenditures up (see Figure 5-3).

- By 2010, the youngest of the baby boomers will be 65 and an elder boom will ensue.

- The diffusion of medical technology has proved to be the most potent cost driver in health care.[14]

- A shift to new, more expensive pharmaceuticals and increase use is driving drug costs faster than other components of national health care expenditures. Employers reported 17.5 percent increases in 2000.[15]

INFORMATION TECHNOLOGIES OFFER NEW TOOLS FOR MANAGED CARE

Health care organizations, in comparison with other industries, have chronically underinvested in information technologies. Internet-enabled IT is lowering the costs of adopting IT for many organizations. It is also helping managed care organizations to manage administrative costs. The health care players who adopted Internet-based IT early on have found the Internet to be a powerful force for change and cost-efficiency, but it can also help improve clinical care by:

- *Preventing errors.* Well-designed electronic systems can confirm that the correct patient is being treated and ensure that the right dose of a medication is administered—and, in so doing, can prevent errors and complications.

- *Improving clinical decisions.* Several studies have shown that information systems can influence decisions at the point of care. One trial showed that using information systems to prompt physicians and "vigorous application

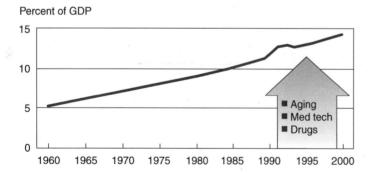

Figure 5-3. Expenditure increases persist.

Percent of GDP

Source: IFTF; Health Care Financing Administration.

of a simple and effective information intervention could save thousands of lives annually."[16]

■ *Improving disease management.* Patients with special needs can be referred to disease-management programs or case-management programs and can be monitored closely through Internet technology, thereby reducing high-cost acute episodes, such as emergency-room (ER) admissions for patients with asthma.

■ *Reviewing quality of care and conveying feedback.* The electronic capture of standardized data elements permits a systematic analysis of clinical practice, benchmarking, and rapid dissemination of the results that can drive adoption of best practices.

The convergence of affordability and usefulness in information technology will support innovation in managed care.

THE NEW CONSUMER DEMANDS MORE

Accustomed to using the Internet for work, online shopping, and stock trading, New Consumers have come to expect a similar benchmark of convenience from their health plans too. They are demanding access to information about health plans on the Internet. They want online administrative services, such as claims processing and precertification, information about enrollment and benefits, referrals, and appointment scheduling. Increasingly consumers are seeking information to help them manage their own health and health care, including information about physicians, consumer-friendly clinical guidelines, and information about treatments.

REGULATION MAY HAVE COST CONSEQUENCES

Regulation is limiting managed care's ability to control costs and coordinate care even as it is mandating information technology that has the potential to improve clinical care.

■ *Electronic data interchange.* HIPAA is intended to improve the efficiency and effectiveness of the health care system by standardizing the electronic exchange of administrative and financial data and simplifying administrative processes. Health plans, providers, and clearinghouses that manage health care data are "covered entities" under the law. This regulation, with fines and imprisonment for noncompliance, is a driving force that is pushing health care plans to adopt electronic data interchange (EDI), irrespective of whether EDI was among their highest priorities. In the short run, costs may be high, but the potential for improving care coordination is great.

■ *Privacy.* In his last weeks in office, President Clinton enacted wide-reaching privacy regulations that could have a strong impact on managed care. The White House estimated that new privacy requirements will increase costs for the nation's providers and health plans by $1.2 billion during the first year alone, and $3.8 billion over the course of 5 years. Other estimates have put the 5-year cost as high as $22.5 billion.[17] Along with HIPAA regulations, these new regulations will cost managed care organizations plenty.

■ *Patients' rights.* The highly publicized federal Patients' Bill of Rights legislation attempts to hold health plans and self-insured purchasers accountable for health care decisions. If a federal Patients' Bill of Rights that increases the liability of self-insured employers were to pass, these employers might drastically change their role in purchasing health care. Experts believe, however, that the real importance of the Patients' Bill of Rights may be more political than practical. Aggressive lobbying by health plans, employers, and providers makes it highly unlikely that a bill assigning such liability to self-insured employers will pass.

INNOVATION SPURS MANAGED CARE TO NEW WAYS OF DOING BUSINESS

Innovation outside of established managed care organizations is fostering innovation within them. Companies marketing health care information, products, and services on the Internet are capitalizing on the discontent with managed care, focusing on consumers, and driving managed care to change. These e-health care companies are claiming functions traditionally performed by insurers, IPAs, consultants, and brokers in both the business-to-business and the business-to-consumer markets. Such companies include Medscape, the purveyor of digital clinical data and medical information; eHealth-Insurance, the online portal for individuals, families, and small businesses seeking health insurance; and the employee-benefits-management companies eBenX.com and Sageo. Although the recession threatens such innovators' survival, it does not affect their ability to bring about long-

term change in health care. They have already made their mark.

Established managed care organizations are responding to the threats of these e-businesses. The old dogs of managed care are expanding their presence on the Web and offering new products that respond to consumers' demand for service. Kaiser Permanente allows patients to make and cancel appointments and order prescriptions online. Destiny Health, Inc. (www.destinyhealth.com) is launching a medical savings account product. Highmark Blue Cross Blue Shield is using the Internet to allow enrollees to construct personalized health plans. The New Economy is certainly teaching old dogs new tricks.

DRIVING MANAGED CARE TOWARD NEW TOOLS

These drivers have gotten managed care moving. The ready availability and potential of information technologies, the demands of the New Consumer, regulatory action, and innovation in the e-health sector itself are driving managed care to develop new methods of care coordination and cost containment during the next 5 years. These new methods will take advantage of information-driven approaches that track costs, guide clinical practice, and engage the consumer in self-management while meeting consumers' demands for greater choice.

POTENTIAL BARRIERS TO IT IMPLEMENTATION

What stands in the way of the managed care industry's adopting information-driven techniques for controlling costs while coordinating care? Consumers' demands for choice and control of their health care, providers' resistance to scrutiny and loss of autonomy, money, the economy, regulation, and technology themselves pose formidable barriers that will hamper managed care's attempts to lay the groundwork for its own reinvention.

CONSUMERS' DEMANDS

- Consumers' fears that they may lose control over their health information due to breeches of privacy and failures in data-security systems may slow the adoption of electronic data-interchange systems.

- Consumers' preference for choice may thwart attempts to channel them to cost-effective providers and plans, thereby limiting purchasers' efforts to use data to control costs and health plans' efforts to guide clinical care.

PROVIDERS' RESISTANCE TO SCRUTINY

- Providers' resistance to scrutiny and their lack of faith in traditional measures of health care performance may prompt them to resist increased pressure from purchasers and plans to provide performance data.

- Providers, being independent and notoriously resistant to change, might balk at consolidation and fail to amass the market share and command of costs and high-quality data necessary to help them negotiate with health plans for favorable payment rates. They may also fail to capitalize on the savings potential of substituting

nurses for physicians or allied health care workers for registered nurses.

MONEY AND THE ECONOMY

- The capital demands of investing in information systems may be significant. As money markets have shied away from health care, managed care organizations and providers alike may find it hard to make the investments in IT required to collect and analyze data and to drive cost containment.

- A softening economy may distract large-scale purchasers and purchasing coalitions from their focus on purchasing high value in health care.

REGULATION

- Ironically, privacy regulations may inhibit the use of Internet-enabled systems to manage care across practice settings. Privacy restrictions could inhibit the flow of information among providers and plans.

- The delay in enacting federal privacy regulations could cause a consumer backlash against HIPAA-induced increases in electronic data exchange and slow the use of Internet-based systems to track and control costs of clinical practice.

TECHNOLOGY

- Information systems, particularly at the provider-group level, may fall short of what is needed to support sound quality measurement and, perhaps more important, improved clinical decision making. The resulting dearth of timely and useful information about quality of performance—particularly for PPOs and provider groups—and the absence of evidence of cost savings for purchasers may thwart the use of value purchasing as a data-driven, cost-control tool.

THE FORECAST: EXPERIMENTS IN REINVENTION

Imagine managed care in a laboratory, running experiments in coordinating care while controlling costs. Managed care, like health care in general, will have begun to invest in IT by 2005, and will be developing new processes to track costs and direct the delivery of care.

Managed care products that offer choices to consumers and help providers deliver better care will thrive. Health care expenditures will continue to rise. There will be stellar examples of improved health care management across the country, but the practice of medicine will not be fundamentally transformed. By the end of that period of experimentation, managed care will be poised to reinvent itself. Thus, the story of managed care will be one of experiments in reinvention.

ALL PLAYERS IN THE HEALTH CARE SYSTEM WILL WORK TO CONTAIN COSTS

After several years of rising premiums, managed care will find itself in a crucible, combined with four reagents—purchasers pushing to control rising premiums, consumers seeking choice, providers demanding better pay, and the health care system generally pushing to invest in information technologies.

Plans will partner with purchasers to contain costs. Although the well-worn methods that managed care organizations have used to date to manage provider costs may not disappear, new models of managing costs will come to the fore. Plans will work in concert with purchasers to make consumers become active participants in health care choices that the consumer will pay for.

Tiered payment systems. Premiums and copays will differ based on cost-efficiency of providers and plans and the nature of the services received. One approach, used in medical savings accounts, is to implement a higher deductible coverage—such as a $2,000 deductible—whereby consumers pay for most of their low-cost, ordinary care. Alternatively, health-plan copayments can be adjusted to be higher when a patient picks a less cost-efficient provider. PacifiCare health plan in California recently announced that it would use this approach for its Medicare HMO enrollees. Thus, patients are free to make a choice. If they believe that a provider is better and worth the added cost, they can choose to incur that cost.

Channeling consumers to preferred providers. Although purchasers have had some reluctance to choose a health plan that places restrictions on network size, this choice may become more acceptable if costs continue to rise. Restrictions will be based on provider and plan performance and consumers will pay more if they choose a provider that has a poorer track record than alternatives. The Leapfrog Group, a coalition of large organizations purchasing health care, has established network restrictions for complex procedures for which there is considerable variation in quality as one of their criteria for choosing health plans.

Redesigning reimbursement. In the coming years, plans will experiment with:

- *Specialty capitation, case rates, and episode-based payment.* There will be moves to paying specialists a capitation payment based on their providing coverage for a fixed number of patients, and paying a specialist a single fee for providing care for a patient's episode of illness, adjusted for severity. Either of these approaches relies on an ability to risk-adjust the payment, so that treating a more severely ill patient or panel of patients results in greater compensation. These approaches also require good methods for monitoring quality and outcomes because of the inherent potential for undertreatment.

- *Paying for best practices.* More institutions will focus on providing highly specialized care, becoming especially adept at particular practices like cardiac surgery, hernia repair, or oncology. These so-called "focus factories" may be the best places for patients to go if they want highly standardized and predictable outcomes because their high volume helps them to hone their skills to deliver highly predictable results. As consumers and purchasers become more aware of the quality *and* cost advantages of this type of provider, it may become more acceptable to direct patients to these centers and to pay preferential fees to those that demonstrate they provide the best care.

- *Paying for electronic visits.* An increasing number of computer-savvy patients want to communicate with their doctors and receive health care

services through the Internet. Physicians have been reluctant because of concerns about privacy, lack of reimbursement, and potential exposure to malpractice litigation. Considering consumers' demand, solutions to these problems are likely to be found. At least two health plans have announced plans to reimburse physicians for limited services provided through the Net. This capacity has the potential to both reduce costs and increase consumer satisfaction.

- *Revising payment for chronic illness care.* Evidence from disease-management programs indicates that monitoring and supporting chronically ill patients at home lead to better outcomes and potential cost savings. The ability to provide this type of care will improve as new technology provides devices such as sensors that can transmit data from remote sites and software that can organize it into meaningful information. These approaches potentially can reduce expensive visits with practitioners and time lost from work for travel. Models for reimbursing providers for such services will increase.

MANAGED CARE WILL ADVANCE DISEASE MANAGEMENT

High-risk patients—patients with a serious, chronic illness who are generally at risk of complications or debilitating infirmity—are the most costly patients to treat, and the patients who benefit most from the comprehensive care that managed care can offer. Designed to treat acute, episodic illness, our standard health care system does not provide well for patients with a chronic disease. It is not designed to monitor patients, nor can it provide the education, behavior modification programs, and continuity of care that are needed to control chronic conditions.

Enter disease management. Motivated primarily by a desire to reduce costs, disease-management programs focus on identifying high-risk patients and then working to implement best-practice protocols. Based on the relatively sparse evidence available, disease-management programs reduce or eliminate the need for hospitalization and ER visits and reduce the costs associated with chronic conditions.

To date, much of the initiative for disease management has come from the vendors of these services and from health plans, but that is changing. As provider organizations consolidate and develop both resources and management capabilities, we forecast that they will compete with health plans to take over disease-management programs. Where they have responsibility for much of the financial risk, they will want to maintain control of the programs implemented for their patients. It is also likely that, during the next 5 years, there will be greater information available about the disease-management programs that work, those that do not, and the cost-benefit ratio of such an approach to care.

HEALTH CARE PURCHASERS WILL RENEW EFFORTS TO CONTAIN COSTS

While employer-purchasers will retain their role in buying health care and negotiating premiums and benefits,[18] they will also move more decisively than they did during the late 1990s and the early 2000s to contain growth of their health care expenditures.

Our experts agree that there will be no dramatic move toward radical forms of defined contribution by 2005. Tax laws make it cheaper for employers to buy health insurance than for individuals to buy it. Employers do not know how to implement an equitable voucher system. There is no rational, easy-to-use individual market for health insurance. Risk adjustment and adverse selection pose knotty problems for insurance companies. In a 2001 survey of public and private employers, very few employers were "very likely" to move to defined contribution during the next 5 years (see Figure 5-4). Instead, our experts say that purchasers will become information brokers, pushing employees to become more informed and more engaged consumers of health care.

Employer-purchasers will not be willing to pay rising insurance premiums and rapidly rising prescription-drug costs for much longer. They will educate employees and reformulate benefits. With easing labor markets purchasers will be able to use the portfolio of cost-containing tools they have at the ready. Those tools include:

- *Shifting costs to employee-consumers.* Employers will reduce premium contributions, reduce benefits, and introduce higher deductibles or higher consumer copayments for care. This approach reduces employer payments directly, and it also makes consumers seeking care more careful in their choices because they will pay more of the bill.

Figure 5-4. Employers are unlikely to switch to defined-contribution health benefits. (Likelihood of employers switching to defined contribution for health

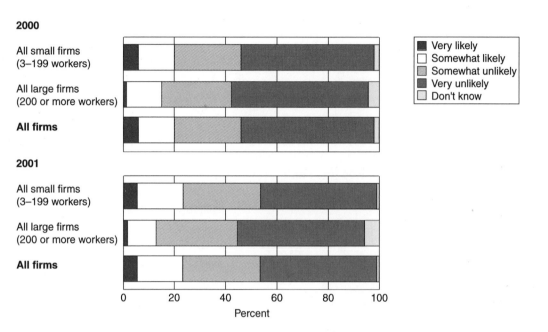

Source: Kaiser Family Foundation/Health Research and Educational Trust, Employer Benefits Survey, 2001.

Managing pharmacy expenditures. Many purchasers will move to three-tiered copays, increase the use of formularies, and educate consumers to use drugs that are less expensive. Some may experiment with new benefits designs, using deductibles rather than copays for prescription drugs.

Purchasing value. For large-scale employers and purchasing coalitions, eliminating plans and providers that are not cost-efficient or cost-effective can make a big difference in the costs of health care. Purchaser groups, including the large automotive companies and the Leapfrog Group, are writing cost-effectiveness requirements into their contracts with plans

and providers, and they pay according to performance.

With all of these "kinder, gentler" ways of controlling costs, purchasers will provide the options—the consumer and provider will choose. Choices will depend on the ready availability of information about cost and performance. Rather than overtly imposing rules and roadblocks, these cost-control methods will use data to guide consumers' and providers' choices.

CONSUMERS WILL KNOW MORE AND SPEND MORE

We forecast that consumers will become more active and better informed by 2005, as they begin to foot a greater share of the bill for rising health care costs. But because they will pay, consumers will also have a more robust array of managed care products, responding to their need for choice, information, and control over their health care. Insurance companies will continue to develop managed care products that provide consumers—both purchasers and patients—with flexibility and savings over conventional indemnity products.

The HCFA projects that consumer out-of-pocket spending on all health care will reach $297 billion per year by the year 2005, an increase of 34 percent over projected expenditures for the year 2000 (see Figure 5-5).[19]

Despite the expenses they bear, consumers have very little information with which to determine the value or quality of the

health care they purchase, relative to its price. The data available by which to assess quality among health care providers are woefully crude. There are increasing efforts, however, to collect data useful for consumers. In many instances, this information is available through Internet companies, such as HealthGrades.com and FACCT.com, through large-scale employers, or through purchasing coalitions like the Pacific Business Group on Health (PBGH). Independent organizations like *Consumer Reports* are publishing ratings of health plans. Access to information is likely to improve gradually, coming first from consumers' assessments of each provider's performance rather than from rigorous measurement of the technical clinical quality of health care. As information systems are further deployed, however, more specific detailed measurement will be possible.

INFORMATION TECHNOLOGY WILL GUIDE CARE DELIVERY

Sparked by HIPAA compliance, the health care industry will take substantial strides toward embracing Internet-based IT by 2005, creating new clinical and administrative efficiencies that have the potential to contain costs. In the short run, investments in IT may drive costs up, but players in the health care industry who have access to capital and make wise investments—either by purchasing new systems or contracting for information services—will have the information instrumental to controlling costs and guiding physicians' decisions in the next phase of managed care.

Figure 5-5. Consumers will pay more.

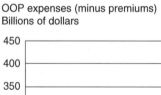

OOP expenses (minus premiums)
Billions of dollars

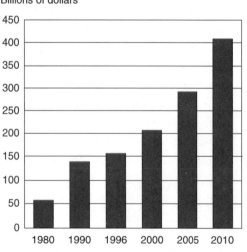

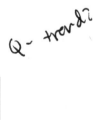

Source: HCFA Office of the Actuary, 2001

Q - what a PPO?
a IPA?

THE HEALTH CARE DELIVERY SYSTEM WILL POSITION ITSELF FOR POWER

Provider Consolidation Moves Downstream.
We forecast that providers will consolidate to achieve economies of scale, particularly to acquire expensive infrastructural components, such as information systems, and to strengthen management. The desire to gain regional market share and bargaining clout in relation to health plans will be the key factor spurring most providers to consolidate.

↑ consolidation

Consolidation of providers may take any of several forms:

- Consolidation of individual physicians and small group practices. This form of consolidation has been a general trend nationwide for several decades, and it will continue in regions that have been slow to develop organized physicians' groups.

- Consolidation of existing group practices and IPAs. The pressure of managed care cost-containment efforts has caused many regional organizations to fail. When the weaker ones close, many of the physicians are absorbed into surviving entities, as was the case after the collapse of Med Partners and FPA Medical Management—both large, national providers' management organizations. The surviving organizations have succeeded financially despite the pressure, and it is likely that they will have greater market share in the future.

- *Hospital closure with consolidation of patients into fewer institutions.* Consolidation can also mean mergers of hospitals to form stronger entities for

bargaining power and efficiency of operations. However, mergers do not always meet their goals successfully, as was proved by the merger of the Stanford University and University of California San Francisco Medical Centers, which dissolved because the merger was poorly implemented and financially disastrous. The experience will continue to be mixed.

THE MIX OF THE HEALTH CARE WORKFORCE IS UNLIKELY TO CHANGE

Despite the potential that redeploying of the health care workforce to ensure that the least expensive, *qualified* professional renders care may have for controlling costs, significant change in this direction is unlikely to occur. Considering that we now train more medical residents than most authorities believe are needed, it is difficult to see how putting allied health care professionals into the mix would not simply add to the workforce rather than substitute for physicians. In the absence of a health care workforce policy in the United States, there is little hope that planning for a different mix of manpower is likely to occur within the next few years.

QUALITY MEASUREMENT WILL HAVE MORE INFLUENCE ON MANAGING CARE

The IOM's report, *To Err Is Human*,[20] alerted consumers and purchasers to the frequency and consequences of errors in medical practice in the American health care system. Although it is unlikely that the quality of health care will improve quickly, the new focus on medical error will help several forces coalesce to encourage an increasing emphasis on

Chapter 5: Managed Care

improvements in quality over the next 5 years:

- *Development of data regarding quality for PPOs and medical groups.* NCQA and others in the business of evaluating health care performance are working to develop quality-measurement tools for PPOs. RAND corporation "Quality Assessment Tools," which will evaluate medical groups, will be available by 2002. Both PPOs and medical groups will be the subjects of quality measurement by 2005, and the results of these measurements will become increasingly available to consumers.

- *Deployment of clinical information systems.* Although the proliferation of tools to foster improved quality of performance is likely to be gradual, they will become increasingly available to practitioners as information systems are installed. Such tools as computerized physician order entry systems accessible by handheld devices, electronic medical records, and clinical databases that physicians can access when making decisions about a patient's care will make quality management more effective and consistent.

- *Studies building a business case for quality.* It seems highly likely that a business case for quality can be built, particularly if the focus is on the prevention of error and its complications—the added work needed to remedy the sequelae of medical errors and the loss of an employee's productivity due to inadequately treated illness.

- *Pressure from purchasers of care.* Large-scale purchasers of health care and members

of business coalitions have experienced the requirements for optimum quality in their own industries, and they are beginning to experiment with "value-based" and "quality-based" purchasing of health care. Purchasing coalitions have begun to put provider payments at risk based on quality. Purchasers will look for evidence that quality pays and differential payment matters.

It is likely that improvements in quality will not have a major impact on cost over the next 5 years because so many factors have to be in place to make high quality an effective driver. However, we forecast that measurement and management of quality of performance will become more prominent as a force driving the shape of managed care.

MANAGED CARE 2005: A KINDER AND GENTLER MANAGED CARE?

The existing degree of dissatisfaction with the current system of controlling costs makes it likely that managed care will modify its "brute force" approaches, relying on information systems and incentives for consumers and providers, and perhaps placing an even greater emphasis on the cost-effectiveness of health care during the coming years. We forecast that information-driven techniques for coordinating care and controlling costs will begin to dominate managed care by 2005.

MANAGED CARE 2010: PATTERNS OF POWER

Managed care will be in transition during the next 5 years. We can conceive of three patterns of market power that could emerge by the year 2010:

- Big Insurance Dominates

- Government Leads

- Consumers Meet E-Health-Care
  Markets

These *power plays* are examples of how the relative power of health care stakeholders could shift to create new market dynamics 10 years from today. These power plays may coexist. They are meant to provide insights about potential market shifts that warrant strategy and forethought.

BIG INSURANCE DOMINATES

Consolidation has created a market dominated by a handful of large health plans. Providers are dependent on these plans and focus on delivering care within the frameworks set by the plans. Those with robust IT systems that demonstrate high performance in delivering care and controlling cost succeed. Health plans that reduce hassles for consumers, possess information systems that track costs, and collect and publish provider performance information will lead the industry. The IT infrastructure is critical. Customer service is Internet-driven, providing easy and rapid access to information and services. Plans are responsive to consumers' needs, offering a variety of insurance products. Yet consumers have little choice among health plans. Since the large-scale consolidation of health plans included the acquisition of e-health care companies, only a few of those companies remain independent and operate in the business-to-business space. A lax antitrust environment has allowed health plan mergers and acquisitions to proceed unhampered. Medicare managed care has become a competitive program and Med-

icaid managed care thrives. Government and large employers are still the dominant purchasers of health care.

Drivers

- Plans and providers consolidate to gain market share and capital.

- Big Insurance makes substantial investments in IT.

- E-health care companies play a subordinate role as they meet with financial failure or acquisition by health plans in the e-health market.

- Lax antitrust regulation allows health-plan mergers.

Barriers

- Data standards fail to evolve in order to facilitate the free flow of information among plans and providers.

- Consumers protect their health information, and privacy regulations constrain the flow of information within the health care system.

- The science of performance measurement in health care fails to provide useful, understandable information about providers.

- Purchasers, dissatisfied with the price of plans and their services, work around them and negotiate directly with providers.

- Providers cannot deliver the data needed to drive care management, pricing, and accountability.

Government Leads

An economic downturn in 2004 triggers a market failure that leads people to lose their health insurance or to drop it. A reduction in employer-based health insurance increases the ranks of the uninsured. The e-health care market fails as a vehicle by which consumers can purchase insurance. Consequently, consumers struggle unsuccessfully in the marketplace for individual insurance. Health care costs and premiums rise in the face of an aging population, advances in medical technology, and soaring pharmaceutical costs. The public decries differential access to health care. Medical technology costs spin out of control, creating an incentive to use technology assessment. These forces push the government to step in. Legislation is signed that expands the Federal Employees Health Benefits Plan (FEHBP) to include private purchasers and purchasing coalitions.

Drivers

- An economic downturn triggers a failure in the employer-paid insurance market, increasing the number of people who are uninsured.

- Health care costs escalate out of control (19 percent of GDP) due to advancements in technology and an aging population.

- The e-health care market fails as a vehicle by which consumers can buy insurance.

- As medical technology costs spin out of control, the public decries differential access to treatments.

Barriers

- The health care-industry lobby opposes governmental regulation.

- The pervasive perception among the public is that government cannot provide high-quality health care because of bureaucracy and lack of expertise.

- Advocates insist that this version of government protection is not adequate because the system is still inequitable as long as consumers with higher incomes can purchase high-end plans.

- Innovation is stunted by government regulation.

- Providers oppose oversight of their activities by the government.

- Negotiating power between purchasers and providers is limited

Consumers Meet E-Markets

In a continuing effort to control their costs, the purchasers of health care—largely employers—shift an increasing share of the health care bill to consumers. At the same time, employers invest in educational programs to enable employees to become more aware of the cost and quality of the health care they choose. Consumers pay for a larger percentage of their insurance premiums than they did just 5 years ago, but they are being offered a growing menu of health care goods and services. As a result, consumers are in the driver's seat in health care decision making. New

Q: How do gov't regs designed to protect privacy
affect quality of care?

Consumers relish taking on this role, as they have taken on the self-determining role in other aspects of their lives, from personal finance and investments to shopping.

Capitalizing on this changing role of the health care consumer, e-health care companies emerge to provide the tools consumers need to make health care decisions—data on the cost and performance of providers, personalized health plans, personal health records, financial transaction tools for purchasing care, and treatment information. Online brokers and health agents assist consumers in selecting care. Privacy regulations that give consumers knowledge about who sees their medical information, and control over access to it, make consumers more confident about the safety of personal health information. By 2010, a consumer-centered, commercial e-health care market thrives.

Drivers

Q - options

- Costs rise relentlessly and employers suffer from "benefits fatigue."

- E-health care companies support consumers' health care decision making with products such as personal health records, medical savings accounts, peer-reviewed treatment information, performance data on providers and plans, e-brokerage services, and e-health plans.

- Privacy regulations are implemented that make consumers more comfortable in using the Net as a vehicle for conveying personal health information.

- New Consumers act on their need for information, choice, and control of their care, and they increasingly use the Net to manage their own health care.

Barriers

- Consumers are reluctant to sit in the driver's seat when it comes to managing their own health care and are slow to fully use cafeteria plans to augment their dwindling health care coverage.

- E-health care companies fail to design sustainable business models and die out as quickly as they emerge, reducing consumers' confidence in the direct health care market.

- High-profile incidents involving violations of the privacy and security of health information make consumers wary of the Net.

- Providers are slow to make the necessary adjustments to capitalize on the Net and to integrate IT into their practice.

- Powerful health care providers and plans successfully lobby against the publication of data about their performance and cost, and consumers' ability to make decisions is hampered by lack of information—slowing the transition to a consumer-centered market in health care.

- Changes to ERISA and employer tax laws are incremental and constrain employers' move to free themselves of the burden of health care benefits.

Chapter 5: Managed Care   63

WILD CARDS

- The quality movement takes off. Sparked by the actions of the IOM and large-scale purchaser coalitions, an intense focus is placed on improving quality and using health care quality data as major criteria for purchasing care.

- Purchasers, plans, and providers begin to quantify meaningful savings attributable to improvements in quality. Thus, the business case for quality is unassailable, and value purchasing and providers' emphasis of improvement in quality become standard health care business practices.

- Universal health coverage is enacted that excises the costs of avoidable morbidity, redundant technology, and unnecessary prescriptions and procedures. It also mandates implementation of Internet-based approaches, such as electronic medical records and tools to support physicians' decision making. These changes promote best clinical practices. Purchasers are off the hook. The pace at which managed care adopts information-driven cost management picks up dramatically.

- A federal Patients' Bill of Rights passes without protections for self-insured purchasers, causing a large-scale move to defined contribution, in which consumers have a voucher to purchase coverage directly. Thus, the pressure that purchasers put on plans and providers to join the information age is eliminated.

- Physicians become sufficiently frustrated about managed care and their level of reimbursement that they yield to unionization and collective bargaining, thereby inhibiting the use of information-driven techniques to hold down the costs of care delivery.

ENDNOTES

1 Gabel, J., L. Levitt, J. Pickreign, et. al. Job-based health insurance in 2001: inflation hits double digits, managed care retreats. *Health Affairs* (September/October) 2001; 20(5):180–186.

2 Kaiser Family Foundation. *National Survey of Consumer Experiences with Health Plans.* The Henry J. Kaiser Foundation, Publication #3025. June 2000.

3 Watson Wyatt Worldwide. Putting Employees in Charge, A Survey of Employers, Health Care Providers, and Health Plans. Catalog #: W-332. Bethesda, MD, 2000.

4 Arthur Anderson and HealthCare Forum. Leadership for a Healthy 21st Century: Creating Value Through Relationship. 1999.

5 Milliman and Robertson, Inc. 2000 HMO InterCompany Rate Survey. Brookfield, WI, 2000.

6 California Medical Association. *The Coming Medical Group Failure Epidemic: Access to Medical Care for Millions of Californians Is in Jeopardy.* Special Report by the California Medical Association. San Francisco, CA. September 2, 1999.

7 Reinhardt, Uwe. Rise and fall of physician practice management. *Health Affairs* (January/February) 2000; 19(1):42–55.

8 Weiss, Marin D., Chairman, Weiss Ratings. Reuters. September 19, 2000.

9 Bodenheimer, T. California's Beleaguered Physician Groups—Will They Survive? *New England Journal of Medicine* 2000; 342: 1064–1068.

10 Trauner, J. Reassessing the plight of physician organizations in California: The uncertain future for IPAs. *Journal of Ambulatory Care Management* 2000; 23:28–38.

11 *Twenty First Century Health Care Consumers.* IFTF. Menlo Park, CA. 1998.

12 Kaiser Family Foundation, *National Survey of Consumer Experiences with Health Plans.* The Henry J. Kaiser Foundation, Publication #3025. June, 2000.

13 Noble, A., and T. A. Brennan. The stages of managed care regulations: Developing better rules. *Journal of Health Politics, Policy and Law* (December) 1999; 24(6):1275–1305.

14 Spetz, J., and L. Baker. *Has Managed Care Affected the Availability of Medical Technology?* Public Policy Institute of California. 1999.

15 William M. Mercer. 15th Annual Mercer/Foster Higgins National Survey of Employer-Sponsored Health Plans. 2000

16 Balas, E. A., S. Weingarten, C. T. Garb, et al. Improving preventive care by prompting physicians. *Arch Intern Med.* (February 14) 2000; 160(3):301–308.

17 First Consulting Group. One huge HIPAA; AHA-funded study sees compliance costs in the billions. *Modern Healthcare* December 18, 2000.

18 Hewitt Associates. *Employers to Face Double Digit Health Care Cost Increases for Third Consecutive Year.* October 2000.

19 HCFA. Personal Health Care Expenditures and Average Annual Percent Change, by Source of Funds: Selected Calendar Years 1970–2008. Health Care Financing Administration, Office of the Actuary. November 1998.

20 Kohn, L. T, J. M. Corrigan, and M. S. Donaldson, eds. *To Err Is Human: Building a Safer Health System.* Committee on Quality of Health Care in America, Institute of Medicine. National Academies Press. 2000.

CHAPTER 6

Health Care Providers

Themes of the Future Delivery System

The mixture of physicians, hospitals, and other providers that makes up the American health care delivery system has never been a well-organized entity. We are a few years into what we perceive will be 15 to 20 years of profound change in the way health care providers are organized. This period of change will occupy all of our forecast period up to 2010, and the outcome of those changes will be of profound importance for the future well beyond 2010. Although patients will be involved in all stages, both as active agents and as passive recipients of change, most of the action will be driven externally by employers, governments, and health insurers, with various players in the system trying to create organizations that will survive and even prosper in the future. Several key backdrops frame this system:

■ *Continued organizational change.* A combination of the demands of employers, the rise of managed care, the recommendations of consultants, and the infusion of Wall Street capital into the health care system has led to a desire for new models of health care delivery. Current providers are trying to make sure that they will be in the game for the long term. Consequently, there has been a rash of mergers, acquisi-

tions, and new initiatives among all sectors of the market. This activity has been as prevalent among nonprofit organizations as it has been among their Wall Street–funded brethren. It presages a slow transition from a world of independent entities to one of more corporate systems. Between here and there have been—and will be—many false starts, poor investment decisions, and organizational disasters.

■ *The role of intermediaries.* Health care plans, disease management companies, case managers, and other management organizations will become much more important in directing patients to providers and in intervening and directing the activities of care providers and patients. There is a possibility that providers will attempt to circumvent the intermediaries and go directly to such end payers as employers or Medicare. There is also a possibility that, as patients become more engaged in their care, they will influence the behavior of these intermediaries as well as that of their providers. Intermediaries supported by integrated delivery networks (IDNs), managed care organizations (MCOs), pharmaceutical companies, and grants to small providers will prove increasingly popular with patients and families, reducing the influence of providers responsible for overseeing the care. The empowerment of patients with other sources of information, such as the Internet, will accelerate this process of provider demotion in the patient's eyes.

■ *An oversupply of hospital beds and a surplus of physicians.* America has far more hospital beds than it uses, and many more than it needs. Whether or not this situation is a surplus to some normative "need," the overall market effect is that providers increasingly will be working in a buyer's market rather than the seller's market that has existed for the past six decades.

■ *Control over medical management* will be the main arena of interorganizational conflict in the medium-term future. Physicians and providers have lost substantial organizational, financial, and clinical control to health plans and payers, but they have been building systems to win back some of that control. Control over medical management will be the central arena in which this power struggle plays out. The shift in locus of decision making away from individual clinicians to other entities will continue. The question is how far and how fast will that shift go, and exactly who will direct medical decision making. During the next decade evidence-based medicine (EBM) will increasingly be used in large organizations seeking the best clinical methodology and guidelines. The cohort shift in the population of

practicing providers will be more accepting of this loss of autonomy. The end result will be more widely accepted guidelines in use, with less variation and therefore better quality.

Assuming these four major themes— overcapacity in the system, continued change among all organizations, the evolving role of the intermediary, and a battle over control of medical management—this chapter forecasts the future roles of intermediaries, the new models of payment to providers and care organizations, and the structure of service-delivery organizations.

INTERMEDIARIES

BACKGROUND: THE CONVERGENCE OF OPEN NETWORKS AND THE DEMISE OF VERTICAL INTEGRATION

The past two decades have produced a dramatic change in the commercial insurance market and we are now seeing the beginning of a similar change in the Medicare and Medicaid systems. HMOs, PPOs, and POS plans, which limit patients' access to physicians and services through financial incentives and gatekeepers, have become the dominant form of health insurance for employees and their families. Similarly restrictive plans have been able to increase enrollment in Medicaid and even in Medicare. However, most enrollment growth has not been in the classic prepaid health plans—the staff- and group-model HMOs—but rather in IPA-based HMOs that use mainstream community physicians and hospitals.

There has been a market shake-up in managed care Medicare products, which have been dropped by many payers in unprofitable areas. Nevertheless, with refinement and modifications, managed care will remain profitable and new products and improved methodologies (e.g., United Healthcare's increasingly customer-service-oriented business model) will keep the larger payers profitable and growing during this next decade. Smaller payers will find alternative niche markets for special groupings of covered lives that are actuarially sound. This process of economic market maturation will reduce destructive cut-throat competition, and increase barriers to entry during this next decade. It will also provide a broader menu of health care delivery options, with each niche that develops.

The growth of IPA-based HMOs surprised many observers who thought that the cohesiveness and internal controls of group and staff plans would give them a competitive advantage over the IPA models. However, IPA models have succeeded in controlling provider costs, meaning that there has been little competitive advantage of the staff-model HMOs. Providing access to the same providers that patients were already seeing has been the IPA models' biggest advantage in selling their products. The shift toward IPA-based HMOs has significantly changed what most pundits thought the managed care landscape was going to look like (see Figure 6-1).

Maturation of the IPA model has been accompanied by some business failures and liquidity problems, arising from the role of IPAs as a "middle man" offering cost controls. This has played out most noticeably starting in 2000 in the California market.[1] During the next decade, the successful IPAs will consolidate and develop systems that add value through the addition of information and services, and gain brand value recognition in the market place as the perception of this value increases.

Virtually all HMOs—with the notable exception of Kaiser Permanente and the few other group- and staff-model HMOs—use the same provider networks, and they pay providers through a mix of discounted FFS and partial forms of capitation. Moreover, as health plans have widened their networks and developed point-of-service plans and direct patient referrals to specialists, their HMO products are becoming increasingly similar to the products of PPOs.

Near the end of our forecast horizon, HMOs will be tackling the balance between the cost savings of prevention and the cost of later care. New technology and clinical information may well bring the time horizon for the payback into the range of annual financial planning. This would increase their ability to focus on prevention.

ISSUES: NOW THAT WE ARE ALL IN MANAGED CARE, WHAT ARE WE GOING TO DO?

Most intermediaries offer a mix of insurance products that provide more or less the same physician networks and similar medical management techniques. They compete on the basis of price to employers, customer service, and benefits to

Figure 6-1. Managed competition: How it was supposed to be . . .

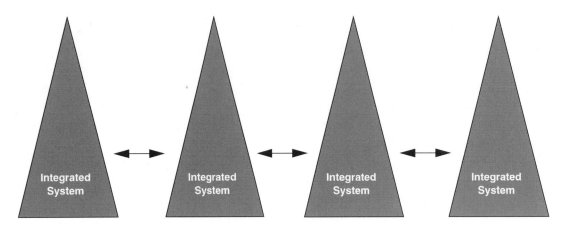

World of:
- competition between vertically integrated systems
- exclusive relationships
- empowered consumers

. . . and how it really is.

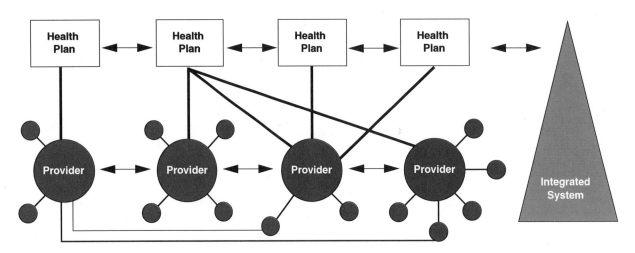

World of:
- horizontally integrated delivery systems
- nonexclusive relationships
- competition among plans and providers
- confused consumers

Source: IFTF.

individual enrollees, particularly in the Medicare market. Most of the savings they have gained were achieved by cutting payment rates to providers, and those cuts have gone about as far as they can for the short term. These plans are coming under three new types of pressure:

- Although intermediaries have been successful in cutting costs, the savings have been achieved by one-time reductions in payment rates. Meanwhile, utilization rates are rising across the board, particularly as these plans have added new providers to their rosters, included different types of populations in their membership such as Medicare recipients, and added new products such as POS. In the latter part of 1996 and through 1998, the "medical loss ratios" (i.e., how much money was passed on to providers) of many publicly traded HMOs began to increase. Yet cutting back on product offerings is not an option, as their employer customers are demanding *more,* not less, variety and choice among provider networks.

- Employers, the government, and accreditation agencies such as the National Committee on Quality Assurance (NCQA) are demanding proof of quality performance. Given the lack of provider differentiation among different health plans, it is hard for them to demonstrate quality—particularly quality as compared to that provided by a competitor.

- It is also increasingly difficult for health plans to avoid a commitment

to treat high-risk populations, both because of such legislation as the Kennedy–Kassebaum Act and because often they are getting a large enough share in any one market that they cannot avoid treating the sicker segments of the community. If insurers cannot avoid expensive cases, their only option is to manage the care of their numbers in a more cost-effective manner without cutting quality. How to do this is a new adventure for virtually every plan in America. Patients have not been able to understand or use HEDIS or other quality measures yet, and employer and business groups will continue to pressure providers to improve the data and make it more understandable.

As patients from every venue enter managed care, the question becomes: Which intermediary model is best suited to resolve the issues of cost, quality, and care management? The attempt to find such models is a key driver for the future of health plans and for health care in general.

FORECAST: INTERMEDIARIES MULTIPLY IN TYPE

What types of intermediaries will patients use? For the insured segment of the population, the mix of indemnity to HMO plans will reverse over this next 10-year period. For enrollees in Medicaid, indemnity Medicaid will become managed care Medicaid, perhaps with slightly better access to providers. The uninsured will rely on the same network of safety-net providers, who will survive with a mixture of state and local funding.

EBM, outcomes statistics, and the reduced variation in clinical care will cause even the FFS patients in effect to receive managed care, but perhaps with more associated personal services. Changes in the technology of care, the inclusion of prevention into care, and the impact of genomics and proteinomics on care will change the definition of managed care. And this will create new roles and new intermediaries during the next decade. Toward the end of our time horizon, we will see the dawning of the age of more general use of medical informatics that will begin to determine the prevention or care needed and define the mix of these that is purchased either out of pocket or under a health plan.

The net result of this forecast is that enrollment in HMOs will increase from 27 percent to 47 percent of all Americans by 2007. Combined enrollment in HMOs and PPOs will cover just over two-thirds of the entire American population (see Figure 6-2). Only the uninsured, a little over half of Medicare recipients, and a few upper-echelon employees—those in our "high-end FFS broker" category—will be outside of managed care.

Health plans will spend the next 3 to 5 years in a constant flurry of consolidation, experimentation, and restructuring. Several dominant strategies will emerge by 2005. Most intermediaries will adopt one or more of these strategies, depending on the geography, philosophy, and availability of organized providers:

■ *The case manager intermediary.* The case manager intermediary divides a population into the well and the sick and permits the well to have free access to virtually all of its loosely organized provider network. Its primary focus is the aggressive medical management of the sick, often parsed out by disease state. It uses a mixture of provider organizations and relies on the development of information systems to track the activities of its loosely organized provider network. The intermediary spends much of its energy in directing the activities of providers and sick patients. Providers are paid in a multitude of ways, usually on a fee-per-episode basis, but must meet or exceed several stipulated specifications regarding costs, quality, and patients' satisfaction in order to keep their contracts. The growth of knowledge has been exponential in recent years. This has or will exceed the capacity of some specialists or intermediaries as individuals to know

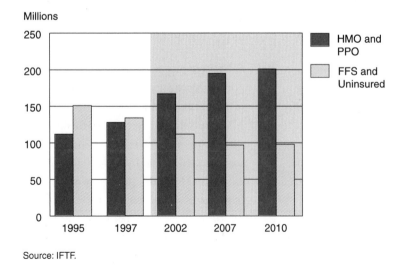

Figure 6-2. Managed Care takes over from "unmanaged care."
(Number of Americans, in millions, in HMOs and PPOs versus FFS and uninsured over time)

Millions

Legend:
- HMO and PPO (dark)
- FFS and Uninsured (light)

Source: IFTF.

everything they could need to know even in one specialized area. The competence of organized subspecialty knowledge systems and the use of artificial intelligence (AI) in organizations may become a more significant competitive factor beginning at the end of this decade.

- *The provider-partner intermediary.* The provider partner allows providers to be responsible for the medical management of the enrollees. The intermediary takes on responsibilities for customer service to members, for marketing its providers' services, and for redistributing risk among its providers. The health plan relies on the use of various risk-sharing vehicles to pay providers, including full and partial capitation, satisfaction incentives, and rewards for customer retention. The intermediary rigorously audits providers to ensure that they manage patients to an agreed-upon standard but relies on the clinicians to develop protocols and demand-management techniques. This model operates successfully only with large provider organizations. Most intermediaries run this type of model in one region and the case-manager model in others.

- *The high-end FFS broker.* For upper-echelon Americans, the remnants of the old FFS system will offer indemnity insurance products or PPOs with very rich benefits and less rigorous utilization controls. Although these plans are unable to compete directly with the more aggressive "case managers" or "provider partners" on price, they are able to select better risks in their enrollee population and charge

relatively high premiums for good customer service and access to high-tech and complementary care. Meanwhile, a slight majority of Medicare recipients remain in the FFS system, which provides access to a provider network that looks just like this one. High-end FFS brokers will be ideally placed during the next decade to be the intermediaries in new specialties that are yet to be defined; these could include genomic-prevention with nutrition programs or pharmacogenomic treatment optimization programs. Such procedures will be possible and arise, but will become part of mainstream medicine at the end of this decade. More general adoption will await knowledge of the value proposition this creates.

- *Direct to provider.* In a minority of cases, large employers in rural markets and a few big employer coalitions are able to bypass the major plans and set up their own administrative systems that allow them to contract directly with providers. The providers are asked to take most of the downside risk from these arrangements and to provide medical management and population care to enrollees. Essentially, the intermediary functions here are shared by employer and provider alike. The financial solvency of this sector will not be strong for the first few years, but by 2005 a small but important portion of the market will be contracting directly with employers.

- *The low-tier safety-net funding recipients.* Most of the Medicaid population and some of the indigent will end up in a provider-partner or a case-management

*Figure 6-3. The "fee-for-service brokers" will lose their dominance.
(Percentage of population in each insurance model)*

Where we were in 1998

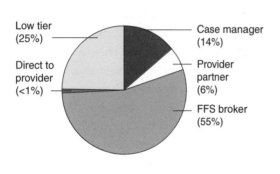

Where we'll be in 2007

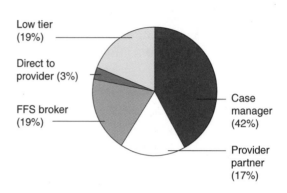

Source: IFTF.

HMO, but some of them—and the majority of the uninsured—will end up in a "no intermediary, no luck" scenario with limited access to care despite the best efforts of safety-net providers. Figure 6-3 shows how much of the population was covered by each type of insurance intermediary arrangement in 1998 and forecasts what that will be in 2007.

REIMBURSEMENT MODELS: BETWEEN FINANCE AND DELIVERY

BACKGROUND

For patients with either Medicare or private insurance coverage, reimbursement for physicians and hospitals was on an FFS basis until the 1980s, when Medicare introduced a prospective payment system (PPS) for hospital inpatient services based on diagnosis-related groups (DRGs). The introduction of

DRGs led to the early movement of Medicare patients from inpatient status to outpatient facilities where services could be charged on an FFS basis. Those outpatient facilities were usually owned by hospitals.

Meanwhile, in an effort to control the cost of health benefits for employees, many employers and employer coalitions moved to HMOs or other managed care insurance products. Insurers, except in staff- and group-model HMOs, slowly began to "push risk" to the providers, either capitating physicians only (partial capitation) while paying hospitals a discounted per diem, or capitating physicians or physician-hospital organizations for all required services (global capitation).

When we naively asked a Boston colleague why the HMO membership rate in Massachusetts was the same as in California, yet the utilization rates in

California for all services were so much lower, he replied, "We have lots of managed care in Boston—it's just FFS managed care." The numbers in Figures 6-4 and 6-5 confirm that theory: the spread of managed care has not meant a significant spread of capitation.

In fact, only about one in ten dollars paid out by HMOs is in the form of global captitation—the classic Southern California model that was developed in the late 1980s. Although capitation is spreading outside of Southern California, it is generally used only for primary care services. Instead, aggressive HMOs have reduced FFS payments to specialists and hospitals and have placed money in risk pools that primary care doctors may share if their overall utilization and

referral rates are below a specified level. The net result has been a transfer of resources from hospitals and specialists to primary care physicians and health plans without much global capitation occurring (see Figure 6-6). Many of the organizational models that hospitals and physicians have designed over the past few years have not been successful because they were designed to treat capitated lives. Even the Southern California providers found that some health plans did not want to pass the risk, and possibly the profits, on to the providers. Those providers who did accept global capitation found that the rates they were paid were restricted by the plans. When providers tried to resist those rate changes, they found that their market power was less than they had hoped.

Figure 6-4. How physicians got paid in 1997
(Percentage of patients with various forms of payment)

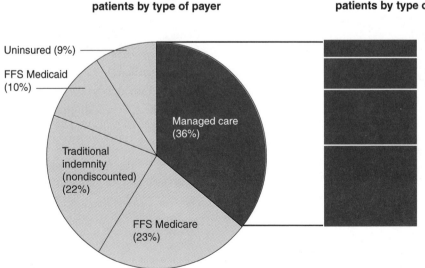

Percentage of patients by type of payer

Uninsured (9%)

FFS Medicaid (10%)

Traditional indemnity (nondiscounted) (22%)

Managed care (36%)

FFS Medicare (23%)

Percentage of managed care patients by type of payment

Capitation for all services (all physicians and hospitals) (10%)

Capitation for physician's own services only (17%)

Discount FFS with a withhold/risk pool (29%)

Discount FFS (44%)

Source: Health Care Outlook Physicians Survey, 1997.

Figure 6-5. How HMOs pay their doctors and hospitals (Percentage of HMOs using various methods for any portion of provider payments)

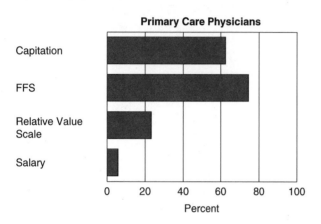

Primary Care Physicians

Method	
Capitation	
FFS	
Relative Value Scale	
Salary	

(x-axis: Percent, 0 to 100)

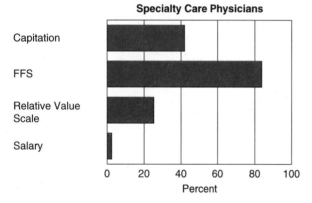

Specialty Care Physicians

Method	
Capitation	
FFS	
Relative Value Scale	
Salary	

(x-axis: Percent, 0 to 100)

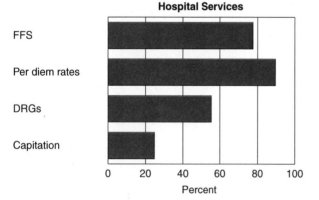

Hospital Services

FFS	
Per diem rates	
DRGs	
Capitation	

(x-axis: Percent, 0 to 100)

Note: Percentages do not equal 100.

Source: Interstudy, using 2000 data.

While mixed payment methods for providers such as discounted FFS, withholds, and partial capitation on the physicians' side and DRGs and per diems on the hospital side remain the norm, they all provide incentives for more utilization. The health plans counteract this by attempting to control utilization externally. Although increases in utilization are still a significant problem for intermediaries, they generally have not responded by passing that risk off to providers in the form of capitation.

There appear to be three reasons for this:

- Health plans that were successful in managing risk could be more profitable than those that pass it off in the form of capitation.

- Providers generally are not organized to take on the risk-bearing function of capitation and have little incentive to so organize in a world where FFS still predominates.

- Patients and consumer groups fear that capitated providers may withhold necessary care, although they fear that FFS encourages providers to overtreat in equal numbers. Several highly visible court cases have fueled this backlash.

The question for the future is whether incentives will continue for utilization and what the current flood of people into HMOs will mean for payment mechanisms for providers. The type of payment will have a great impact not only on providers' behavior but also on how providers organize themselves.

Figure 6-6. How premium payments get divided up: The PPO world versus the HMO world

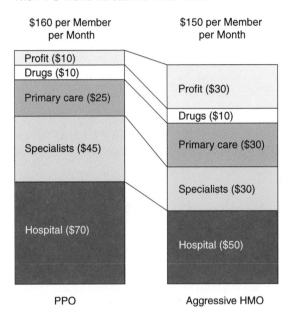

Note: These figures are hypothetical.

Source: IFTF.

Figure 6-7. Fee-for-service will fade, but capitation is not its only successor. (Share of physicians' revenue coming from different payment schemes)

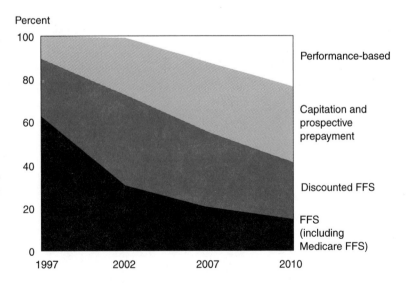

Source: IFTF, based on data from IFTF, Louis Harris & Associates, Interstudy, and American Medical Association.

FORECAST

It is likely that neither global capitation nor discounted FFS is sustainable in the long run. FFS is inherently inflationary, and capitation raises fears of undertreatment among consumers. We believe that eventually a new way of paying providers will emerge. But over the rest of this decade a version of the current system will develop that shifts toward more capitation because of the flood of people into HMOs. Global capitation will most likely double in prominence as the number of HMO recipients increases, but it will never cover much more than 10 percent of patients. Meanwhile, Medicare will start to introduce episodic prepayment for many of its components, including outpatient care, and increasingly will replace the current FFS system. Figure 6-7 presents a forecast of how dollars for care will flow to physicians.

Out of this mixture, a separate type of payment system will develop. Plans and intermediaries will devise reimbursement systems that give providers incentives to deliver care in a manner that improves quality, customer satisfaction, patients' tenure in the plan, and outcomes, as well as productivity and cost-effectiveness. We dub this system "performance-based" reimbursement, as payments will depend on the provider's performance on a string of relevant algorithms. By the latter part of the decade, this system will be the single most important way of paying provider organizations, although the old methods will still be a prominent part of the system. Pay for performance will be more rapidly adopted toward the end of the decade where there is enough cost-efficiency to allow the pay to providers to increase. At what point does the cost of

Chapter 6: Health Care Providers   77

the necessary informatics fall below what can be afforded in capital to provide the required cost-efficiencies of the care delivered? The way in which this plays out will help determine if rewarding quality will be anything other than a minor form of reimbursement in the next decade.

Care Delivery Organizations for the Next Decade

Background

The chaotic upheaval of the American health care system that started in the early 1990s is driven by several forces. The most important of them is the search for stability. Individual physicians and smaller organizations have looked to the large hospitals and health plans to buffer them through tough times. Larger groups and hospitals have allied and merged with each other in an attempt to develop bargaining power against the health plans, which have also been merging to amass bargaining power over providers. There have also been attempts to change organizational structures and processes in order to make patient-care management more effective, but so far that goal has been elusive. On an international comparative basis, the United States has high resource use and provider salaries, with fewer hospital beds and shorter stays than other OECD countries. This was associated with outcomes that were in the bottom half of measures and ranking. Toward the end of our time horizon, this poorer comparative performance can be expected to improve as the benefits of our medical informatics and technology bring efficiency.

Several types of provider groups have looked to for-profit companies for

capital, although the investor-owned sector is a small, barely growing minority of hospitals (about 14 percent) and an even smaller minority of physicians. It does not appear yet that there is anything fundamentally different about the way for-profit groups are behaving. However, there is investment money available for people trying to create new types of provider organizations, many of them focused on disease management or specialty care.

The market behavior of nonprofit hospitals is currently deviating from their for-profit competitors. There has been a trend, after mergers of nonprofit hospitals, to use the reduced competition to increase pricing more aggressively than the for-profit hospitals.[2] This is likely a short-term effect that will correct itself during the next decade.

Issues

Through all the activity of the past several years, most physicians who were independent have stayed independent and most hospitals have joined systems more in name than in terms of substantially changing their organization and governance. But the driving pressures of reimbursement reductions and the certainty that the challenges of tomorrow will be different from those of yesterday are driving continued reinvention in every provider organization. What changes this reinvention might produce are less certain than ever, and at present several models exist in different stages of evolution. They include:

- *Vertical integration.* A combination of providers and health plan, usually developing in an altered form of staff HMO (e.g., Lovelace Health System in New Mexico).

■ *Horizontal integration.* A combination of several similar organizations, such as independent hospitals, in one system (e.g., Catholic Healthcare West, Promina in Atlanta).

■ *Integrated delivery systems or networks.* A combination of physicians with hospital services and other types of delivery systems in one organization, typically by hospitals' purchasing physician practices but sometimes by physicians' acquiring hospitals (e.g., Advocate EHS in Chicago, Mullikin Medical Centers in Southern California).

■ *Virtual integration.* A combination of various care-delivery services provided by separate organizations that offer services under contract to each other and are organized seamlessly (no good examples yet!).

■ *Centers of excellence.* Single-specialty organizations that provide a defined service, either as a subcontractor to another provider or directly to a plan (e.g., MedCath in cardiology, M.D. Anderson Cancer Center).

The dominant issue for delivery organizations is which model will prove flexible, resilient, and profitable enough to survive the turbulent decade ahead. Intermediaries and end payers will demand not only cost-effective and efficient processes but also the ability to manage patients and coordinate care among a range of institutions.

FORECAST

We do not believe that any one organizational form will emerge by 2005 to replace the individual practitioner and large teaching/community hospital model that dominated medical care from the 1930s to the early 1990s. In order to satisfy the demands of intermediaries and patients, different types of organizations will use various models, each of which will provide a substantial percentage of care in at least some regions of the country. In the early 2000s, versions of each of these models are being built with more or less aggressive intentions by entrepreneurial physicians and businesspeople. They include:

■ *The hospital-centered system.* The series of large hospital mergers in the mid-1990s were intended to create a model that provides all services in a metropolitan area across a range of facilities. The range includes inpatient, outpatient, diagnostic, and ancillary facilities, as well as physician multispecialty clinics, usually owned by or closely aligned with the system. These systems will employ many clinicians, either directly or under a contractual umbrella. Many of the systems will be based around AMCs, which will have problems making the transition to this more comprehensive approach, particularly in relation to their faculty and the physician practices with which they contract.

Fundamentally, the primary problem for AMCs is their organizational origin as inpatient care centers. The cultural inertia of the principle underlying the former system, which required them to "fill those beds,"

Physicians in Group Practice

During the past 30 years, there has been an explosion in the total number of physicians in group practices, with an increase from 28,000 in 1965 to 207,000 in 1998—more than three times greater than growth in the overall physician population. What still surprises many people, however, is that more than 40 percent of all office-based physicians still deliver care in individual or two-physician practices. Furthermore, only 60 percent of office-based physicians are in group practices of three or more and, of those, about 70 percent are actually in small, three- to six-doctor practices. A practice of that size is probably too small to develop effective contracting and management skills during the next 12 years.

Despite all the press coverage and expectations, only 56,000 office-based physicians are in multispecialty groups of more than 100 members—the type of group best suited to accept global capitation. That is less than 13 percent of all office-based physicians and less than 10 percent of the market of physicians delivering patient care. Most physicians have not reorganized into large multispecialty group practices to counterbalance the forces of consolidating health plans.

Younger physicians, however, are more interested in group practices and other employment opportunities than they are in setting up their own individual practice. In a comparison of age-matched California physicians with less than 9 years in practice, the rate of practice ownership declined from 53.3 percent in 1991 to 42.4 percent in 1996.[3] Overall, between 1983 and 1995, employed physicians increased from 25 percent to 45.4 percent of all practicing physicians.[4]

Of this new influx of physicians into employee positions, most are joining existing group practices—they are not starting their own groups. These young physicians are looking for security. They will continue to swell the ranks of group physicians, but it will take time before they alter overall physician demographics.

The growth of group practice will not be driven purely by the influx of new physicians, but they will certainly be the greatest influential force. Our core forecast projects that the percentage of patient-care physicians in group practice after their residency training will increase from 46 percent in 1996 to between 57 percent and 62 percent in 2005 and will reach between 63 percent and 67 percent by 2010 (see Figure 6-8).[5] A historic shift will therefore occur in the next 3 to 8 years that will place the majority of patient-care physicians in groups. However, a substantial minority of physicians (150,000 to 200,000) will continue operating in solo and two-physician practices until 2005 and are likely to continue practicing that way, especially in more rural areas.

will cause many to falter. Nonetheless, in many areas of the country the large capital reserves of these systems and their significant presence in the market will ensure their survival. This is particularly true where their brand name (e.g., Johns Hopkins) is sufficient to ensure their presence in intermediaries' networks.

■ *The virtual physician-group cooperative.* This is an evolved form of the IPA—the most common current organizational form for physicians. Although IPAs originally were thought of as a transitional model on the path to "real" medical groups, they will continue to be an important factor to 2005 and beyond. Their ability to use information technology and their contractual flexibility to coordinate services will enable virtual groups to enter into contracts with several health plans. In many cases, the "real" medical groups at the core of these networks will be neither large nor cohesive. The organization will be created from independent physicians with a natural set of referrals, on-call coverage, and clinical respect for each other. A management services organization (MSO) will help them make contracts with plans for business, with hospitals, and with other providers for services, and often will help them assume risk. The MSO will also help to identify and negotiate with providers whose utilization or quality is inadequate. IPAs will remain as an umbrella organization for these physicians, and within them there will be a range of activity, including attempts to build groups. Nonetheless, almost all small groups and individual physicians

*Figure 6-8. More physicians and many more group physicians
(Number of physicians in group practice)*

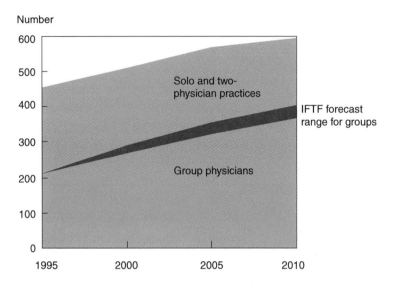

Source: IFTF, based on data from American Medical Association.

will find that, as a contracting vehicle, the virtual group provides them with a substantial proportion of their patient revenue stream.

■ *The corporate physician practice management (PPM) corporation.* The trail of for-profit PPM companies to Wall Street that started in the early 1990s will continue through this decade. The main growth in this area has and will come from the PPMs that accumulate existing smaller practices, including purchasing physician groups abandoned by former staff- and group-model HMOs. While pressures from Wall Street will cause many of those corporations to fail, several will develop a common platform across their groups that is similar to the mix of corporate and franchise-owned operations seen in other industries. Consid-

ering the administrative inefficiency of most physicians' practices, there is no reason that these economies of scale should not show some savings. Achieving greater returns may prove difficult over the longer term.

■ *The single-specialty carve-out.* In some specific disease areas, single-specialty groups and networks of specialists will market their services either directly to payers or to other providers such as hospital-based systems or multispecialty groups that need particular expertise. A proliferation of networks will provide specialty disease management services for cancer, cardiovascular disease, nephrology, and AIDS (acquired immunodeficiency syndrome), among others. Some multispecialty groups that do not have sufficient volume will refer their patients in some disease categories because they cannot support nearly as large a specialty panel as can a single-specialty network. Patients needing specialty care will appreciate being able to go to these networks, which usually will allow them a wide choice of physicians. Some of these organizations will provide all comprehensive specialty services in a particular specialty area, such as cancer treatment, whereas others will provide niche support services, such as patient monitoring and education, that are used in combination with services provided by other organizations.

■ *The remnants.* Changing an 80-year-old health care system that has been supported by government subsidies for the past 30 years is not going to be accomplished quickly. Some

Chapter 6: Health Care Providers 81

independent hospitals, such as profitable community hospitals in some suburbs and cash-strapped public hospitals in inner cities or rural areas, will not find partners or be incorporated into a bigger system. Many of the remaining individual and small-group practice doctors will still be doing what they have always done until their retirement. In that regard, much of the present system will remain in the health care system of the future.

MEDICAL MANAGEMENT: THE NEW ARENA OF ACTIVITY

BACKGROUND: FROM MANAGED CARE TO MANAGING CARE

While all of these arrangements on the intermediary side, the payment scene, and in provider realignment are continuing, the number of people employed in the health care industry and the utilization of pharmaceuticals and technologies continue to increase. At the same time, consumers and physicians in tandem frustrate the attempts of case managers to significantly reduce utilization. Meanwhile, the health care industry has been rocked by the "realization" that it is the care of the sick that is expensive. Serious attempts are now being made to manage and establish routines for the care of the chronically ill in the expectation that this effort will save money overall, particularly in substituting preventative maintenance for adverse acute events. This is called *disease management*.

Because of the inability of health plans to control providers and the projected

potential of disease management, control over the management of medical care will continue to develop as the key arena of activity—and conflict—in health care into the middle of the next decade.

The cost to Medicare for the postacute care of beneficiaries over 85 years of age has been the fastest-growing expense for Medicare over the last 30 years.[6] These pressures for supportive services for those with age-related clinical impairments and disabilities are a further pressure on Medicare managed care. This is therefore a likely focus for future disease or condition management activities in the next decade.

ISSUES: A NEW IDEA MAKES SENSE AND TROUBLE

Medical management—active management over the full care of patients and populations—is currently applied sporadically if at all. The main issue is to what extent medical management will spread and be applied more comprehensively. In some respects this movement is taking the health care system from a state of managed care to one of "managing care." That active management component involves not only changing how physicians and clinicians manage patients, but also how health systems monitor and look after patients, including how much they encourage and support self-care.

The issue of medical management involves to some extent at least five parties: health plans, providers, employers, patients (and their representative associations), and the government. All of these groups are wrestling over decisions surrounding the creation of clinical pathways and protocols, specifically, what should be done and what should be measured. Intermediaries and providers are most concerned with control over adherence to those pathways and protocols. The main arena of conflict concerns who enforces the behavior of patients and clinicians: Will it be the intermediaries or provider organizations?

Still, the main question for the health care *system* is how much of the care delivered is actively managed. That question will be broken down in two steps that will categorize the population by their health status. How important will the management of disease states be for the acutely sick and chronically ill, and how much impact will demand management have on the generally well?

The most important question behind all the protocols, the process management changes, and the disease-specific approaches is whether they will make any difference to cost, care quality, and outcomes in the long term.

FORECAST: MEDICAL MANAGEMENT FOR THE CHRONICALLY SICK

Conflicts in deciding which treatment protocols will apply to whom will stay visible as a political issue during the next decade. Intermediaries, providers, and others, including specialty societies and quality organizations (like NCQA), increasingly will issue multiple and conflicting guidelines. In addition, states and the federal government will

continue to be involved in legislating lengths of stay for particular procedures and occasionally will demand minimum staffing levels and mixes in different types of medical facilities as well. However, during the next decade the focus of activity will shift from *designing* guidelines to *enforcing* their use.

Neither plans nor provider organizations will clearly dominate or appropriate the role of controlling utilization. For instance, the provider-partner strategy mentioned earlier essentially assumes that providers will take on that role, whereas in the centralized case-manager strategy the intermediary keeps that role. In either event, the prerogative of medical management will shift away from the independent physician. Both internal managers, working as part of a clinical team within provider organizations, and external managers, working for intermediaries, will assume increasing authority over physicians and patients in three areas:

- Managing physicians and physicians' organizations' adherence to protocols, guidelines, and pathways to ensure consistent application of best practices.

- Creating systems that extend care pathways across the continuum of care to all facilities where patients receive care—the descendant of current case management.

- Managing patients' compliance with their treatment regimens, particularly in the case of pharmaceutical use, and educating and motivating them to better self-care.

Whereas there remains great variation in medical practice patterns in the 1990s, the spread of guidelines will have a significant impact on medical practice and patient management for the chronically ill by 2005, and a sporadic but discernible effect on practice variation by 2010. Most chronically ill patients will be under some type of disease management program by the end of the decade, and there will be hints of measurable improvements in outcomes. The use of demand management by advice nurses in contact with patients via the telephone and the Internet will be commonplace by 2005. However, the struggle over who controls patients' and physicians' behavior between the intermediaries and providers, and among and within the different provider organizations, will not be resolved by 2010.

There will be ample evidence by 2005 that individual patient management programs for the more severely chronically ill will improve health outcomes in the short term, deliver more consistent and higher quality care, and save a small amount of money. However, there will be no clear evidence that overall cost savings are realized systemwide by the development of these programs, and their impact on the overall costs of American health care will be hard to ascertain.

WHAT HAPPENS TO HOSPITALS?

THE DEATH OF THE HOSPITAL?

To borrow from Mark Twain, reports of the demise of American hospitals have been much exaggerated. The growth in

numbers of hospital beds stopped in the early 1980s, slightly before the move of Medicare Part A to the DRG-based PPS. Since then, reimbursement and medical technology have been pushing care out of inpatient settings. Beds have closed, from a high of slightly over 1 million in 1983 to approximately 830,000 in 1999 (see Figures 6-9 and 6-10).

The rate at which inpatient utilization of beds has declined has been much faster than the rate of closures, and hospitals *themselves* have closed at a very slow rate, somewhere between 30 and 80 a year, from a high of 5,800 in 1980. Despite all the rhetoric about the surplus of hospitals, not much has changed, and in 1997 there were still 5,000 of them. In their 1999 survey published in 2000 the AHA noted that in the United States there were 5,890 registered hospitals, of which 4,956 were community hospitals with 829,575 staffed beds remaining available.[7] Of these nearly 5,000 or so community hospitals, 2,238 are in systems and 1,310 are in networks, leaving 28.4 percent freestanding still in 1999. This statistic will continue to reduce over the next 10 years.

So many hospitals have survived during what has been regarded as an unfriendly era partly because facilities and beds have been converted to day-surgery and 23-hour stay units, and staff time has been converted from inpatient to outpatient care. But it's also because closing beds and particularly hospitals themselves is very difficult for a variety of business, political, and social reasons. Nonetheless, hospital occupancy has fallen quite rapidly across the country since the early 1980s to an average of

Figure 6-9. Hospital beds are slowly disappearing.
(Total beds in community hospitals*)

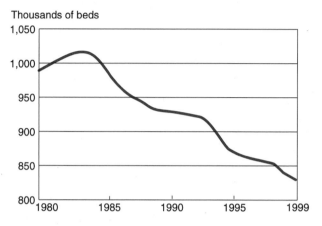

Thousands of beds

*AHA hospital definitions cite community hospitals as "all nonfederal short-term general and other special hospitals." This *includes* AMCs, for-profit hospitals, and state and local government hospitals that match the category. It excludes federal hospitals, long-term hospitals, hospital units of institutions, psychiatric hospitals, and several other specialized long-stay hospitals.

Source: American Hospital Association.

Figure 6-10. Occupancy has also fallen.
(Average hospital occupancy rates in community hospitals)

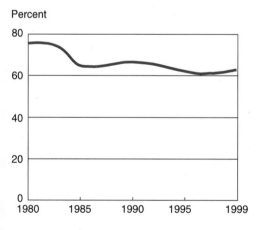

Percent

Source: American Hospital Association.

diagnosis to be treated will be managed in the outpatient setting. Those patients with two or more diagnoses will remain receiving inpatient care in a traditional hospital. This will refine the inpatient role of hospitals into the provision of care for even more high-acuity patients and resource-intense care. The United States already leads the world in this trend. Adjustments in reimbursement to reflect this change will be needed to keep hospitals solvent during the next decade.

In the mid-1990s, even those areas that previously had been exceptions to the general trend started experiencing lower occupancy rates. For instance, occupancy rate percentages in New York City fell from the high 90s to the 80s by 1997. In contrast, some parts of California had already seen occupancy rates below 50 percent by the mid-1990s. Meanwhile, the increased needs of the comparatively sicker patients occupying inpatient beds have led to a significant increase in staff per bed over the past 15 years (see Figure 6-11). Rather than there being merely a *relative* increase in the ratio of employees to beds because beds were closing and those remaining in them needed more intensive treatment, there has been an *actual* increase in total hospital employees (see Figure 6-12).

Overall, the future of hospitals is murky. A combination of technological advances, managed care, and changes in Medicare reimbursement policy[8] means that the underlying demand for inpatient services will continue to fall. Community hospitals appear to be weathering the storms of the early 1990s by venturing into other services and reengineering their inpatient delivery services in a way that's allowed

63 percent in 1999 (see Figure 6-10). Increasingly, with carve-outs, specialty care, and outpatient care capabilities improving, those patients with just one

Chapter 6: Health Care Providers   85

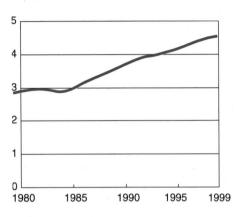

Figure 6-11. Sicker patients and fewer beds mean more staff per bed. (Full-time equivalents per hospital bed in community hospitals)

Source: American Hospital Association.

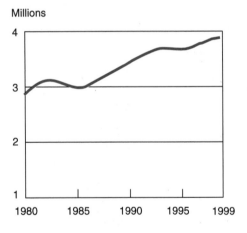

Figure 6-12. There are also more staff in total. (Full-time equivalents in community hospitals)

Source: American Hospital Association.

them to become more profitable in the mid-1990s. Average operating margins for community hospitals rose from 2.7 percent in 1990 to 4 percent in 1994, where they've hovered with little fluctuation since. Reported profit margins for hospitals increased from 4 percent in 1991 to 5.5 percent in 1996, only to fall off again in 1997. But these numbers are only estimates of true performance, because many hospitals use their strong investment portfolios to subsidize losses.[9]

Their larger siblings, the AMCs, are applying the same tactics. AMCs have been getting subsidies from the government, including DSH payments and GME subsidies, which have maintained their profitability over recent years. Furthermore, all hospitals are getting a greater share of their revenues from outpatient care and other services, and many plan to become more heavily involved in those services by making the leap from hospital to "health system."

The overall financial success of American hospitals is uneven—one-third of hospitals are failing, one-third are just getting by, and one-third are doing extremely well, particularly those that enjoy a geographic monopoly.

ISSUES

Despite the past 15 years of downsizing, pressures from Medicare, and the growth of HMOs and other aggressive health plans that have cut hospital days for their members, more than 35 percent of the health care dollar is spent on hospital services. That's a little more than the 34 percent they consumed in 1960, but down from the high of 41.5 percent in 1980. Moreover, hospitals remain a big chunk of the health care landscape: they are the biggest employers in health care and usually are major employers in their communities.

Among health care institutions, hospitals enjoy the greatest ease in raising and retaining capital. The increased number of for-profit hospitals, even though they still only account for 14 percent of all hospitals, has made for even greater access to capital. Hospitals and hospital-centered systems used this capital to buy physician practices, all types of ancillary providers, and each other in the late 1990s. But in the next 10 years some fundamental questions about hospitals will be answered. Most of them concern organization and ownership:

■ *The for-profit, nonprofit divide.* Of all hospitals in the United States, 3,000 remain nonprofit and another 1,250 are publicly owned, usually by counties[10] (see Figure 6-13). But the rise of the big for-profit chains, notably Columbia/HCA, which consolidated several smaller for-profit chains between 1993 and 1996, showed some market advantages for investor-owned hospitals. Consequently,

several nonprofits began to convert to for-profit status—usually by selling out to Columbia. Only nine converted in the decade from 1983 to 1993, but 93 converted from 1994 to 1995. A combination of more aggressive regulatory scrutiny by attorneys general in several states and some bad publicity about Columbia slowed the trend in 1996. Columbia reversed its aggressive strategy of acquiring and converting nonprofits in the late 1990s, and the trend toward for-profit status appears to be slowing. But the valuation Wall Street has put on investor-owned hospitals is so much greater than the amount nonprofits can raise to buy them[11] that the incentives to become for-profit will remain strong. So this issue is not going away.

■ *The tax status of hospitals.* Though only a small minority of hospitals are for-profit, several studies have shown that most nonprofits act like for-profits in several ways with only marginal differences in their costs, the amount of charity care they deliver, and the way they deliver services. Furthermore, the fact that nonprofit hospitals—many of which own for-profit subsidiaries—advertise on TV, compete aggressively with each other, and otherwise look much like any other corporation is increasingly attracting politicians' attention. Given the tax advantages state governments bestow on nonprofits, might this status be withdrawn or amended in the future?

■ *The prevalence of hospital systems.* Many hospitals have announced or activated plans to become part of a larger system,

Figure 6-13. There are more for-profits, but not that many more. (Community hospitals by ownership)

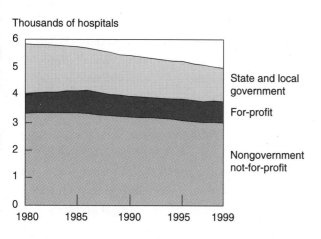

Thousands of hospitals

State and local government

For-profit

Nongovernment not-for-profit

Source: American Hospital Association.

even in the nonprofit sector. Usually this means a hospital enters some form of alliance with others; these arrangements vary from a nominal affiliation to full-blown mergers of assets—although most start with the former. Some 445 nonprofit hospitals were involved in some form of merger and acquisition in 1995 alone,[12] yet most hospitals still behave as if they were independent. Even in "merged" systems, there are often different boards and competing interests that don't look like a typical corporate organization. Some hospitals are taking an alternate track and staying independent. How prevalent will these systems be in the future, and what will they look like?

■ *Which services will be under the hospital umbrella?* The early 1990s saw hospitals trying to get into the business of offering physician services. But now most faculty practices have been "integrated"—with success akin to Stalinist collectivization—and many hospitals are suffering financial trouble with the private physicians' practices they've bought. Will we see a return to these health systems' offering only traditional hospital services—possibly employing hospitalists but not primary care physicians? Or will they be a base for creating truly integrated care delivery? And if they manage to create the latter, will they take the opportunity of Medicare PSN legislation to bypass health plans and sell insurance directly to individuals and employers?

■ *The future of the AMC.* Over the course of the past 30 years, AMCs have increasingly delivered large amounts of routine care in addition to serving as

centers of specialized tertiary care, teaching, and research. In fact, they have used their care services as revenue generators that subsidize their medical schools. They've also expanded their residency programs, both in their home-base hospitals and at other teaching hospitals in their regions. But this expansion is under attack on multiple fronts. Medicare, which subsidizes GME to the tune of about $80,000 per residency place per year, is planning to reduce those subsidies by 25 percent over the next 5 years. Moreover, while Medicare has been willing to pay the premium that AMCs charge to cover their generally sicker mix of patients, private health plans have become increasingly reticent to do so—and have played AMCs against each other as suppliers of big-ticket procedures. As a result, AMCs are redesigning themselves. Many have merged with crosstown rivals to cut competition in specialty services. Others have developed regional health networks. Still others have struggled with a low-paying mix of patients and reduced state and local funding, and several are being spun off by their owners—usually universities—to other nonprofit or for-profit organizations. What will these battleships of the medical care system look like in the future? Will they still be flexible enough to play a role in health care service provision?

Besides the issues of ownership and organization, there are a couple of broader issues about the future of hospitals.

■ *How many hospitals, how many beds?* We've seen a steady decline in the number of hospitals and beds. But declining faster is the number of occupied beds as more and more procedures move outside the inpatient ward. How many hospitals and beds will there be to serve the presumably sicker inpatient population?

- *How much money and will it matter?* Since 1985, a smaller share of overall health care spending has gone to pay for hospital services each year, apart from one blip upward in 1990. The money instead has flowed into home health care, SNFs, ambulatory surgery centers, and all the other facilities that have accepted the exodus of patients. Part of that flow is inevitable as technology permits less invasive procedures. But part of it has to do with the intricacies of Medicare financing, which has rewarded early discharges from hospitals to SNFs and home health visits. Now that Medicare is getting serious about the cost explosion in these areas and private health insurers are increasingly putting providers at risk for a continuum of services, it may make sense for hospitals to keep patients in hospitals a little longer if it prevents other expenses later. But the bigger question is: If we're moving to a system of more integrated patient care, does hospital spending *per se* matter as a separate category?[13]

- *A reduction in variation in hospitals.* The reduction in variation in the delivery of clinical care by physicians reduces costs and improves quality. Similarly, the variation in architecture, operational methods, and organizational structure will be measured for efficiency and benchmarked. This

will increasingly lead to reduced hospital operational variation during the next decade, with a growing appreciation of the "best of breed" in operational methodologies. This may be an opportunity for larger systems to implement more broadly and gain operational advantages during the next decade.

FORECAST

Given the complexity of the issues regarding hospitals and their increasingly intertwined relationships with the rest of the health care delivery world, not all of the issues will resolve themselves by 2010. Generally, we do not expect radical change in terms of either mass hospital closures or significantly less money spent on inpatient services. This will be more a period of gradual attrition. But eventually the number and organization of hospitals will look quite different.

Hospitals and beds will continue to close, but not much faster than the slow pace we're currently seeing. Beds will close a little faster than hospitals, with occupancy rates falling faster still. For example, hospitals will close beds at a faster rate in the next 5 years than they will thereafter—our forecast is about 2 percent of all beds closing each year from a 1997 level of 850,000. In 1999, there were still 5,000 community hospitals with 830,000 beds in the United States, and 71.6 percent were in networks or systems.[14] In 2002 there were roughly 800,000 beds and there will still be more than 670,000 in 2010 (see Figure 6-14). Hospitals themselves will close much more slowly. Even if they close at twice the rate at which they've been closing for the past 15 years, there will still be 4,300 hospitals in the year 2010; the actual number will probably be closer to 4,500. This rate in part reflects the difficulty of closing the big white building and in part reflects a transformation of many to smaller, more patient-centered facilities. Hospitals will still perform most of their activities without using their inpatient beds. However, in the very long run, many hospital systems will hang on to their bed licenses, waiting for the baby boomers to supply the demand for inpatient care after 2015.

In terms of ownership, about 1,000 hospitals will remain city-, county-, or state-owned facilities (down from 1,300 in 2000), and about 2,400 will be traditional independent nonprofits (mostly community or religion based). The tax status of nonprofits will come into debate but is unlikely to change significantly. In 1999 there were 747 investor owned for-profit hospitals in the United States. A minority—about 300 of the nonprofit hospitals over 10 years—will convert to for-profit status in order to gain better access to capital, leaving about 25 percent as for-profit hospitals (1,100) by the year 2010. But most hospitals will stay nonprofit because of their religious mission, increased scrutiny from regulators about those conversions, and eventually waning interest from Wall Street in investing capital in an industry that cannot easily create fast growth in earnings.

Tracking hospitals' membership in systems is very complex, and several different definitions of "hospital system" will make the rounds over the next few years. But the AHA will likely count individual hospitals, and their owners will at least try to make them look independent and community based. So the official figures will look something like the Department of Labor's counting of "firms" and "establishments" where one firm can encompass many establishments. We estimate that around 35 percent of hospitals are currently in a multihospital system that shares a common overseeing board if not common ownership. This is likely to increase to 60 percent by 2002. As this happens, there will be continual increases in the sizes of various systems, particularly on a regional basis. However, by the time the merger and consolidation wave plays out it's likely that several will have fallen apart, and the number of hospitals in systems will be back down to 50 percent or lower by 2007. The majority of the systems that exist after 2005 will be more "real" than virtual and more corporate: a single management structure will

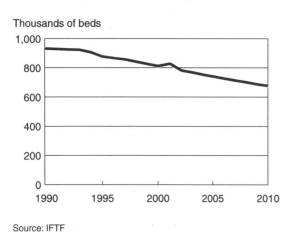

Figure 6-14. Hospital beds will keep slowly disappearing.
(Total beds in community hospitals)

Thousands of beds

Source: IFTF

have final authority over the activities of all its hospital facilities—including the authority to close them down.

A similar pattern will play out as hospitals move into other services. Most will continue to be in the business of ancillary services such as providing home health care. Most hospitals will retain arm's-length relationships with other services, especially those provided by physicians. A minority of the systems will become successful long-term employers of virtually all their doctors. Most will enter into looser relationships with virtual medical groups, single-specialty groups, and individual physicians. The pattern will vary greatly depending on the region, with more successful hospital-based integration with physicians in the Midwest and South than in the West or Northeast but with intense variation within each region. Successful integrated systems in regions outside of the large metropolitan areas in the West and Northeast will have the best chance of successfully starting PSNs and providing insurance coverage direct to employers— becoming the truly vertically integrated system. But the hospital-based system going direct to employers will remain a minority, even in regions where hospitals remain dominant as compared to medical groups and health plans.

AMCs will continue to face financial pressure from all angles. In response, they will continue to merge or at least will find ways to reduce local and regional competition in tertiary and quaternary care and extreme subspecialty procedures like transplants. They will face slow but steady reductions in their Medicare GME subsidies and increas-

ingly will be forced to withdraw residents from other teaching hospitals. The problem of uncompensated care will increase, and the margins earned on Medicare will decrease, especially for outpatient services. But the political strength of the major AMCs means that they will continue to receive reimbursement from Medicare that reflects their mix of sicker patients. It's unlikely that many will take any option other than merging clinical services with their neighbors, but some may look to enter for-profit chains, and the possibility of severe downsizing or even bankruptcy will exist for a few. Those that are in the public sector and have the worst payer mix—those with a high HMO penetration in their region and situated in a poor inner-city area—are the most likely not to survive.

In terms of overall spending—their share of the health economy—hospital services will stabilize at approximately 32 percent of health spending after 2002, falling from the current level of 34 percent. That will come as a combination of more aggressive health plans and the new lower Medicare reimbursements squeeze the rate of spending increases. Since the early 1980s, hospital costs have increased at just under 1 percent less than growth in total national health spending, and we expect that pattern to resume by the early part of the next decade. Total spending will increase from around $424 billion in 2000 to $560 billion in 2005 and $660 billion in 2008 (see Figure 6-15). By 2010, hospital spending will be about 30 percent of NHE, but the distinction between hospital services and other classifications will become increasingly irrelevant as

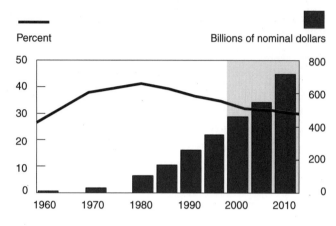

Figure 6-15. Hospital spending—still a big deal, but proportionately falling slowly (Spending on hospital services 1980 to 2010 as a percentage of all health spending and in nominal dollars)

Percent | Billions of nominal dollars

Source: IFTF; Health Care Financing Administration.

leaving most Americans in a Cadillac-style top-tier plan, which doesn't enforce change on a recalcitrant delivery system.

■ Medical management proves to be easier than we thought. After some research, clinicians identify what are the right courses of action for virtually all disease states and use information technology–enabled care processes to quickly ensure the best practice of care for most people. Practice variations decrease dramatically and outcomes improve considerably, resulting in measurable savings for the system by 2010.

■ A new edition of the North American Free Trade Agreement (NAFTA), including the recognition of foreign medical degrees and residency training, allows the entry of some 100,000 Mexican, South American, and Canadian physicians. Supply is so great that patients, plans, and government take advantage of the newly available medical talent and seek care at lower prices with emphasis on better patient service. The privileged position of the physician in American culture fades.

some care is reintegrated into hospital facilities from nursing homes and other facilities.

The underlying change in technology—especially interventions and pharmaceuticals that reduce length of stay and admissions—means that inpatient days will drop continually. That's the main story for hospital services over the next 13 years, as it has been for the past 13.

WILD CARDS

■ Physicians leave *en masse,* either retiring at an accelerated rate or finding opportunities outside of medical practice. The physician surplus disappears, and the clout that health plans have over suppliers evaporates.

■ The consumer revolt against the HMOs and their descendants reaches fever pitch. Employers back down,

■ PSNs and direct-to-employer strategies work and take up a considerable market share.

■ New epidemics and new diseases require more hospital beds.

■ Hospitals become supplier parts of truly integrated systems. Their management closes facilities and beds quickly. The supply of inpatient beds reaches market equilibrium by 2005.

- Unexpected adverse events may create the opportunity for political intervention during the current process of major change in health care. This may lead to the loss of variability and the injection of political forces and process into the changes (Clinton Care).

- Improved prevention and new outpatient treatment and care significantly skews the prior flow of patients with

specific diseases such as heart disease, cancer, or stroke so as to impact the existing health care system structure adversely. Currently vulnerability lies in cross-subsidies and long-term capital allocation based on prior projections of use and reimbursement as well as on current incidences of disease. None of these are stable or certain in the future.

ENDNOTES

[1] Robinson, J., Physician organization in california: crisis and opportunity. *Health Affairs* (July/August) 2001; 20:4.

[2] Melnick, G., et al. Market power and hospital pricing: Are nonprofits different? *Health Affairs* (May/June) 1999; 18:3.

[3] Burdi, M., and L. Baker. Unpublished 1996 survey of California physicians compared with age-matched cohorts of physicians, extracted from the 1991 Robert Wood Johnson Survey of Young Physicians.

[4] *AMA News.* January 20, 1997, 40:3.

[5] This forecast assumes that there is no change in the current number of residents, and that all physicians retire at the same rate, regardless of whether they are in an individual, a two-doctor, or a group practice. The lower estimate assumes that all new patient-care physicians will enter group practice and that the number of hospital staff does not increase substantially but rather is consistently replaced. The upper estimate further assumes that 10 percent of the physicians in individual and two-doctor practices join group practices over the next 7 years.

[6] Lubitz, J., et al. Three decades of health care use by the elderly, 1965–1998. *Health Affairs* (March/April) 2001; 20:2.

[7] 1999 data from *AHA Hospital Statistics,* 2000.

[8] Reinhardt, U. Spending more through cost control: Our obsessive quest to gut the hospital. *Health Affairs* 1996; 15:2.

[9] Levitt, L., et al. *Trends and Indicators in the Changing Health Care Marketplace Chartbook.* Menlo Park, CA: The Henry J. Kaiser Family Foundation, August 1998.

[10] 1995 data from *AHA Hospital Statistics,* 1996.

[11] Johnson, R. Nonprofit hospitals: Bargain prices? Letter to *Health Affairs.* (July/August) 1997, 16:4. Describes why conversions make sense from Wall Street's perspective.

[12] Hollis, S. Strategic and economic factors in the hospital conversion process. *Health Affairs* (March/April) 1997; 16:2.

[13] The Congressional Budget Office clearly doesn't think so and declined to make projections on hospital spending in its 1997 forecast.

[14] 1999 data from *AHA Hospital Statistics,* 2000.

CHAPTER 7

Health Care Workforce

Future Supply and Demand

Despite unending speculation about the evolving structure of health care services, there has been little fundamental change in the way health professionals are organized and the way they interact with each other. For physicians, the number and variety of contractual arrangements has increased significantly, as has the oversight from intermediaries in terms of utilization review. But there has been little change in the way most physicians practice medicine. Furthermore, physicians remain the central figures in American health care with nonphysician providers poised to play a more critical part in the delivery of health care services but as yet unable to significantly penetrate the system. Although nurse practitioners (NPs), physicians' assistants (PAs), and other health care providers may possess skills that appear to be well suited to the demands of an environment with a greater focus on cost containment and managing health behaviors, their roles have been limited by their small numbers and the still significant clout of the medical profession. However, changes in the relative supply of new providers and their emerging roles may alter the landscape more drastically over the next 10 to 15 years than has occurred in the past 30 years. These changes in many ways will determine how quickly and in what way new service delivery forms develop in the future.

PHYSICIANS

Roughly 170,000 physicians are currently in medical training, with 16,000 new students graduating from medical school every year (see Figure 7-1). Adding international medical graduates (IMGs) to this equation, the physician pipeline is spewing out close to 23,000 physicians from residency and fellowship programs every year. Given that approximately 75 percent of IMGs remain to practice in the United States and that 7 percent of physicians choose administrative and research careers, an estimated 19,500 new physicians enter patient care each year. Over the next decade, the number of retirees is expected to increase from an estimated 8,000 to 13,000 annually, leaving a net annual increase of between 11,000 and 6,000 in the number of practicing physicians.

Assuming there is no change in the current production of physicians, and barring significant immigration or other policy changes, this influx will increase the supply of nonfederal patient-care physicians from 450,000 to 600,000 by 2010, or 219 physicians (excluding residents and interns) per 100,000 population (see Figure 7-2). Assuming historical patterns of specialty choice in which 70 percent of trainees enter specialties,

Figure 7-1. Physicians in the pipeline

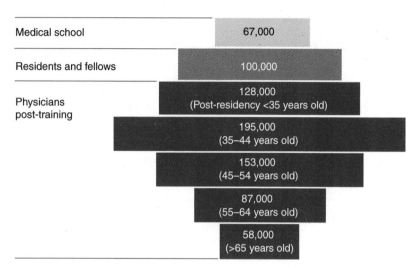

Medical school	67,000
Residents and fellows	100,000
Physicians post-training	128,000 (Post-residency <35 years old)
	195,000 (35–44 years old)
	153,000 (45–54 years old)
	87,000 (55–64 years old)
	58,000 (>65 years old)

Source: IFTF; Association of American Medical Colleges, 1997; American Medical Association, 1996.

Figure 7-2. In excess: Physician supply and estimated requirement (Including residents and interns)

Total supply of nonfederal patient-care physicians

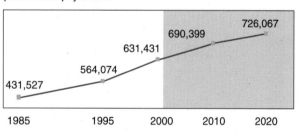

1985	1995	2000	2010	2020
431,527	564,074	631,431	690,399	726,067

Nonfederal patient-care physicians per 100,000 civilian population

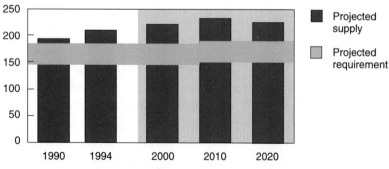

■ Projected supply

▨ Projected requirement

Source: IFTF; Bureau of Health Professionals, American Medical Association, Council on Graduate Medical Education.

the specialist-to-population ratio is expected to reach 152 per 100,000 population in 2010, whereas the generalist physician-to-population ratio will remain stable at 67 per 100,000.

WHY SO MANY DOCTORS?

Over the past 25 years, the patient-care physician-to-population ratio has increased 65 percent from 115 to 190 physicians per 100,000 population, with specialists increasing from 56 to 123 per 100,000 population. Several factors have contributed to the growth in physician supply. In 1970, amid dire predictions of a physician shortage, the federal government provided financial incentives to medical schools to expand their capacity and foster the immigration of physicians trained in foreign medical schools. Between 1970 and 1994, the number of medical students educated in the United States grew by 65 percent and the number of residents increased by approximately 100 percent. However, when the shortage threat dissipated, not all policies were adjusted accordingly. From 1988 to 1994, although the annual number of medical school graduates in the United States remained flat, the number of residency positions increased by more than 80 percent. As a result, there are now 1.45 first-year residency positions for every medical graduate. The excess positions have been filled by IMGs.

PHYSICIAN SURPLUS— OR PHYSICIAN SHORTAGE?

In the latter half of the 1990s, the Pew Health Professions Commission, the AMA, the Bureau of Health

Professionals, and the Council on Graduate Medical Education (COGME) all projected an oversupply of physicians overall, an inadequate to marginally adequate number of primary care physicians, and an enormous oversupply of specialists. The media tracked residents who were completing training and entering practice and reported that their numbers exceeded openings. The typical "unemployed" new physician was a specialist; reports often featured the job searches of anesthesiologists, radiologists, and pathologists. Other specialists obtained jobs in undesired situations and locations, while others were able to find only part-time positions. The IFTF joined the chorus proclaiming a glut of doctors, and once-popular specialties were unable to fill postgraduate training programs with graduates from the 125 United States medical schools.

In a report released in February 2001, however, the Council on Graduate Medical Education—the same COGME that had continued to predict a surplus of specialists at the end of 2000—announced that the nation faced an immediate and projected shortage in a wide range of specialties that, with one exception, pediatricians, would be needed to treat an aging population already experiencing the chronic conditions brought on by genetic predisposition, unhealthy behavior, and environmental factors.

Prior to 2001, how did the supply of physicians compare to the projected needs of the population? Pooling results of four different requirement models, the Council on Graduate Medical Education (COGME) estimated that in the year 2000 the United States needed 145 to 185 physicians providing patient care per 100,000 population: 60 to 80 generalists and 85 to 105 specialists (see Table 7-1). Looking out further, they projected that the need for all types of physicians would increase moderately, reaching between 150 to 190 per 100,000 population in 2010. Each of these models assumed varying levels of managed care penetration (between 20 and 66 percent), various generalist-to-specialist staffing ratios (based on staff- and group-model HMOs, which vary from 88:50 to 56:81), and current patterns of utilization.

The main differences in the projected requirements are for specialists, as each model assumes a slightly different competitive environment in the future. However, even the highest estimates of specialist demand were well below the projected supply of 152 per 100,000 population. The situation for primary care physicians was a little less clear.

Table 7-1. Projected physician supply and demand, as envisaged in 2000 (Physicians per 100,000 population)

Year 2000	Supply	Requirement
All physicians	203	145–185
Generalists	63	60–80
Specialists	140	85–105
Year 2010		
All physicians	219	150–190
Generalists	67	60–80
Specialists	152	90–110

Source: IFTF; Council on Graduate Medical Education.

The number of generalist patient-care physicians was, and still is, expected to remain stable at 67 per 100,000, a number sufficient in some scenarios but inadequate in others. With some specialists providing more primary care (see below) and the slowdown in primary care as a gatekeeper in managed care, the forecast was an adequate supply of primary care providers through 2010.

The apparent oversupply of physicians prompted questions regarding the appropriateness of current medical education policy, particularly at the graduate level. Many advocated that the number of residents trained in the United States should be reduced to give preference to graduates of American medical schools. In 1999, the Pew Health Professions Commission went even further, recommending the closure of 20 to 25 percent of the nation's medical schools. But even if drastic changes are made to reduce the number of new entrants, and new regulations make it more difficult for foreign medical graduates to practice in the United States, many of the physicians who will supply the future market in the United States are already in the pipeline. Medical training takes so long that any changes in either medical education or policy will not be felt in the market for at least another decade.

TOO MANY SPECIALISTS?

In addition to being in excessive supply, there is an uneven distribution of physicians by specialty in the United States. Despite the shift to more outpatient care and the emphasis HMOs place on the role of the primary care physician as gatekeeper, primary care doctors still represent roughly the same percentage of all physicians as they did back in 1970 (44 percent). In fact, if we remove the primary care subspecialties and consider just general primary care, the percentage of primary care physicians has actually declined from 43.2 percent in 1970 to 38.2 percent in 1997. Why? Because, as Figure 7-3 shows, the money still goes to specialists.

Although the number of physicians *trained* as general practitioners is unlikely to affect the proportion of primary care providers in the near future, more of the specialist physicians are likely to be providing primary care. In a 1997 survey of physicians conducted by Louis Harris & Associates, nearly half of specialists reported spending at least 25 percent of their time providing primary care, and 22 percent of specialists said they will be providing more primary care in the future. Even though specialists are not flocking to formal retraining programs, they are following the market's prompting. The share of all physicians *self-reporting* as primary care providers was a full 16 percent higher in the 1997 survey than in the 1994 survey (46 percent versus 30 percent)—and we know this is not due to a large increase in the number of primary care physicians being trained.

Throughout the 1990s, the projections were for an excess of physicians in 2010, primarily among specialists and predominantly in the medical and surgical specialties. The tragedy here was thought to be twofold: not only would there nationally be an underuse of highly skilled specialty doctors, but also the money expended for a large portion of their training would have come out of

Figure 7-3. Median net income

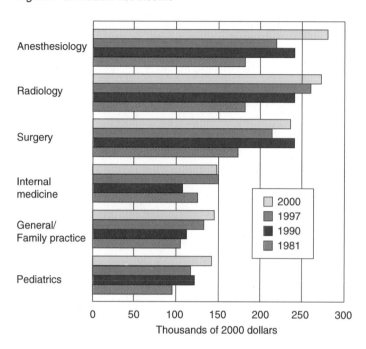

Source: Association of Medical Colleges, 1997; American Medical Association; Center for Health Policy Research. Medical Group, Managed Care, 2000, Managment Association, 2001.

the public purse. Basically, this would be a waste of valuable resources whichever perspective one assumes.

Some suggested that the excess of specialists might nudge some physicians to practice as clinical investigators, filling the ranks of a depleted cadre of physicians engaged in clinical research and the conduct of clinical trials. Others might assume new roles within chronic-disease management organizations. As the number of Americans suffering from chronic disease increases, these organizations will assume total care for defined populations of patients with diabetes, congestive heart failure, and cancer, and they would seek highly trained specialists to develop and manage their programs.

REASSESSMENT OF PHYSICIAN SUPPLY AND DEMAND

COGME's reported present and projected specialist shortage has not been confirmed uniformly by other studies, and at least one unpublished study contradicts the COGME report's projections for California. Nonetheless, while recognizing regional differences that may be extreme, on balance the *demand*, and presumably the need, for specialty care exceeds the supply, presently and in the next 15 to 20 years. The reasons for this are varied, unpredictable, and in part unintended consequences of organizations and processes of the health care delivery systems of the preceding decade of "managed care." Although multiple forces were in play, in our opinion five stand out as critical factors:

- The increasing complexity of medical practice promotes specialization to achieve best outcomes (e.g., following acute myocardial infarction, stroke, Whipple procedure for pancreatic cancer).

- New medical technologies may replace prior care, but many new technologies are additive, in that they expand the spectrum of available interventions (e.g., thrombolytics in stroke, stents in coronary artery disease, implantable ventricular assist devices in congestive heart failure).

- In a new era of consumerism in health care, the public demands specialty care. Better informed and more health-conscious consumers rebelled against PCP gatekeepers, but probably more important was the consumer's perception that specialty care was superior. For example, this led to legislative action to allow choice and access to specialty care.

■ For physicians, "managed care" brought disincentives to continue in the practice of medicine, which promoted unprecedented numbers to choose early retirement or positions that did not involve direct patient care. This dissatisfaction was not lost on aspiring college graduates, as reflected in the decline in applications to American medical schools.

■ Although demographic projections were accurate, assessments of the impact of the changes in the relative frequency of diseases they imply did not anticipate the medical interventions that would become available to manage the inevitable chronic diseases of an aging population. Health care is a service industry, and as more service is required to meet demand the workforce will expand proportionately or nearly so.

The history of supply and demand of our physician workforce for the past 50 years has been one of alternating cycles of mismatches and overcorrections. Most likely, we have entered yet another one. However, this particular cycle may prove more resistant to correction and therefore more lengthy than in the past. The impacts of our national economy, genomic medicine and preventive care among many possible future trends are unknown and difficult to predict. However, the present and projected shortage of many specialist physicians is almost certainly real if we assume that the richest nation in the world will continue to demand the best health care that those who have access to it can afford.

POOR GEOGRAPHIC DISTRIBUTION

Geographic maldistribution of physicians, generalists as well as specialists, has characterized American medicine in the past, present, and likely future. The reasons for urban concentration of the physician workforce relate to lifestyle, family considerations such as educational resources, cultural opportunities, level of income, access to continuing medical education, and availability of newer medical technologies and resources. For certain specialties and subspecialties, the population and resources of a metropolitan location are essential and always will be.

The issue for people living in areas with low physician-density is access to care. Not only may the closest physician be located several hours away, but the practice may be so busy that the doctor cannot take on additional patients. For many people, these are effective barriers to obtaining necessary medical care in a reasonable amount of time. In the absence of timely medical attention their health suffers accordingly.

Financial incentives have had only a limited effect in attracting physicians to rural areas where the professional isolation, long working hours (especially for on-call duties), and cultural isolation have acted as strong deterrents. In fact, the number of areas in the United States with physician shortages is greater now than it was 30 years ago. The most successful efforts to retain physicians have actually relocated GME training to these underserved communities. Once trained in these areas, physicians are more likely to stay and practice, regardless of where they went to medical school.

Medicare's decision to reimburse physicians for rural telemedicine consults could lead to greater use of this technology and thus, to a certain extent, combat the professional isolation of a rural practice. However, the social and cultural isolation will continue to deter physicians from locating in rural areas, and the medical access problems faced by these communities will remain unresolved in 2010.

INADEQUATE DIVERSITY

In addition to the uneven distribution of physicians across specialties and geographic areas, ethnic minorities are poorly represented in the medical profession. Nationally, African Americans represent 12.6 percent of the general population but only 3 percent of physicians, and Hispanics represent 10 percent of the general population and only 4.6 percent of physicians. The racial and ethnic maldistribution is even more stunning in regions with diverse populations. For example, in California, Hispanics constitute 31 percent of the general population but only 5 percent of practicing physicians.

Because of cultural and language differences, underrepresented minorities prefer to, and when possible do, obtain care from physicians with similar backgrounds. These physicians in turn play a major role in providing care to minorities, especially to those residing in underserved low-income communities. If the physician workforce does not mirror the ethnic and racial diversity of the population to be served, it is more likely that minority populations will not have access to essential health care services. In the absence of significant

policy change directed at recruiting minority physicians, their underrepresentation in the medical profession will continue and will be further exacerbated in regions where minorities are becoming a greater proportion of the general population.

NEW ROLE FOR DOCTORS

The New Inpatient Specialist

There are two new and emerging roles for physicians in the health care arena. The first is the "hospitalist" or "intensivist." These physicians work full time in the hospital, providing all of the care to the inpatients of office-based physicians. They are distinct from the radiologist, anesthesiologist, and pathologist who also work full time in the hospital. Most hospitalists are general internists, 10 to 15 percent are critical care doctors (hence the term "intensivists"), and 5 and 10 percent are family practitioners and emergency room physicians.

Hospitalists are perceived to be more efficient than office-based physicians, not only because of their greater familiarity with the inner workings of the institution but also because they are more capable of effectively managing inpatient care. Because they are constantly in the hospital, they are able to monitor patients more closely, which leads not only to the ordering of fewer tests but also to better patient outcomes. Furthermore, because hospitalists have the authority to discharge, patients do not have to wait for their physicians to conduct their morning or evening rounds—they can be discharged at any time, which leads to higher satisfaction and shorter lengths of stay for patients.

Chapter 7: Health Care Workforce

There is some question regarding the continuity of care that is provided when the oversight for patients' health is transferred among providers. In one sense, transferring the care of a patient to a hospitalist is akin to referring a patient to a specialist—and all of the questions regarding continuity of care that are raised with specialists also apply to the hospitalist. What is new, however, is the movement of this phenomenon into the arena of general hospital care and the transfer of authority for the patient from the primary physician to the hospitalist.

There are an estimated 5,000 hospitalists currently providing inpatient hospital care. Assuming that the average hospitalist can care for 15 to 20 patients at any one time and considering the need for on-call duties and time off, it is estimated that the smallest functioning unit will be four hospitalists caring for approximately 50 inpatients. Over the next 15 years, the greater efficiencies provided by the hospitalist will lead to increases in their employment in hospitals with at least 80 medical beds. They will also begin to work in SNFs. It is estimated that most nonsurgical inpatients will be cared for by hospitalists by 2005.

The Medical Manager

The second new training path for physicians leads to a business-savvy MD. Frustrated with their diminished autonomy in a managed care environment and intent on keeping an upper hand, many physicians are retraining, either in business schools or in health care administration, and are seeking employment managing other physicians. It is difficult to quantify the exact number of physicians seeking this form of retraining because many pursue this avenue through correspondence courses. However, as HMOs and pharmaceutical companies enter the medical management arena, they will be seeking physician administrators who not only understand the health issues but also have the business acumen to manage their colleagues and their patients. The demand for these dually trained doctors will increase as forces trying to alter physician behavior realize that the best way to do that is to employ someone who is respected by physicians—and to that end, nothing beats a colleague.

RENEWED EMPHASIS ON CLINICAL INVESTIGATORS

The number of clinical investigators and the proportion of time that academic physicians devote to clinical research declined steadily in the 1990s as one unintended consequence of "managed care." The academic community and the NIH are aware of this trend and have instituted corrective measures and strong incentives, fully recognizing the critical role of committed investigators in conducting the clinical research that leads to advances in health care. The subject has multiple facets, but suffice it to state that a once-projected surplus of specialists did not swell the ranks of clinical investigators but rather failed to do so because of the demands that revenue-producing clinical practice placed on academic physicians.

NURSES

In many ways, the nursing profession is the most qualified to respond to current changes in the health system. Nurses' training focuses more on the behavioral and preventive aspects of health care than does that of physicians. Their skills are increasingly in demand in an environment that is moving more toward outpatient care and requires its health care providers to function as teams and assume managerial responsibilities.

REGISTERED NURSES

Registered nurses (RNs) are the largest single group of health care providers in the United States, numbering over 2.2 million. Hospitals are their primary place of employment. As the acute care hospital takes a backseat to other venues of care, one might predict that RNs' primary place of employment will disappear. However, despite the substantial rise in outpatient activity, two-thirds of RNs continue to work in the hospital setting. This ratio has remained steady over the past 15 years with only a slight decline since 1992. In fact, Linda Aiken at the University of Pennsylvania has shown that total hospital employment of all nursing personnel has declined, but the number of full-time equivalent (FTE) hospital RNs actually increased between 1984 and 1994 by 27.6 percent, increasing the RN-to-patient ratio by 29.4 percent. However, when adjusted for case-mix severity, the ratio increased by only 0.3 percent, indicating that the increases in RN hospital employment barely kept pace with the increased case-mix severity. Other hospital nursing staff such as licensed practical nurses (LPNs) and nursing aides have been reduced in absolute terms, suggesting that the staff-to-patient ratios for these nurses have not kept pace with the increased case-mix severity. RNs are providing more of the care for a sicker population of patients.

Based primarily on 1996 projections by the Division of Nursing, Bureau of Health Professionals, the previous edition of the IFTF forecast stated that the future supply of RNs would be adequate to meet increased demands (Table 7-2 and Figure 7-4). This forecast assumed the movement of RNs from hospital-based care into ambulatory care settings, nursing homes, subacute nursing facilities and community health clinics. Allowances were made for projected closings of hospitals and hospital beds and a sicker population of in-patients. In 1995, the Pew Health Professions Commission also anticipated a surplus of nurses and recommended a 20 percent reduction in nursing programs. Although there were murmurs even then about the possibility of a nursing shortage, the majority view, with which we were in agreement, believed that the nursing supply would meet demand through 2010. We weren't misinformed but we were wrong, nonetheless—wrong, because we failed to anticipate a rapidly dwindling number of applicants to schools of nursing and a mass exodus of nurses from acute care settings because of poor working conditions. At the beginning of 2001, the existing and projected shortage of nurses was characterized as a national disaster of crisis proportions and the number one concern among health care leaders and hospital administrators.

In June 2001, a poll released by the American Hospital Association found serious shortages in the workforce with 168,000 open positions, three-quarters for RNs, with a vacancy rate of 11 percent.

Table 7-2. Projected RN requirements by employment setting, 2000–2010

	Total	Hospitals	Nursing Homes	Ambulatory Care	Public/ Community Health	Nursing Education	Other
2000	1,969,000	1,231,800	128,200	134,200	364,300	37,800	72,500
2005	2,095,000	1,305,200	138,000	142,600	387,200	41,500	80,200
2010	2,232,000	1,386,100	152,600	150,700	411,000	45,500	87,400

Source: Projections by Division of Nursing, Bureau of Health Professionals; Health Resources and Services Administration; U.S. Department of Health and Human Services, March 1996.

Multiple factors account for the present and future shortage of RNs overall and most significantly among nurses choosing to work in hospital settings. The major impact has fallen on hospitals—on the acute care nursing units in the emergency department and in the operating room. As hospitals' reimbursements, revenues, and margins have been squeezed by private and government payers, patient-to-nurse ratios have increased, nursing salaries have fallen behind other sectors, overtime (in many cases "mandatory") has increased, and job satisfaction has plummeted. Stress, irregular working hours, declining working conditions, low morale, and frustration at providing suboptimal care collectively have amplified the shortage as disaffected nurses leave their jobs, some to work in other health care settings and some to work for vendors, insurers, and managed care organizations.

High school graduates, particularly females, no longer view nursing as an attractive career when compared to other opportunities within health care or in other service industries. The young adult public is aware of the angst within the nursing profession, and therefore chooses other careers with better pay and more satisfying work. Enrollment in nursing programs has fallen by a cumulative total of 25 percent over the past six years. The result: a declining entry of new nurses and a rapidly increasing exodus of practicing nurses.

NURSE PRACTITIONERS

The nurse practictioner (NP) is a registered nurse who works as a primary health care provider, focusing on health

Figure 7-4. Projected supply of RNs, 2000–2020

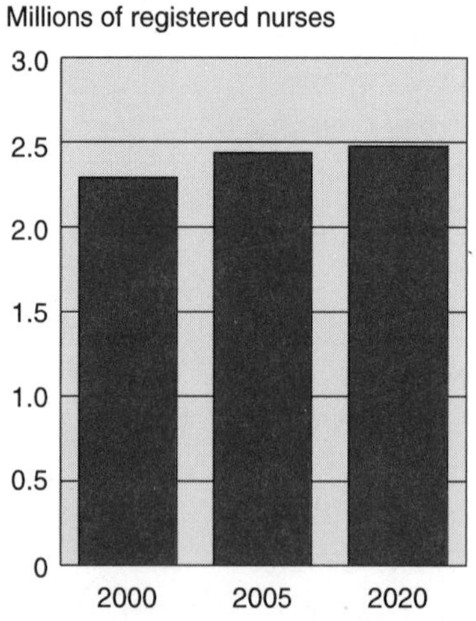

Millions of registered nurses

Source: Projections by Division of Nursing, Bureau of Health Professionals, Health Resources and Services Administration, U.S. Department of Health and Human Services, March 1996.

Chapter 7: Health Care Workforce

promotion and disease prevention as well as the diagnosis and management of acute and chronic diseases. Unlike RNs, 90 percent of NPs work in outpatient settings, one-third of which are private practices or HMOs. Although only nine states permit NPs to practice independently of physicians, over two-thirds of NPs have primary responsibility for a specific group of patients within either a team or a panel situation. More than 85 percent have the authority to prescribe pharmacologic agents. One in ten has hospital admitting privileges, and one in three has hospital discharge privileges. In some circumstances, NPs function as physician substitutes, and in others they serve as complements, providing health prevention, education, and counseling.

There were approximately 71,000 nurses with NP training in 1996, about half of whom are actually practicing as NPs. In the late 1980s and early 1990s, the expectation that there would be insufficient numbers of primary care providers fueled an increase in both the number and capacity of NP training programs. Approximately 40 percent of currently practicing NPs deliver primary care and 80 percent of graduates are specializing in this area.

The future supply of NPs will undoubtedly increase as the demand for their services grows and the number of training programs increases. Based on current training capacity, there will be at least 6,000 graduates every year. As demand rises, some of the nurses who are trained but not practicing as NPs may reenter the profession. Estimating conservatively, 125,000 NPs will be practicing by the year 2010.[1]

PHYSICIANS' ASSISTANTS

Physicians' assistants (PAs) are health care professionals licensed to practice medicine under a physician's supervision. This new category of health care professional emerged in the 1960s, partly in response to the supply of experienced hospital corpsmen and combat medics returning from Vietnam and looking for work. In 1970, there were only 237 practicing PAs. Between 1990 and 1997, the number of new graduates increased 134 percent from 1,195 to 2,800 per year. In 1998, there were approximately 31,000 PAs in clinical practice and by 2005 there will be about 50,000. Approximately 7,400 students are enrolled in PA programs with 3,700 graduates annually, a class size that has more than tripled since 1990.

PAs' precise scope of practice varies across the country according to each state's medical practice act. They all require physician supervision, but in some states this supervision must be on-site and in others it can be provided from a distance. PAs provide basic health care services that 20 to 30 years ago were provided by the physicians themselves—and in many cases still are. These tasks may include taking medical histories and performing physical examinations, ordering and interpreting lab tests, diagnosing and treating illnesses, assisting in surgery, prescribing or dispensing medication, and counseling patients. PAs can legally prescribe drugs in 39 states.

Approximately 43 percent of PAs work in primary care settings, but there is a steady increase in surgical subspecialization, in which only 22 percent of all PAs currently work. Roughly one-third of PAs are employed in hospital settings, 40 percent in physicians' offices, 10 percent in clinics, 7 percent in HMOs, and the rest in nursing homes, correctional institutions, and federal agencies.

In 1998, just under nine out of every ten PA graduates were employed as PAs in less than a year. The growth in PA jobs is projected to increase by 22 percent annually between 1997 and 2005—9 percent faster than the overall job-growth rate in the United States. Based on current training capacity, it is projected that at least 68,000 PAs will be in practice by the year 2010.[1]

FUTURE EMPLOYMENT

In this cost-cutting era, health plans, hospital systems, and medical groups are looking at diverse combinations of providers as part of their cost-control strategies. The roles of many health professionals overlap to a certain extent but the scopes of practice for nurses and PAs most closely resemble that of physicians. To what extent will nonphysician personnel be employed in the future and in what capacity?

Staff- and group-model HMOs, which have the greatest incentive to employ the most efficient mix of personnel, exhibit great variation in their employment of nonphysicians, ranging from a low of zero to a high of 67 per 100,000 enrollees. It's therefore difficult to forecast future requirements with any certainty based on expected growth in managed care. There is evidence that some staff-model HMOs are using non-

physician providers as substitutes for primary care physicians, but this practice is not widespread.

Large multispecialty group practices and physician groups that are heavily capitated are another source of employment for NPs and PAs. The correlation with size suggests that smaller practices are unable to take advantage of the cost savings offered by nonphysician providers. Furthermore, even though studies indicate that nonphysician providers increase physician productivity and incomes, professional resistance certainly affects physicians' decisions. As an example, physicians are more likely to employ PAs, who cannot function independent of a physician's oversight, than NPs.

In the short term, the greatest impediment to wholesale use and integration of nonphysician personnel into provider networks is lack of supply. If all large multispecialty group practices restructured with a ratio of one NP or PA for every two physicians—which some capitated primary care groups aim to do—there would not be sufficient personnel to staff them. If training programs were expanded sufficiently now, it is possible that by 2010 the supply of nonphysician providers could increase to fulfill the demand.

However, beyond the supply issues there are several barriers to the widespread involvement of nonphysicians as direct-care providers.

■ State laws somewhat arbitrarily limit the care that nonphysician providers

New Roles for Pharmacists

Pharmacy benefit organizations

Disease management

Interviewing and instructing customers and patients (inpatients and outpatients)

Joining teams in hospitals, clinics and managed care organizations

Outpatient vaccinations

Head positions in planning organizing and conducting clinical trials

Administrative positions within the pharmaceutical industry

---

may give by restricting pharmaceutical prescribing, requiring on-site supervision, and requiring case-by-case physician approval of services that are ordered. Organized medicine has a strong incentive to lobby and maintain such restrictions.

■ The perception of lower-quality care, regardless of its merit, not only limits consumer demand for access to nonphysician providers but also may make health plans skittish about using them more aggressively in cost-cutting efforts.

■ The salaries of nonphysician providers are approaching those of newly trained physicians. Although these income gains are the results of hard-won battles, in an era of a glut of physicians and quality consciousness, medical groups and hospitals may prefer to hire a newly trained physician over an NP or PA.

Overall, we expect to see greater but sporadic use of nonphysician providers in the next 10 years. NPs with extensive pri-

mary care experience will compete with general practitioners in certain markets. Many physicians will still not be working with nonphysician providers in 2010.

PHARMACISTS

In 1995, the Pew Health Professions Commission projected a surplus of pharmacists and recommended a 25 percent reduction in pharmacy programs. Although we did not include pharmacists in our first forecast, given trends at the time we would have agreed with the Commission. However, 6 years later pharmacists are overwhelmed and a shortage of 10,000 registered pharmacists exists and is worsening steadily. In many chain pharmacies, the major provider of outpatient drugs, pharmacy technicians now do routine tasks formerly performed by pharmacists. So why the shortage?

In the 5 years between 1992 and 1997, the number of prescriptions increased 50 percent and this growth will continue as more people take more prescription medications. The second principal reason for the current and projected shortage of pharmacists is that they are assuming new roles (see sidebar) beyond dispensing prescriptions. The incentives to obtain an advanced degree in clinical pharmacy (PharmD.) have drawn recent pharmacy school graduates away from their traditional role as mixers and dispensers of prescription drugs. The shortage is real, but with rapidly rising starting salaries and governmental support for increasing the number of entering pharmacy students, the mismatch between supply and demand may be corrected much sooner than nursing and medicine reach that goal.

WILD CARDS

- Americans opt out of managed care when policy changes in 2001 offer them MSAs at a considerable tax advantage. Freed from the hassles of managed care, physicians once again find solo and small-group practice affordable and rewarding.

- Although skeptical at first, patients find their experience with NPs and PAs exceptionally positive. Patients demand to see these health care providers on a regular basis; state laws are changed, allowing greater freedom from physician oversight; nurses assume key managerial roles in managing care.

- NPs, supported by effective practice guidelines and computerized data on treatment protocols, replace physicians as the patient's first point of entry into the medical care system.

- Frustrated by the power of large health plans and insurers, physicians embrace unionization. It becomes increasingly difficult for health plans and insurers to enforce compliance with cost-control efforts.

- With exceptions legislated by a few states, nonphysician clinicians (advanced practice nurses, physician assistants, and pharmacists) have been limited as to scope of practice, autonomy, reimbursement for patient care activities, and equivalence with physicians. With a projected shortage of primary care and certainly specialty care physicians, these restraints may be modified substantially, with consequently more rapid growth in entering students than currently anticipated.

ENDNOTE

[1] Cooper, R., et al. Current and projected workforce of nonphysician clinicians. *Journal of the American Medical Association* (September 2) 1998; 280:9.

CHAPTER 8

Medical Technologies

Effects on Care

New medical technologies are one of the key driving forces in health care. Beginning in the 19th century, medicine has made great strides in verifying the germ theory, creating aseptic surgical techniques, discovering antibiotics, developing anesthesia, and imaging the inside of the body. The impact has been huge: improving public health, extending our life span, saving lives, and heightening quality of life. The related cost impact has been equally large, especially in the United States, where new medical technologies are enthusiastically embraced as they become available.

Here we examine nine medical technologies that will affect patient care over the next decade. We describe the technology, then discuss the magnitude and areas of impact as well as the barriers to change where applicable. We've excluded some of the leading-edge developments that, because of the long lead time needed to bring them to market, will result in new technologies beyond our 10-year time frame. The technologies we focus on here are:

- rational drug design
- advances in imaging
- minimally invasive surgery
- genetic mapping and testing

- gene therapy
- vaccines
- artificial blood
- xenotransplantation
- use of stem cells

Even after a medical technology or technique has been discovered, developed, approved, and commercialized, it may take years for it to be disseminated widely. Similarly, in many clinical areas state-of-the-art knowledge is slowly adopted in community practice. We conclude with a discussion and forecast of the process of procedural technology transfer in health care.

We interviewed experts in many different disciplines and selected technologies that we forecast to be major advances evolving over the next decade. Although gene therapy is unlikely to have a role in the mainstream of medical management by 2010, by virtue of intense interest in its potential and a myriad of ongoing clinical trials, we determined that gene therapy will be a high-impact technology. In the nine descriptions that follow, we were selective in certain areas because a thorough review of the topic was beyond our intent of highlighting a particular technology for its future impact.

RATIONAL DRUG DESIGN

Most drugs on the market today have been discovered in random screens of naturally occurring products or from analog development programs—once a time-consuming manual process. Although today's robotic systems can screen millions of compounds in a year's time, this method of random trial and error is inefficient: of 10,000 agents tested, 1,000 typically show bioactivity, 100 are worth investigating, 10 go to clinical trials, and only one reaches patients on the market. Most current pharmaceuticals were chanced upon after years of this research by trial and error. Occasionally, researchers came across something that was not only safe for human use but also beneficial. The chemicals identified from these experiments were discovered as they existed in nature. Happily, we are no longer just searching randomly in nature to find therapeutic chemicals. Now scientists are *designing* thousands every day.

Rational drug design is the development of new chemical or molecular entities by looking at the physical structure and chemical composition of a target—a molecular receptor or enzyme—and designing drugs that bind to those molecules, turning them on or off. Drug designers use physical chemistry to identify qualities of the specific agent that initiates a pathology; once a known chain of events is identified, designers attempt to intervene at a particular point with a specific method. Designers use several strategies and methods:

- *Structure-based design.* The central assumption of structure-based design is that good inhibitors must be complementary to their target receptor. The two-step process begins by determining the structure of receptors and then solving the 3-D jigsaw puzzle of matching molecular structures by using specially developed computer programs.

- *Molecular modeling.* This technique looks at the physical structure of a receptor and creates the model of a compatible chemical entity by using computer imaging. This can be done with incredible precision down to the level of DNA coding. With the help of computed chemical algorithms, designers can build—first virtually on the computer, then "wet" in the lab— the molecule of perfect chemical fit.

- *Virtual reality modeling.* This is a form of computer-enhanced molecular modeling. It includes features such as a force feedback handle that permits tactile manipulation of a 3-D image of the candidate molecule model's orientation.

- *Combinatorial chemistry.* This technique allows drug researchers to produce quickly as many as several million structurally related compounds, which they then screen to find those that are bioactive and possibly have therapeutic value. The chemical attributes of those molecules are known, and the chemists working with them expect certain biological activity. With the development of more reliable and rapid screening tests, thousands of related chemicals can be tested in parallel processes for reactivity with a complement of human antibodies on a mass scale.

- *Pharmacogenomics.* See below, p. 120.

Rational drug design will shorten the drug discovery process. New chemical and molecular entities will get to clinical trials faster as the random and unpredictable time for discovering a compound by chance is replaced by these more predictable design processes based on the structure and complexity of the pathogen.

Because rational drug design may result in too many promising new chemical entities and not enough resources to test them all, prioritization and stratification of candidate products will be an important area of concern.

MAGNITUDE AND AREAS OF IMPACT

Rational drug design will have impact in a number of therapeutic areas. Chief candidates are:

- *Neurologic and mental disease.* Drugs are being created that fit the receptors for various neurotransmitters, potentially to modify neuronal activity and influence the function of the nervous system in different areas where neurological and mental pathology are manifested.

The Pace of Change in Drug Design

The pharmaceutical and biotechnology industries have enthusiastically adopted the techniques of rational drug design. Five years ago, few pharmaceutical companies were heavily invested in rational drug design. Today, entire biotechnology companies have been formed primarily to carry out structure-based design, and most major pharmaceutical companies have structure and computational groups as part of their drug discovery effort. In 5 years, rational drug design will yield a rich crop of new candidate molecules for clinical trials.

- *Antiviral therapies.* Protease inhibitors designed to combat viral disease will be an important area of development. Every virus uses proteases to chop proteins into amino acids, which the virus then uses as building blocks. Targeting and inhibiting these enzymes could lead to the creation of the first truly effective antivirals. In the next 10 years, rational drug design will create antiviral therapies to combat diseases like human immunodeficiency virus (HIV), encephalitis, measles, and influenza.

KEY BARRIERS

One of the key driving forces behind rational drug design has been the increasing power of computers. The techniques and processes involved in rational drug design are highly information intensive and well suited to computer processing. The pace of drug design advances is regulated in part by the availability of research teams that combine knowledge of biochemistry with that of computer technology.

As researchers seek to combat more complex pathogens, they need to develop drugs that interact with their targets in more specific ways. With increased specificity and complexity will come increased costs in developing the proper new chemical entity.

As drug design can create an embarrassment of riches in terms of screened candidate compounds, much progress will need to be made in evaluating and prioritizing the candidates.

Unnatural Natural Products

Antibiotics that are in current clinical use are compounds made by antibiotic-producing bacteria and fungi—researchers have accepted the natural products that nature provided. Now, using recombinant DNA technology, "unnatural" natural products can be produced by combinatorial biosynthesis using genetically altered strains of a bacterium such as *Streptomyces*. Instead of isolating and testing a single natural product, thousands of novel biosynthetic molecules, a new class of antibiotics, can be obtained and screened. One such product may prove to be a powerful neuroregenerative agent that could be used in conditions such as Parkinson's disease, multiple sclerosis, Alzheimer's disease, and stroke.

Drug-Producing Animals and Plants

Transgenic animals and plants can be engineered to produce proteins that act as drugs. These living drug factories can be grown from animal embryos injected with human DNA. Transgenic animals can be cloned, and an entire herd can be created in a single generation. A transgenic ewe can produce milk containing an antienzyme, and its use in treating asthmatics is now in clinical trials. A transgenic drug industry has been born as yet another product of biotechnology. Among plants, tobacco has ideal characteristics for mass-producing bioengineered proteins, augmenting the current production of specific proteins in vats of bacterial cultures.

ADVANCES IN IMAGING

Imaging technologies present an enhanced visual display of tissues, organ systems, and their functions. They reveal the structural and functional aspects of organs, allowing clinicians to localize specific functions or conditions noninvasively.

Imaging has four elements: aiming energy at the area of interest; detecting or receiving that reflected or refracted energy; analyzing the data with computers; and displaying those data with technology that allows the clinician to view and interpret the information. Advances are taking place in each of these areas that will open up new functions for imaging technologies.

■ *Energy sources* currently used for imaging include X rays, ultrasound, electron beams, positrons, magnets, and radio frequencies. There is a constant trade-off in the energy sources used: on one hand, the more powerful the energy source, the more deeply it can penetrate and the more detail it can reveal in the image; on the other hand, powerful beams can injure tissues and organ systems. The same ultrasound energy that reveals "baby's first picture" to expectant parents also can, at a higher energy level, smash kidney stones in an electrolithotropter. Energy source technology is advancing as scientists find ways to more narrowly focus an energy beam to avoid damage to adjacent tissue. Research also is being conducted on alternate energy sources such as thermal differences in order to minimize residual damage.

■ *Detector technology* is advancing along two dimensions. First, digital detectors benefit from the trends in microelectronics toward smaller and smaller features on devices. The resolution of those detectors is improving constantly. The first commercially available "megapixel" detector (able to detect an image that comprises a grid of 1,000 by 1,000 pixels, discrete elements of the image) became available more than a decade ago. By 2005, detectors that can resolve 6,000 by 6,000 pixels will become available. Second, there are advances in contrast media. These are chemicals that, when introduced into the body, enhance the contrast between light and dark regions of an image in specific ways—for example, by highlighting areas of

Mini-MRIs and MRNs

An important trend in MRI technology is the design of increasingly smaller scanners with much lower capital and operating costs. The key: smaller and less costly magnets. Mini-MRI units will be available for dedicated uses in orthopedics, neurology, and mammography.

Magnetic resonance neurography (MRN) can identify the site of damage to a peripheral nerve by detecting increased signals at sites of nerve entrapment and trauma. It can also show the process of peripheral nerve degeneration and regeneration, the first imaging modality to do so.

■ *Infrared* imaging technology may allow accurate assessment of implanted coronary stents. Known as ocular coherence tomography (OCT), it will identify factors leading to restenosis.

■ *In vivo molecular imaging*—the imaging of gene expression in humans—is likely in the next 5 years. The technology is already being used in animals, and its potential (e.g., for determining whether a transgene gets to the tumor site and whether it expresses and if so for how long) will be invaluable in assessing the effects of many forms of pharmaceuticals and gene therapy.

malignant tissues or tissue abnormalities with more blood flow. Work is proceeding on contrast media that have organ, tissue, and cellular specificities.

■ *Analysis of the images* is the next function in which there are rapid advances. Computer analysis of the masses of data from high-resolution detectors gets faster and better with increases in raw computing power. Breakthroughs in algorithms and techniques, such as neural networks, will speed the conversion from 2-D to 3-D images, improve pattern recognition through better detection of edges and other features of images, and ease the manipulation and enhancement of digital images.

■ *Display technologies* are getting bigger, faster, and cheaper. There is spillover to medical imaging from a range of applications that require high-quality images. Improvements include larger displays, higher resolution, richer and more meaningful contrasts, and deeper color.

MAGNITUDE AND AREAS OF IMPACT

Advances in imaging are combining in several areas. *Electron-beam CT* scanning—in contrast to conventional CT scanning that uses X-ray beams—offers substantial improvements over old technologies. It allows for rapid acquisition of an image, reducing the discomfort patients experience from remaining immobile for the duration of a conventional CT scan. While this technology can detect calcium in the wall of the coronary artery, showing atherosclerosis, it does not show whether there is narrowing of the blood vessel. With the development of new contrast agents, electron-beam CT will be able to show visuals of the arteries themselves, making this technology competitive with MRI, although MRI has the additional value of showing blood flow.

Positron Emission Tomography (PET)

PET was developed and applied clinically to the central nervous system for the diagnosis of epilepsy and brain tumors. It became the gold standard for determining myocardial viability and myocardial blood flow, but it found only limited application to other organ systems. Within the past 5 years the introduction of multislice imaging, 3-mm resolution, and 3-D resolution has revolutionized the field and made whole-body PET imaging one of the most exciting developments in imaging for the diagnosis of metastatic and recurrent cancer. For recurrent cancer of the head and neck, a notoriously difficult area to image using current technology, PET has shown an accuracy of greater than 95 percent in detecting recurrent disease. Although it is being used to stage many cancers, because the current technique uses glucose uptake as the marker, this highly sensitive detector lacks specificity. Within the next decade tumor-specific marker molecules will be labeled with positron emitters to provide more specificity, at which point whole-body PET scanning will be faster, less expensive, more widely available, and the most accurate and rapid means of detecting cancer that has spread beyond the primary site or has recurred.

Harmonic imaging will overcome a number of barriers in ultrasonography. About one-third of all patients are "difficult to image," which means that a patient's body wall anatomy, for a variety of reasons, is difficult to "see" through. Specifically, someone who is obese or extremely muscular or someone with narrow rib spacing is often difficult to image. Smokers and people who have had radiation therapy can also fall into this category for cardiac imaging, and for OB/GYN a variety of impediments of the abdomen can cause difficulty.

Harmonic imaging improves the quality of images in these patients. Ultrasound generally works as follows: sound waves are transmitted into the body at a relatively low frequency and are detected by a receiver that is tuned to the same frequency. In harmonic imaging, the receiver is tuned to a higher frequency than the transmitter so that the clinician detects the harmonics, or the frequency-multiples of the echoes, that are produced inside the body itself. Higher frequency waves produce images with better resolution. Applications of harmonic imaging include better prediction of heart attacks by allowing the clinician to visualize blood flow through the myocardium.

The recent introduction of cine ultrasonography and refinement of microbubbles as a contrast agent will greatly enhance the imaging potential of ultrasound, including a new role in highly focused therapy by intentionally exploding "loaded" microbubbles at specific sites, such as a liver tumor.

Functional imaging, which provides information about how a tissue or organ system is operating, will go far beyond the capabilities of conventional MRI, CT, and ultrasonography, which now provide only *structural* information about tissues and organ systems. PET has long been capable of metabolic imaging—detecting patterns of energy use in the body. High-resolution PET will offer pinpoint accuracy in these images, which will render many invasive diagnostic procedures such as surgical biopsy obsolete. Functional MRI is used to determine location of neurological functions such as memory and reasoning in the brain, giving us the first look at how the brain works. In many respects, neuroimaging has revolutionized the study of behavioral neurology and cognitive neuroscience. Future applications of functional MRI will be in the study of disease and the body's response to treatment—for example, changes in the pattern of neural activity in the brain of schizophrenic patients being treated with new drugs.

Because developments in computing power have increased image display speed and improved the quality and content of digital data, *image-guided surgery* is becoming a mainstream procedure. Image-guided surgery is a new kind of minimally invasive surgical intervention. It improves on endoscopic and endovascular surgical methods by allowing the clinician to see a computed functional image superimposed on the surgical instrument's location and other relevant information. The current combination of nearly real-time imaging and functional mapping will result in real-time, high-contrast, and high-spatial-resolution images.

Overall, imaging technologies will improve the diagnostic process immensely. Clinicians will use these technologies to look at the form and function of organs that were once examined only by surgery, reducing the need for invasive diagnostic procedures.

KEY BARRIERS

There are few barriers to the development of new imaging technologies, which benefit from the continual progress of computing power. Simple economics will limit the application of some technologies. Historically, imaging technologies have been additive—new technologies do not replace old ones but rather supplement their use. In a cost-constrained health system, more restraint will be exercised on the use of new imaging systems. Comprehensive analyses of cost-effectiveness, including the full life-

cycle cost of the equipment, will become commonplace.

MINIMALLY INVASIVE SURGERY

Also called minimal or limited-access surgery, minimally invasive surgery was made possible by the introduction of fiber-optic technology, miniaturization of improved instruments and devices, image digitization, navigational systems for vascular catheters, and a sudden awareness that image-guided surgery was the wave of the future. Early examples of minimally invasive surgery were arthroscopic knee meniscectomy, endovascular obliteration of intracranial aneurysms, coronary angioplasty, and laparoscopic cholecystectomy. More recent innovations are image-guided brain surgery, minimal access major cardiac operations, and the endovascular placement of grafts for abdominal aneurysms. Over the same period of time, open surgery biopsy has been replaced by fine-needle aspiration of many tumors, which is gaining general acceptance for use on tumors of the breast and thyroid gland.

The movement toward minimally invasive surgery has promoted the proliferation of ambulatory surgicenters. The consequent major reduction in the volume of surgical procedures performed in hospital facilities has achieved a remarkable reduction in the length of stay, as patients having procedures previously requiring hospitalization enjoy more rapid recovery and return to full activity because of the lowered morbidity of the less invasive operations. In areas where minimally invasive procedures have replaced their more disruptive antecedents, short-term as well as long-term outcomes have been the same or, in most examples, better, with a high level of acceptance and satisfaction by patients. In the case of invasive procedures, less *is* better.

MAGNITUDE AND AREAS OF IMPACT

To begin at the top, brain surgery has been a major beneficiary of image-guided technology. Operations requiring access to areas of the brain beneath the surface are conducted by using navigational systems and image guidance through small openings in the skull. Even more dramatic has been the impact of endovascular surgery, the creation of a group of innovative interventional radiologists. Using current technology—digitized image guidance, catheter navigational systems, and an array of implantable materials—endovascular surgeons can treat almost all intracranial aneurysms and many arteriovenous fistulas. Moreover, subsequent open surgical procedures can be facilitated by preoperative blockage of blood flow to the tumor or congenital arteriovenous malformation.

All endovascular surgery has advanced and matured rapidly in the past decade. The practitioners of the art fall into three broad categories with a slight degree of overlap. The first, interventional neuroradiologists, deal with vascular pathology of the brain and spinal cord. In addition to the procedures described earlier, these neurointerventionalists can lyse blood clots in cerebral arteries and veins, dilate intracranial arteries narrowed by pathologic vasospasm, and open partially or completely occluded arteriosclerotic arteries that restrict blood flow to the brain.

The second and largest group of endovascular interventionalists are cardiologists whose major procedure is coronary angioplasty. With advances in intravascular stent technology and the introduction of pharmaceuticals that inhibit the principal cause of restenosis—postangioplasty proliferation of subendothelial smooth muscle in the arterial wall—percutaneous angioplasty will further reduce the indications for open operations for coronary artery bypass grafting. Two recently reported studies have established the superiority of coronary angioplasty with stenting plus administration of a platelet glycoprotein inhibitor (abciximab) for unstable angina and acute myocardial infarction.[1,2] The effect will be a significant broadening of indications for angioplasty over radical (conservative) management of coronary artery disease. Cardiac interventionalists can also correct cardiac arrhythmias, treat selected cardiac valve disorders, and, by using improved technology, close congenital septal defects.

The third group of endovascular surgeons operate in sites other than the central nervous system and the heart; for example, they place endovascular prosthetic devices for the treatment of abdominal aortic aneurysms, create therapeutic vascular shunts, and perform angioplasty of narrowed arteries in the trunk and extremities.

Laparoscopy has truly revolutionized the practice of abdominal surgery for procedures on the gastrointestinal tract and female organs. The most recent addition to the laparoscopic surgeon's growing list of operations is bilateral adrenalectomy. Further advances will incorporate telepresence technology, which permits a surgeon to operate remotely, robotics, and 3-D imaging. Technological advances are proceeding with unprecedented speed, placing pressures on practicing general and gynecologic surgeons either to seek additional training or to drift into obsolescence with out-of-date skills.

Future refinements in minimally invasive surgery will expand the present scope and range of procedures. New arthroscopic procedures, wider use of image guidance in operations on the head and neck, and innovations in limited-access procedures for spinal and thoracic diseases are evolving; within the next 5 years they will be accepted practice. These advances will be aided by interventional MRI, currently used for liver and kidney biopsy, with its shorter acquisition time and 3-D capability.

For patients with acute stroke, interventional MRI will be a major addition to the surgical process. Pharmacologic brain protection will extend the viability of ischemic brain and prompt transfer to a dedicated MRI facility will permit immediate assessment of the brain's viability and blood flow. When appropriate, occluded vessels can be opened by endovascular intervention under the guidance of MRI. By the year 2010, large population centers will have "vascular institutes" that are serviced by emergency transportation networks. Vascular institutes will facilitate rapid movement of heart attack, stroke, and other acute vascular accident victims to

an institute staffed around the clock by endovascular surgeons who can prevent the death and disability that today's technologies cannot. Current gaps in ancillary pharmaceuticals will be closed by products emerging from the biotech industry. The development of stent grafts that can be used in cervical vessels and at branchings will extend their application at sites currently beyond the reach of endovascular technology.

KEY BARRIERS

- The American public wants big automobiles, SUVs, and RVs but minimally invasive, or, even better, noninvasive surgery. The appeal and marketability of minimally invasive operations have the effect of pulling these technologies into the health care system in advance of adequate technology assessment, including evaluation of cost-effectiveness. Adverse outcomes can and do result from prematurely applied minimally invasive procedures, the rash of common bile duct injuries inflicted by inadequately trained laparoscopic (cholecystectomy) surgeons being one example. The consequences could be restrictive legislation that would have the effect of creating major barriers to innovative clinical trials of this promising technology.

- Insurers restrict or deny payment for new minimally invasive procedures by declaring them experimental and therefore not a covered benefit.

- Currently, mechanisms for transfer of procedural technologies into the practicing medical community are barely adequate, bordering on inadequate. As computer-enabled procedural technologies evolve at an ever-increasing pace, their successful penetration into the delivery system will be restricted unless better models for teaching practicing physicians to use these technologies are designed and implemented.

GENETIC MAPPING AND TESTING

Until recently, most genetic tests were used to detect rare and singular conditions. Many of these single-gene disorders become clinically apparent during infancy and childhood whereas others, such as Huntington's disease and polycystic kidney disease, are of adult onset. Genetic tests are used to detect carrier states, in relation to marriage and conception, and for prenatal diagnosis and counseling, e.g. for Down's syndrome.

The special field of clinical genetics has evolved from observations of familial occurrences of inherited disorders to the use of the tools of human molecular genetics. Genetic tests have become available for more common and more complex diseases, many with onset in adult life. With the identification of cancer susceptibility genes and of genes leading to neurogenetic disorders including Alzheimer's disease, the Human Genome Project provided the engine that propelled the rapid identification of a wide range of genes that can cause complex diseases such as diabetes, cancer, and heart disease, in which both genetic predisposition and environmental and behavioral factors combine to reach a critical threshold for causation. These

gene discoveries provide the basis for genetic susceptibility testing—recognition of a predisposition to disease—and with it unprecedented opportunities to intervene with strategies for prevention, avoidance, or modification of the predisposed condition. Abruptly, clinical genetics assumed a role whose importance was only imagined a decade ago.

With the possible exception of stem cell biology, no scientific discipline is advancing more rapidly than medical genetics. It seems that each week one or more disease-associated genes are identified and added to the genomic database to fuel a parallel growth of diagnostic and screening tests. To date, clinical tests have been developed for almost 500 human genetic disorders, a number that will continue to grow.

The National Cancer Institute has established three primary goals with regard to genetic testing: (1) identification of every major human gene that predisposes individuals to cancer; (2) clinical application of these discoveries to people at risk; and (3) identification and remedial attention to psychosocial, ethical, and legal issues associated with inherited susceptibility. A secondary goal is developing an informatics system to collect, store, analyze, and integrate cancer-related molecular data with epidemiologic and clinical data.

PHARMACOGENOMICS

Pharmacogenomics, a particular application of genomic information, is the science that defines how an individual responds to drugs. Basically, a drug may be safe or dangerous depending on the

The Ethics of Genetic Testing

When the importance and future ramifications of genetic testing became clear, a number of panels were convened to look at the technical, social, and ethical issues. The Task Force on Genetic Testing was created by the National Institutes of Health—Department of Energy Working Group on Ethical, Legal and Social Implications of Human Genome Research to make recommendations to "ensure the development of safe and effective genetic tests, their delivery in laboratories of assured quality, and their appropriate use by health care providers and consumers." The task force called on the Secretary of Health and Human Services to establish the Advisory Committee on Genetic Testing and to apply "stringent scrutiny" when a test can predict future inherited disease in healthy or apparently healthy people, is likely to be used for that purpose, and when no confirming test is available. The National Center for Human Genome Research has set aside funds for consideration of ethical, legal, and social implications of human genome research in which genetic testing has the central role.

Related to pharmacogenomics is tissue fingerprinting (i.e. testing of tissue rather than a person) to determine whether a specific drug will be effective. The best example is the testing of breast cancer taken from a patient for the presence of HER2 amplification: if the gene is amplified, a drug, Herceptin, will be effective, and if not, the drug will be ineffective. This example illustrates the reclassification of a condition, in this case breast cancer, according to genetic (molecular) features and at the same time provides an example of prescribing a treatment based on a distinguishing molecular abnormality.

MAGNITUDE AND AREAS OF IMPACT

Genetic susceptibility testing for cancer of the breast, colon, and prostate has moved into clinical reality, and in each instance the hereditary pattern of disease provided the initial search for the identification of the critical gene or genes.

genetic profile of the individual, most often having to do with the function or nonfunction of an enzyme responsible for the metabolic fate of a drug. For a particular drug to be effective (a different question than its safety), an individual's genetic profile is equally important. Testing for these drug effects is one use of genetic testing.

Pharmacogenomics has two broad applications. First, for individual patients, pretreatment testing will predict safety and efficacy of a particular drug or class of drugs. Second, for the pharmaceutical industry pharmacogenomics will have profound effects on preclinical drug development and equally impressive consequences on the design and conduct of clinical trials. The initial application of drug-related genetic testing will concentrate on the safety of the drug for individual patients.

More complex genetic disorders, such as childhood asthma and late-onset Alzheimer's disease, suggest either a polygenic inheritance, in which more than one gene is responsible for the disease in a particular individual, or genetic heterogeneity, in which different combinations of genes produce the same condition in different individuals. Of even greater complexity are the conditions currently being studied in the emerging field of neurogenetics, where genes that increase susceptibility to schizophrenia, manic-depressive illness, and depression are studied to find out how they interact with nongenetic (environmental) factors to trigger the onset of the recognized

Chapter 8: Medical Technologies

disease state. In these psychiatric disorders, identification of the specific genes may give clues for designing pharmacologic interventions. The discovery of genetic susceptibility provides the basis for initiating preventive measures, whether through pharmacologic means or counseling. The new term "genometrics" has been applied to the discovery of a gene or genes responsible for a trait and to defining precisely the trait controlled by each gene involved in complex multifactorial illnesses.

Within a few years, our present methods of genetic analysis, sophisticated though they seem, will be viewed as time-consuming, labor-intensive, expensive, and myopic in scope and application. New technology will use microchips designed to interrogate DNA or RNA samples for sequence or expression information. The molecular arrays for these microchips can be synthesized cheaply, rapidly, and efficiently by using methods borrowed from the semiconductor industry. With fluorescent methods for the detection of DNA and RNA targets, hybridization will occur in a special chamber, and the resulting signals will be detected by scanning microscopy in a matter of minutes. Current applications of this microchip technology will revolutionize the fields of diagnostics and genomics. Within the next decade, cancer tissue will be analyzed for differences in gene expression, and in another 5 years specific therapies can be assigned to individuals with identified cancer genotypes. Tumors of a particular type will be re-classified by genotypic profile (genetic fingerprint) and once they are classified, individualized treatment will be quite

specifically administered based on pharmacogenomic information. Applied to genetic testing, microchip technology will have predictive power for disease and disease predisposition that heretofore was almost unimaginable.

KEY BARRIERS

Practicing clinicians—generalists and specialists alike—lack the knowledge base to practice genomic medicine. Genetic testing, particularly the predisposition genetic testing for late-onset disorders in adults, requires a multidisciplinary approach. People seeking such testing need appropriate pre-test education and genetic counseling and post-test follow-up care. Before testing is done, the person must be informed that other factors, genetic and nongenetic, may influence onset and severity of the condition, and that in many situations testing is probabilistic rather than deterministic. Potential consequences must be understood, as must the clinician's inability to guarantee confidentiality despite all safeguards and legislative protections.

Genetic testing has a predictable future based on technological potential. This potential could be constrained, delayed, or lost entirely through several possible developments: the desire in prenatal testing to enhance specific attributes of offspring; technology's advancing too rapidly for rational assimilation and application because of an understaffed clinical genetics workforce; premature availability of self-administered testing kits as a consequence of unregulated commercial interests; and ethical roadblocks imposed because of misuse of genetic information contrary to public policy (e.g., sterilization of people afflicted with a serious heritable disease to prevent genetic transmission to offspring).

With proper safeguards, genetic testing will revolutionize prevention and treatment of many conditions and diseases, but without these safeguards the possibilities for mass confusion, misapplication, discrimination, and lawful or unlawful commercial exploitation are sobering.

GENE THERAPY

In 1997, a blue-ribbon panel of experts sharply criticized the rush to initiate clinical trials of gene therapy before an adequate scientific base was established. The consequence was a slowdown in clinical applications and a return to basic research in several critical areas: better vectors or delivery vehicles to ferry corrective genes into target cells; more precise targeting of genes to specific sites and tissues; and enhancement of gene expression following entry into the target cell. The widely publicized and criticized death in 1999 of a patient undergoing gene therapy initiated sweeping improvements in dealing with human subjects of clinical research, not only in gene therapy trials but also in human research generally.

Nevertheless, revolutionary advances in gene therapy are preparing medicine for an epochal shift to an era in which genes will be delivered routinely to cure or alleviate an array of inherited and acquired diseases. Gene therapy can be defined as "a therapeutic technique in

which a functioning gene is inserted into targeted cells of a patient to correct an inborn error or to provide the cell with a new function." The successful delivery and insertion of a functioning gene leads to the expression of a therapeutic protein of some kind that will supplement or replace a defective gene or treat the effects of acquired diseases like cancer. Somatic gene therapy, discussed here, affects only somatic cells—the kinds that are neither sperm nor egg.[3]

Current methods for gene therapy use directly harvested cells, cultured cell lines, genetically modified cell lines, and viral vectors, such as modified retroviruses or adenoviruses. In the *ex vivo* approach, cells from specific tissues are removed, cultured, and exposed to viral or nonviral vectors or DNA containing the gene of interest. After insertion of the genes into these cells, the cells are returned to the patient. In the *in vivo* approach, viral or nonviral vectors— or simply "naked DNA"—are directly administered to patients by various routes. A third approach involves the encapsulation of gene-modified cells and the reversible introduction of an encapsulated cell structure into the human body.[3]

A challenge for genetic researchers is to develop methods that discriminately deliver enough genetic material to the right cells. Most gene vectors in current use are disabled mouse retroviruses. Retroviral vectors offer the most promising prospect for the transfer of useful gene sequences into defective tumor cells because they target only dividing cells and have the potential of long-term expression. They are considered safe and

Chapter 8: Medical Technologies   **123**

effective gene delivery vehicles and are attractive because they are designed to specifically enter cells and express their genes there. Retroviruses splice copies of their genes into the chromosomes of the cells they invade, and the integrated gene is then passed on to future generations of cells. Since cell entry by a retrovirus occurs only when cells are actively dividing, this feature is exploited in rapidly dividing cells such as bone marrow but is not suitable for other tissues, such as muscle and lung. Unfortunately, retroviruses are somewhat indiscriminate and have been known to deposit their genes into the chromosomes of a variety of cell types, prompting research into viral envelope alteration in hope of increasing target specificity. The specificity of the envelope—how the vector is "packaged"—ensures the appropriate receptors are triggered.

Other viral vectors are also being explored. These include adenoviruses and adenoassociated viruses, herpes viruses, alpha viruses, vaccina virus, and poxviruses. Each virus has a potential therapeutic niche established by its attributes and behavior. The next most commonly used vector after retrovirus is the adenovirus, a DNA virus that, though capable of entering dividing as well as nondividing cells, has produced disappointing results. Adenoassociated viruses have an appeal because they cause no known diseases in humans and they integrate their genes into human chromosomes. But because they are small, they may not be able to accommodate large genes. Herpes viruses do not integrate their genes into the host's DNA, but they are attracted to neurons and may be useful in neurological therapies.

Liposomes are yet another potential vector under examination. These synthetic lipid bubbles can be designed to harbor plasmids—stable loops of DNA that multiply naturally within bacteria—into which therapeutic genes are inserted. A synthetic liposome-like vector, the lipoplex, can bind firmly to cell surfaces and insert its DNA package into cells at a significant rate. Mixing lipoplexes with DNA has become a standard technique for inserting genes into cultured cells.

Although currently undeveloped for clinical use, two new viral-based vector systems hold out the possibility of advancing toward the ideal delivery system for directly supplying cells with healthy copies of missing or defective genes. Both systems have the capacity to alter quiescent cells, such as the mature stem cells that generate the immune system. These viral vectors, HIV and simian virus 40 (SV40), share the preceding characteristics. Although HIV is a human pathogen whose use will be restricted at least initially to advanced cancers, origin from a human source may confer an advantage. SV40, an adenovirus, can be rendered harmless, is capable of infecting several resting and dividing cell types, is easy to manipulate, and is stable and nonimmunogenic; it appears to be as benign as any available viral vector and has the added attribute of being directly injectable into target tissues. Some investigators foresee the development of hybrid vectors that build on the best features of viral and nonviral vectors.

MAGNITUDE AND AREAS OF IMPACT

Current clinical trials are investigating the genetic treatment of several cancers and genetic diseases, such as cystic fibrosis and hemophilia. Gene therapy has succeeded in treating the symptoms of patients with cardiac and lower extremity ischemia, and several children with severe combined immunodeficiency diseases are surviving as a direct result of treatment.

One of the most significant developments in this field is the application of this methodology to gene marking in the study of the biology of cancer. Close to 1.4 million Americans will be newly diagnosed with cancer this year alone, and the treatments currently available—surgery, radiation therapy, and chemotherapy—cannot cure 50 percent of those diagnosed. Although gene therapy was originally targeted toward single-gene deficiency diseases that are recessive and relatively rare, about 80 percent of the current clinical trials now focus on cancer.

For treating cancer, a variety of approaches are being attempted. Some involve imparting cancer cells with genes that give rise to toxic molecules. When these genes are expressed, the resulting product then kills the cancer cells. Genetic marking of marrow cells used in similar *ex vivo* therapies permits physicians to monitor the effects of different cancer-purging methods. Another research focus is on the correction or compensation for acquired genetic mutations, particularly of the oft-mutated tumor suppressor gene p53.

Yet another field of cancer research is immunotherapy. Immunotherapeutic research concentrates on how tumors evade detection and attack via the immune system, how they spread away from their sites of origin, how they gain a new blood supply, and how they evolve and spread.

A different form of genetic marking is used in immunotherapy, also called vaccine therapy. Immunotherapeutic vaccinations tag cancer cells with certain genes that make them more visible to the immune system. One method being widely tested involves modifying a patient's cancer cells with genes encoding cytokines—the communication proteins of the immune system's *B* and *T* cells—to draw an attack from the immune system. Unfortunately, this method will benefit only patients with robust immune systems and not those with advanced cancer.

KEY BARRIERS

Despite encouraging results, the field awaits answers to many unresolved questions. An area where enormous progress has been made, but where much more is needed, is developing gene-delivery vectors. Virus-based vectors have been the most efficient for inserting genes into cells in the laboratory, but in clinical applications the results have in some cases been short lived, and there have been unwanted side effects.

In addition, the field needs to develop animal models to test the biological and clinical efficacy of the new vectors and procedures. As a result, gene therapy may take longer to reach patients than originally predicted. The progress of gene therapy also depends on adequate technical, financial, and training resources, and demands close interaction between academics, clinicians, and private-sector companies.

Private industry is playing a critical role in promoting the development of innovative medical technology. These companies have millions of dollars at risk: they have to choose technologies, knowing that the ultimately successful approaches are likely to require complex assemblies of new chemical tools and procedures. For industry, a necessary incentive is the award of exclusive protection of innovative breakthroughs. Limited access to enabling technologies for gene therapy—such as vectors—because of time-consuming and expensive licensing processes, could lead to prohibitive commercial burdens that would delay progress in the field.

In June 1999, there were 313 clinical studies involving gene transfer, of which 277 protocols involved new therapeutic applications with most (193) intended for patients with cancer. The same advisory group that in 1995 accused the scientific community of overselling the present benefits of gene therapy stressed the extraordinary potential of gene therapy for the long-term treatment of human disease. The lack of more efficient gene vectors was singled out as the major barrier to attaining better clinical results.[4]

With the intense ongoing activity in vector development, we project that within 10 years a number of efficient gene delivery systems will be in clinical use. Vectors that have both site- and cell-type specificities will deliver genes to treat a wide range of conditions in most, if not all, organs. The potential of using genes and gene products in novel strategies is an incredibly powerful incentive to pursue gene therapy as the equal of the future's most effective therapeutic modalities.

VACCINES

Since Jenner conferred smallpox immunity with inoculations of cowpox in the early 19th century, vaccines have been administered globally as preventive measures for acute diseases, such as diphtheria, smallpox, and whooping cough, and have been used to avoid acute infection by creating a low-level immune response that remains as an acquired immunity. In the history of public health, vaccines have proved to be among the most effective disease prevention tools. Some diseases, such as smallpox, polio, and measles, have been eradicated or brought under control through mass vaccination programs.

The current use of vaccines includes any preparation intended for active immunization of the recipient. Until recently, vaccines were prophylactic—their sole objective was preventing a specific infectious disease. They were therefore directed against the causative infectious agent. More recently, vaccines have been used against noninfectious diseases. Patients with certain cancers have been vaccinated—either prophylactically, to prevent the emergence of micrometastatic tumors, or therapeutically, to boost the immunologic cytotoxic response to the tumor.

Vaccines can have preventive or therapeutic uses. *Preventive* vaccines permit the vaccinated individual to develop immunologic responses that prevent or modulate subsequent infection or disease. Recently developed *therapeutic* vaccines use new recombinant DNA technology to provide genetic therapy to patients who already have a disease. The key to using this technology is specificity for tumor cells or for an infectious agent such as HIV or tuberculosis.

The application of molecular biology to the identification of virulent genes has led to a fundamental understanding of the pathogenesis of virulent microbes. With the molecular tools of the new genetics, the genes responsible for the organism's virulence can be identified and isolated. The molecular genetic definition of virulence has exciting and highly promising implications for vaccines. Given the side effects of antibiotics, including the emergence of resistant bacteria, novel strategies for controlling infectious diseases are evolving. One of the most promising strategies, that of using molecular microbiology and whole-gene sequencing to develop candidate vaccines, will be the wider use of gene-specific vaccines.[5]

Recent therapeutic vaccines are designed to attack certain chronic infections. Early cancer vaccines had few successes but with the new knowledge and technology ushered in by molecular biology, medical, and recombinant DNA technology, anticancer vaccines are gaining increasing attention. This resurgence of interest in therapeutic vaccines reflects a new and broadened understanding of the immune system and its elements.

Vaccines have been effective in treating melanomas and renal cell carcinomas, two cancers that are unique in their responsiveness to the immune system. Vaccine therapies for cancer that stimulate the immune system and do not involve surgery, radiation, or cytotoxicity could become the least traumatic mode of treatment for particular cancer patients. A vaccine can activate the immune system by delivering a tumor antigen or by eliciting a nonspecific immune system response. Such a nonspecific response would simply boost the activity of the immune system, resulting in greater overall immune activity.

MAGNITUDE AND AREAS OF IMPACT

Prophylactic vaccination to prevent cancers caused by viruses would prevent an estimated 850,000 cases of cancer each year, roughly 11 percent of the global cancer burden. Examples of such viruses and their secondary cancers are Epstein-Barr virus and nasopharyngeal cancer, human papilloma virus (HPV) and cancer of the cervix, and hepatitis B virus and primary liver cancer. Because cervical cancer is diagnosed in 16,000 women in the United States each year, the impact of a vaccine for HPV will be substantial. In addition, a live attenuated HIV vaccine may be a realistic projection by 2005, or even sooner.

A novel new vaccine against rotavirus, a major cause of childhood diarrheal disease mortality in developing countries, which causes an estimated 600,000 deaths worldwide each year, is a live oral rotavirus vaccine. Incorporation of this vaccine into routine immunization could reduce severe rotavirus gastroenteritis by 90 percent.

Could some diseases currently believed to have a noninfectious cause be the direct consequence of an infection by an unidentified or unrecognized agent? If the recent connection of *H. pylori* infection to gastric carcinoma and lymphoma and the putative role of infectious prions with Alzheimer's disease are a prelude to the future, the answer is a resounding "yes." Among immediate candidates for such an etiologic connection are other cancers and rheumatoid arthritis. By the year 2010, prophylactic and therapeutic vaccines will compete with rational drug design for airtime.

KEY BARRIERS

Clinical trials of HIV vaccines will be controversial and politically charged. Traditional approaches to vaccine development, such as "whole killed" or attenuated virus methods, raise special safety concerns with HIV because a faulty vaccine that actually infects a recipient would have lethal consequences. Realistic research goals for HIV vaccine may focus on a product that can inhibit progression to disease or lower viral load in infected persons instead of preventing actual infection.

ARTIFICIAL BLOOD

Blood transfusions are given for two reasons: (1) to increase oxygen-carrying capacity, and (2) to restore intravascular volume. Intravascular volume can be restored by other fluids, such as crystalloids and colloids, which are free from

the risks of transmitting an infectious agent. Thus, increasing oxygen-carrying capacity is rapidly becoming the *sole* indication for blood transfusions, which in most cases is done by administering packed red blood cells. The only major risk of blood transfusion, assuming the absence of human error in the pretransfusion process, is transmission of an infectious agent that has eluded detection by the battery of screening tests currently performed before a unit of blood is cleared for use. The principal concerns are the HIV and hepatitis viruses and more recently the prion diseases, notably Creutzfeld-Jacob disease. Availability of donated blood in the United States has become a problem. Severe shortages of blood and blood products have affected several metropolitan areas, and in the near future continued short supplies are predicted from coast to coast.

Historically, the armed services have tried to develop artificial blood for military use under wartime conditions and in natural disasters. The features of an ideal blood substitute would be ready availability, safety, long shelf life, efficacy, and compatibility across all blood types. Interest in artificial blood peaked in the 1980s because of the seriousness of transfusion transmission of HIV and hepatitis infections, but the current and projected shortages of donated blood have created a new level of urgency in developing suitable blood substitutes.

MAGNITUDE AND AREAS OF IMPACT

Hemoglobin-free fluids carrying dissolved oxygen have been approved for clinical use but because of their inability to achieve desired oxygenation of tissues these products have been used sparingly in practice.

Hemoglobin-containing products have been produced by using outdated human blood or bovine blood. A serious drawback of these hemoglobin products has been kidney damage caused by the splitting of hemoglobin into fragments that were shown to damage the kidneys. Human hemoglobin can be chemically stabilized to avoid this splitting, and refined blood substitutes based on human hemoglobin are now in advanced clinical trials. The obvious problems are the supply of outdated blood and the risk, although reduced, of disease transmission.

A new company, Somatogen, has produced a recombinant hemoglobin using *E. coli*. The recombinant hemoglobin acts like human hemoglobin, and the synthetic process can be programmed to produce a product with an ideal oxygen-release curve free from adverse features such as the hypertensive component of free hemoglobin. The recombinant hemoglobin, like stabilized human hemoglobin, has a half-life of 24 hours. Because four companies have products in the final stage of testing, Food and Drug Administration (FDA) approval of a satisfactory blood substitute may soon be granted. Further refinements of synthetic hemoglobin molecules will lead to a near-ideal substitute for blood by 2010. This fluid will have a shelf life of 1 year or longer; obviate the need for cross-match (i.e., be a universal source of blood); and carry no risk of infection. Such a product will be used routinely

for cardiac bypass procedures and renal dialysis as well as for transfusion.

KEY BARRIERS

- Public's reluctance to accept an artificial product that is perceived to be less valuable.

- Resistance from an entrenched blood-bank industry.

- High cost of artificial blood due to manufacturers' need to have an early return on investment in product development.

XENOTRANSPLANTATION

Xenotransplantation—the transplantation of cells, tissues, and whole organs from one species to another—had its modern beginning in the early 1960s with the transplantation of kidneys from chimpanzees to six human patients. But these xenotransplants, and later other grafts of solid organs across species, resulted in immune rejection after brief periods of normal function in the new host. In contrast, allotransplantation—transplantation within species—of bone marrow and solid organs from related and unrelated human donors has become highly successful because of satisfactory, although still less-than-ideal, means of avoiding immune rejection, principally by using immunosuppressive drugs and avoiding major histoincompatibilities to the extent possible.

MAGNITUDE AND AREAS OF IMPACT

The number of patients meeting strict criteria for receiving transplants of kidneys, lungs, livers, and hearts currently

Chapter 8: Medical Technologies   129

exceeds the supply of suitable donor organs. In the past 10 years, the number of solid-organ allotransplants has increased slightly more than 50 percent, with the greatest increase being in lung transplants. Over the same span of time, the number of names on the waiting list for all organs reached 75,000, in 2000, and more than 5,000 potential recipients died while awaiting a suitable donor organ. Availability of a suitable donor organ poses a particular problem for infants and children because of organ size, and for ethnic minorities because of a lack of suitably matched donors.

As indications for organ transplantation have broadened, waiting lists grown, and waiting times for suitable human organs lengthened, research on xenotransplantation has accelerated by using new knowledge and methods of molecular genetics, transplantation biology, genetic engineering, and transgenic technology. Current xenotransplantation research focuses on the pig because of its size and favorable biologic factors.

The basic strategies fall in two areas: combined transplantation of bone marrow and the solid organ; and modification of the animal serving as the source of the organ. Both strategies are designed to avoid acute rejection. Combined transplantation, considered a high risk but an equally high-reward strategy, depends on first successfully grafting the foreign bone marrow into the patient, thus permitting later successful transplantation of the solid organ. The strategy more likely to be successful is genetic modification of the pig using transgenic technology. Introduction of a

new gene requires 14 months, but this time will be shortened in the future. The short-term goal will be to use organs from modified pig donors to bridge a human recipient for a matter of months while awaiting a suitable human organ, and this may be possible within the next 2 years. The use of pig organs as bridges will teach critical lessons essential to the creation of transgenic pigs whose organs can be transplanted for permanent replacement, an ideal that should be attained within 10 years. Humans are presently living with xenotransplants of nervous tissue mechanically transplanted to the brain for the treatment of Parkinson's disease, so the feasibility of organ xenotransplantation is not far-fetched.

Transplantation of organs has been one of the great medical advances of the century and the one modality that treats a chronic disease successfully by replacing the diseased organ. The present limitation of solid-organ transplantation is the availability of donor organs, and for both social and economic reasons, current waiting lists do not reflect the true need for organ transplants in our population. The applications of xenotransplantation go beyond eliminating the waiting lists for solid organs as they are now used. Chronic conditions, such as diabetes and Parkinson's disease, can be successfully treated with xenotransplants, and xenotransplants of cells and tissues can be used to transfer genes and their gene products for the treatment of genetic diseases, such as hemophilia, and acquired conditions, such as cancer. Pediatric organ transplants could be used in the treatment of congenital heart disease and as a prophylactic measure in the patient with Wilm's disease. The potential is incredible.

KEY BARRIERS AND INDICATORS

The principal scientific concern relates to disease transmission between animals and humans. The pig is known to harbor an endogenous retrovirus, but there is no known transmission of any infection or disease from pigs to humans. In theory, any infectious agent could be bred out of the donor animal, but the threat of disease cannot be dismissed entirely, nor can the successful treatment of a transmitted infection be assured. Preliminary vaccination of the organ recipient is a feasible option that could confer additional protection. Another concern is excessive inbreeding, and one goal of creating herds of pig donors is to use as little inbreeding as possible.

Two issues will need to be addressed: the economic consequences of applying a new technology on a scale that today would seem to be vast but which is not precisely predictable, and the ethical and public policy implications of resource allocation and equity.

STEM CELL TECHNOLOGIES

Embryonic stem cells (ESCs), also called pluripotent stem cells, can generate all other types of cells in the body and therefore hold great promise for replacing or repairing tissues and organs damaged by disease. Although they were known to exist in humans, their incredible plasticity and myriad potential uses seemingly burst onto the scene in 1999, the year that the journal *Science* declared stem cells

the year's major scientific advance. In the years since stem cells have vied for the public's attention with the likes of gene therapy, new drugs, and other medical advances. Particularly contentious has been the debate over the ethics surrounding use of embryonic tissues.

Stem cells also reside in virtually every tissue and organ throughout adult life, and although small in number and difficult to recover except in the bone marrow, they do exist; they are known generally as *adult stem cells*, to distinguish them from ESCs. Adult stem cells, too, can be coaxed into cells of a different lineage or type, but their plasticity is restricted and they cannot reproduce indefinitely outside the body in the same manner as ESCs, hence their relatively more limited potential. The principal attraction of adult stem cells concerns their immunologic compatibility if the donor and the recipient are the same person, and certain cells in the bone marrow have this potential. Another approach for the avoidance of the immune rejection would be the creation of universal stem cells lacking critical antigens, and this possibility is being pursued.

Molecular signals have been identified that determine the future path of differentiation of an uncommitted stem cell (ESC), and comparable molecular signals can promote dedifferentiation of committed cells. To date, stem cells can be coaxed to become cartilage, bone, blood cells, muscle, fat, neurons and related cells in the nervous system, and heart muscle. Other cell types, such as liver and pancreatic islet cells, can be produced under appropriate conditions *in vitro*, and there seems little doubt that all cell types, including those in complex organs, such as the kidney, can be produced as well.

Building organs rather than tissues has engaged the involvement of tissue engineers, who envision scaffolds composed of biodegradable polymers that can be populated with specific cells to create semisynthetic tissues and organs. Skin and bone have been the initial successes, but more complex tissues and organs will follow shortly. Creating an internal network of blood vessels is entirely feasible and prototypes have been created in several laboratories.

Magnitude and Areas of Impact

The magnitude is huge, really huge. Damaged heart muscle could be patched with cardiomyocytes grown from the patient's own cells, diabetics could be implanted with clusters of pancreatic islet cells that will respond to glucose levels appropriately, and patients with Parkinson's disease could be treated successfully by dopaminergic neurons grown in special stem cell laboratories.

These and similar examples are entirely feasible within 5 years, possibly even sooner. The more difficult task of building solid organs to supply the rapidly expanding demand of patients with life-threatening organ failure will require more time for development, and although prototypes may become available as bridges to definitive conventional organ transplants before the end of the decade, fully functional replacements for livers, hearts, and kidneys are unlikely to become available until after 2010.

Barriers

The principal and most predictable barriers to forging ahead with the development of embryonic stem cell technologies may be political and ethical. The political barrier has some relationship to the controlling party at the federal level, but at present there is sufficient support for embryonic stem cell research and application among moderates of both parties that this may not be an issue regardless of who is in the White House. The ethical barrier to using ESCs is rooted in religious dogma and in the objections of ethicists who emphasize the risk of misapplication. Both forces have powerful and articulate representatives, and, although embryonic stem cell research will advance regardless, legal and legislative hurdles could delay its impact on the health of individuals who could benefit from the advances that may be possible.

Wild Cards

- Managed care organizations develop the analytical tools to make rational trade-offs among different therapeutic modalities. Because of their cost-effectiveness, drug therapies offset a large share of medical costs. Drug spending as a share of total health spending increases from 9 percent to 20 percent. Meanwhile, overall health expenditures decline.

- Drug-resistant strains of staphylococcus and tuberculosis become commonplace, not just in developing countries but also in more affluent parts of the world's population. This spurs a renaissance in antibiotics research, but not before millions of lives are lost.

■ Image-guided surgery from remote locations—telesurgery—becomes a common practice mode for procedures such as laparoscopies and chalecystec-tomies. Global centers of excellence develop for those procedures, driving many local specialists out of business.

ENDNOTES

[1] Cannon, P., et al. Comparison of early invasive and conservative strategies with unstable coronary syndromes treated with the glycoprotein IIb/IIIa inhibitor tirofiban. *New England Journal of Medicine* 2001; 344:1879–1887.

[2] Montalescot, G. Platelet glycoprotein IIb/IIIa inhibition with coronary stenting for acute myocardial infarction. *New England Journal of Medicine* 2001; 344:1895–1903.

[3] Ronchi, E. Biotechnology and the new revolution in health care and pharmaceuticals. Special Issue on biotechnology. *Science Technology Industry Review* 1996; 19:19–44.

[4] Jenks, S. J. Gene therapy: Mastering the basics, defining details. *Journal of National Cancer Institute* 1997; 89(16):1182–1184.

[5] Moxon, E. R. Applications of molecular microbiology to vaccinology. *Lancet* 1997; 350:1240–1244.

CHAPTER 9

Information Technologies

Will Health Care Join in the Information Age?

Over the next decade, health care in the United States will at last be dramatically affected by the revolution in communications and information technology that has been in process for the past 20 years. Most information technologies, which have become a familiar part of the business landscape, are outgrowths of the increased power and reduced costs of microprocessors and lasers and the consequent cost reduction in both data processing and computer memory. Indeed, most businesses in the United States are now filled with networked personal computer (PC) technologies (see Figure 9-1) that have migrated into households within the past 10 years (see Figure 9-2).

Although health care industry spending on information technology was estimated to be as much as $21 billion in 2000,[1] health care has lagged behind other industries in adopting technology-enabled processes and has not experienced the dramatic changes in practices seen in finance, retail, distribution, and other industries. No health care company has used technology to change the way of doing business as dramatically as Wal-Mart changed retailing, for instance, or Charles Schwab transformed securities brokering. But it's clear that changes in information technology will continue to be one of, if not *the*, prime catalyst of health care change over the next 10 years. Can we then expect a shift toward the prevalence of automated customer service, electronic information exchange, and real-time data analysis that's commonplace in those other industries? As health care tries to assimilate currently available technologies, new types of, and uses for, information technology are emerging at a rapid and increasing pace. How will health care adapt to incorporating a host of new technologies over the next decade?

There are two key fundamentals. The first is to understand the underlying cutting-edge technologies that will emerge from other industries and that will enjoy mass diffusion by 2010. The second is to understand which aspects of health care will be most affected by these technologies.

BASE TECHNOLOGIES

All of the applications and new processes that will change health care's use of information depend on developments in base technologies. The most important underlying technologies are listed below, with brief explanations of what they do now and what developments are likely.

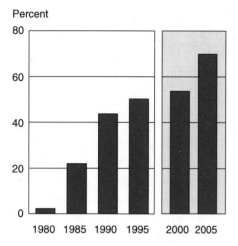

Figure 9-1. More and more PC usage by the workforce
(Percentage of workforce using personal computers)

Percent

Source: IFTF; U.S. Bureau of Labor Statistics.

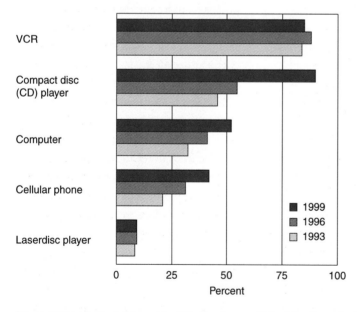

Figure 9-2. Technologies in the home take off.
(Percentage of United States households with . . .)

Source: IFTF; Louis Harris & Associates, Television Bureau of Advertising, Recording Industry
Association of America, International Recording Media Association.

- *Microprocessors.* A microprocessor is the "brain" within computers that executes their functions. Moore's Law suggests that, as has been true for 30 years, microprocessors will continue to double in power every 18 to 24 months. This means that by the end of the decade, PCs will have a processing capacity some 20 times faster than they have today, and powerful processors will be found in virtually every manufactured product, including clothes, furniture, and buildings, as well as cars and consumer electronics. Medical devices and information systems will also benefit from increased processing power.

- *Data storage.* Enabled by the development, in the late 1980s, of cheap lasers—the key to both compact discs and large-capacity optical storage systems—data storage capacity has fallen in price to the point where technology planners believe that it will soon be nearly free. Consequently very large data sets, such as entire film outputs from years of MRI use, can be captured and stored. Those files are then accessible for searching, processing, and analyzing.

- *Wireless technology.* Handheld wireless devices, also known as palm-top devices, allow a clinician access to computerized patient records without requiring him to stay in one place. Their flexibility and functionality can fit seamlessly into a clinician's workflow. Many medical schools are giving new residents handheld devices as both a study aid and part of their clinical toolbox, and analysts predict that 20 percent of physicians will be using handheld devices by 2004.

■ *Networking bandwidth and data compression.* Networks that permit information transfer among computers have exploded in prevalence, speed, and utility. With higher-bandwidth networks and with new techniques in compressing data so that more information can be saved in the same amount of computer storage, larger amounts of data will be transferred at higher speeds among more users. Health care providers, especially radiologists and others working together on large-image files, will benefit from this trend.

■ *Information appliances.* The most common information appliance is the computer, but increasingly the components and functions of computers will appear in telephones, televisions, and other devices. The class and number of information appliances will accelerate dramatically.

■ *Intelligent agents.* Software programs that find and retrieve information over a network that is likely to be helpful to an end user, even though the user doesn't know where that information is coming from, will grow in popularity. Current intelligent agents are somewhat crude, but over the next few years their filtering and retrieval ability will increase dramatically.

■ *Security and encryption.* The transmission of medical and financial information will depend on the full distribution of encryption technologies that permit secure transmission of data. The underlying technology for encryption is developing fast, but the procedures ensuring that all trans-

missions are secure will be difficult to implement.

■ *Internet and the World Wide Web.* Although the Internet as we know it will scarcely be recognizable in a decade's time, its current incarnation provides a common format for viewing, exchanging, and transacting information of all kinds that is transferable among different computer systems. In particular, the volume of transactions conducted over the Internet—as opposed to the simple one-way sharing of information—will increase dramatically.

■ *3-D computing.* Data visualization is the use of computing to represent huge volumes of data in three dimensions on one computer screen. The ability to move, shape, and analyze data in ways that support decision making will enable managers to view activities, classes of transactions, and entire organizations in whole and in detail at the same time.

■ *Databases.* A new class of both relational and object-oriented databases will increase the capacity to store, present, sort, and analyze data over the next decade. Even though these new database systems will be incompatible with older "legacy" databases, a considerable amount of older information will be extracted from those databases by using techniques called "data warehousing" and "data mining."

■ *Sensors.* The real world can connect with computers by using devices such as digital video cameras or blood pressure monitors. A key change of the

Chapter 9: Information Technologies 137

next decade will be the fall in the cost of sensors, making sensors an integral part of many computing devices and information appliances. Their great diffusion will allow the monitoring of events that previously went unreported or were very costly to track.

Given the progress made so far and the massive international commercial investment in information technology research and development, we can expect continued rapid advances in and diffusion of these basic technologies over the next decade. For health care, which has been behind the curve, both the application of currently available information technologies and the development of new technologies will combine to cause dramatic change.

THE ISSUES: THE DIRECTION IS CLEAR, THE PACE UNCERTAIN

While it's possible to imagine some incredible impacts of information technology on health care, the implementation of new information systems is a task barely begun. There are all kinds of organizational, financial, and educational barriers preventing adoption of different technologies and all kinds of difficulties with their use when they are adopted. Several major information system ventures in health care have failed, particularly clinical information systems. The planned exchange of information over dedicated local networks (like the Community Health Information Networks of the early 1990s) also went nowhere despite much effort. The next decade will see much greater change than in the last. But we need to be clear about what we're projecting.

Information systems in health care are used for administrative, clinical, and financial purposes. Most systems have elements of all three activities, but administrative and financial transactions are already much more automated than most clinical ones. For example, about half of all claims are sent electronically, whereas well under 5 percent of physicians use computers to record all clinical information for an average patient. A similar difference exists among hospitals using computer systems to automate their admission and registration functions but paper charts to record nursing activities. The adoption of electronic transactions varies dramatically by sector for the same type of transaction, with physicians' offices typically being the least automated.

Given that information systems will be used to convert health care from paper to electronic recording—but at a different rate depending on the activity and organization—there are some key questions: How fast will different types of technologies diffuse? What kinds of organizations will use what types of technologies and for what purposes? Who will pay for them and who will benefit? While there will be no part of the health care system that doesn't see change caused or enabled by information technology, we believe that four major areas will see the greatest impact.

THE FORECAST: FOUR BIG EFFECTS IN HEALTH CARE

Although health care will use information technology in a variety of ways, we think the most important effects will be in four main areas:

- process-management systems
- clinical information interfaces
- data analysis
- telehealth and remote monitoring

PROCESS-MANAGEMENT SYSTEMS

Provider and Plan Management Systems Go Electronic

The first major area where information technology will affect health care is in the automation of basic business processes among providers and intermediaries and their customers. These processes include provider network contract administration, communications between different organizations over administrative issues, such as patient eligibility and claims submission, and the business and medical protocols used in customer service centers. These developments occupy the broad category of "electronic commerce."

Electronic commerce is being encouraged by cheaper and more flexible technologies, such as transactions conducted over the Internet and other open and cheaply accessible computer networks. But the major driving force behind the adoption of electronic commerce in health care is the combination of mandated standards for electronic data exchange and the regulatory incentives to use them legislated in the 1996 Kennedy–Kassebaum Act (Health Insurance Portability and Accessibility Act, officially known as HIPAA). While the low-hanging fruit of insurance and administrative simplification standards have seen final rules published, several areas have been controversial and have not yet been finalized. Consensus

has been impossible in the area of privacy, and particularly in regard to the National Individual Identifier for patients. Congress failed to enact legislation governing such standards by August 21, 1999. The original deadline for the Secretary of Health and Human Services to publish the final standards for privacy of individually identifiable health information was February 21, 2000.

Several prominent functions are starting to be performed electronically. These include claims submission, eligibility verification, coordination of insurance benefits between providers, utilization review and precertification, materials management, pharmacy claims, and utilization review and receipt of lab tests. So the technology-enabled processes that manage the everyday interactions of health plans, providers, and patients are changing dramatically—and quickly.

These administrative links between providers and plans will be complemented by better use of computing and telephony links among plans or providers and their members and payers, including employers. Telephone-based customer service centers with human staffs are likely to remain the largest single example of this interaction, but other links will be emblematic of this convergence of technology and process. These include automated enrollment by using interactive voice response (IVR) or the Internet, administrative information and health information delivered by a combination of phone, mail, and computer, and even the development of online insurance markets. These secondary electronic commerce developments will become mainstream after 2005.

Chapter 9: Information Technologies

CLINICAL INFORMATION INTERFACES

The EMR has been an elusive promise of technology for at least a decade.[2] The concept is that all medical information about a patient should be stored electronically to be accessed whenever, wherever, and by whomever needs it, and that data need be input only once. That system would loop information back from the patient to the physician, pharmacist, and case manager, permitting medical management in real time rather than retrospectively. This ideal would require ubiquitous use of information technology. But as Figure 9-3 shows, as late as 2000, few physicians used the Internet in their everyday clinical practice for more than research and reference information.

Nonetheless, many of the components that would support an EMR, such as databases, networks, and computers, are being put into place. Furthermore, the past few years have seen the development of sophisticated software tools that support clinical practice. What has been missing to jumpstart the EMR is an easily usable interface that helps clinicians get information into and out of computer systems as fast as they can write on paper, or that at least gives them a payoff for investing in the system's use.

Over the next decade, ubiquitous information appliances, sophisticated decision support systems, and voice recognition will create interfaces with computing systems that are much more clinician-friendly. Consequently, we're likely to see more input of clinical observations into electronic databases and more information being fed back from these systems to clinicians at the point of care. The clinicians' interface will link to most areas of health information systems but will follow a close codevelopment with aspects of clinical databases and analytical tools. So we will be moving closer, incrementally, to an EMR.

The rate of change toward prevalent use of the EMR will depend on the economics driving the adoption of these systems, which currently can cost up to $50,000 per clinician. While the price of the systems will fall, most of the cost actually resides in the implementation and education that is required. Currently the initial training alone is estimated to be at least 48 hours per physician.[3] Of course there are advantages to using EMRs that are also measurable in cost terms, including faster access to data, lower rates of

Figure 9-3. Eighty-five percent of physicians use at least one

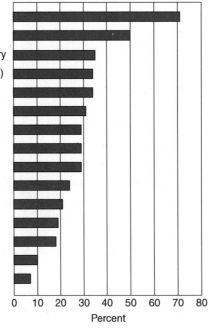

General medical research and news
Access guidelines or protocols
Submitting claims and claims status inquiry
Diagnostic reporting (order or lookup data)
Access pharmaceutical information
Information technology support
Communicate with patients (by email)
Eligibility authorizations
Purchase medical products
Referral authorization
Receive payments, earned remittance
Electronic medical records
Data analysis
Document patient encounters
Order and verify prescriptions

Percent

Source: Health Technology Center, Internet Use by Medical Groups, 2001.

Chapter 9: Information Technologies

retesting as is required when original results can't be found, and often more accurate care as in the case of fewer adverse drug reactions.[4]

Both the increased importance of non-physician clinicians and the fact that younger physicians have greater experience with computers will drive this increased use of clinical information technology. Many health care organizations are also developing into an economic size and type that gives them the financial and management resources to automate clinical activities. Many organizations have announced plans to implement clinical information systems for clinician use. Their reasons stem partly from pressure from intermediaries and end payers for better reporting and partly from a belief that improving the clinical process will give them a competitive advantage in the future. The economic value of automating the clinical process will drive its adoption particularly in payment environments that reward lower costs, such as capitation.

In order to encourage physicians to use this technology, more effort will focus on finding ways to educate and encourage physicians to change their behavior. The pursuit of that goal will lead to greater study of the clinical decision-making process as a whole and the best way to use information technology to influence decisions at the time they are made.

However, the dissemination of clinical information systems into the daily practice of clinicians will be a slow process. Clinicians will start to use computers more as part of their regular work, including accessing and recording

patient information, usually in a hybrid paper/computer approach. But the ideal of the EMR will not come about easily. A number of other information systems challenges, such as a lack of capital and continued resistance from clinicians, will mean that only a small percentage of physicians and clinicians will be conducting their practice using fully computerized medical records until later in the decade.

Within the move toward information systems that clinicians can integrate into their daily work, two models are developing for the future EMR. One will focus on giving clinicians access to clinical information, such as lab results, transcripts, and demographic data, that is currently already available over information networks. These systems will accept physicians' input in any way they can, including voice, handwriting scans, and free text. These systems will concentrate on presenting as much relevant data to the clinician as possible and getting this implementation widespread quickly.

The other approach will also try to provide these data but will go the extra mile to have physicians input their notes in a structured format, either using check boxes or menus or allowing them to type. The system will then use natural language processing technology to codify and assign values to their words. The idea is to capture and analyze physicians' clinical assessments of patients, as that's where the most valuable information resides. The codifying of that clinical assessment will permit better analysis for outcomes studies, provider profiling, and eventually for assessing the value of interventions in close to real time—

potentially changing the model of how information about clinical practice is disseminated. This model demands far more involvement from clinicians and more resources from their organizations and will probably diffuse more slowly. After 2010, these EMRs may include expert systems that support clinicians' decision making and incorporate many of the analytical tools now being developed on the database side discussed below.

DATA ANALYSIS

The analysis of health care data is a growth industry. In the next few years, more data will be collected from diverse input sources, including clinicians, patients, other clinical data sources, and administrative and claims data systems. We are already seeing improvements in the use of databases and data warehouses to store and link disparate data streams; likewise, the ability of analysts to visualize and deconstruct complex data sets is improving. Both data mining and database design will improve dramatically in the coming decade, but the most important aspect of this technology will be sophisticated data manipulation. Two related trends in data manipulation are likely to emerge from this core technology, both involving attempts to better understand the impact of clinical interventions and in particular how clinical interventions affect outcomes.

In the shorter term, a great deal of effort will be aimed at pulling clinical information from what are largely administrative data sets. A new group of sophisticated "data jockeys" will give

plans and providers the tools to learn much more about patients' clinical outcomes from particular interventions. This trend will lead to:

- Better decision-making support for internal and competitive analysis, which will be aided by improved computing that permits 3-D visualization of complex data sets.

- Better understanding of patients' likelihood of future illness.

- The ability to adjust payments to plans depending on the relative risk of illness of an enrolled population. This "risk adjustment" will be based in part on a much wider use of patients' self-assessment to understand their own health status.

Medicare has started to use risk-adjustment algorithms to change the amount it reimburses health plans, considerably increasing the importance of data analysis. Clinicians attempting to understand the costs of care for their patients with different acuity levels won't merely be seeing theoretical savings down the road but instead will have to manage the care they deliver in order to receive those savings. Data mining is already being used by retail companies, computer marketers, and professional basketball teams—we expect dramatic growth in this type of analysis in medical care over the next few years.

In the longer term, more codified and analyzable clinical data will be available directly recorded from the clinician–patient interface. The data will probably include patients' genetic information and not only will provide greater understanding about patients' experiences and outcomes but also will better monitor the performance of both clinicians and patients. The emergence of online analytical processing will permit close to real-time analysis of the key information, such as the result of a particular intervention. This is in contrast to the retrospective analysis that's done today, and will be an addition to, and an improvement on, the analysis based on data mining of administrative data sets described in the previous paragraph. However, analytical processing of clinical data will not be more than a fringe activity until a majority of clinicians are using EMRs. That will take several years and won't be prevalent until well after 2005.

Some of this data analysis will be made publicly available through regulatory agencies and bodies like the NCQA, which accredits health plans. Consequently, the ability of more organizations and individuals to access information about the type and quality of care provided will increase later in the decade.

TELEHEALTH AND REMOTE MONITORING

Combining Case Management, Patient Information Systems, and Remote Monitoring

In the long term, the impact of all these technologies will be greatest on patient care. There are three main trends that will converge in their use of interconnecting technologies to provide remote care. The trends are case management, patient information systems, and remote telemetry.

Case Management Gets Automated

Plans and providers will use automated techniques to case manage patients. Most use of case management will concentrate on the process of disease state or chronic care management. Disease management organizations, whether providers or intermediaries, will use protocols, clinical information, software, and infrastructure that have been developed to support that process. The protocols will make use of mathematical models that assess appropriate treatment for specific conditions and data collected on individual patients. The data will be manipulated both to improve the treatment options of the individual patients and to add to larger databases. Case managers will use medical records and protocols to track and assess treatment patterns, and the growth of call centers will help deliver that information to patients.

Empowered Patients Get Informed

Some of the same technologies that providers will use for medical management will also have an impact on patients independently. Patients will use them for a variety of health information activities that will include shared decision making, psychosocial support groups, disease-specific information research, physician and provider assessment, information about alternative medicine, and patient self-care support tools, such as software that tracks diet and treatment regimens. Empowerment of patients via information gathering will center on use of the Internet and other online services, IVR, CD-ROMs, video, and television, including video-on-demand over cable and satellite networks.

Most of the activity already happening in this area has been inspired by patients and is somewhat anarchic in nature. That won't change any time soon, but there will be significant entry of plans, providers, and other actors into this arena who will try to impose a more structured use of information sources so that they can guide and track the treatment of their patients.

One problem we foresee is that the chronically ill and elderly tend not to have the necessary technology in their homes. In general, while half of American households had Internet access in 2000, that access is much more likely to be in households with higher income and better education (see Figure 9-4). By the year 2003, 63 percent of American households will have appliances with processing power equivalent to a PC, increasing to 65 to 70 percent by 2006 (see Figure 9-5). There is, however, a significant possibility that America's information have-nots will not get access to the services associated with these technologies. Surveys of Internet use taken in 2000 show that only about 11 percent of Internet users were age 65 years or older.[5]

Access to information technology will be an area of public policy contention in the next few years, and possibly of some marker activity as manufacturers get the capacity to introduce Internet-like services in lower-cost devices, such as network computers, game machines, and TVs, and as these become affordable for everyone. If these appliances can be used for accessing online information, there's no reason to believe that they won't be nearly as common as color TV, with more than 95 percent of households having the processing and communications power of a current top-end PC by the end of the decade.

Sensors Boost Remote Telemetry

The final piece of the puzzle needed for remote care to really take off is the monitoring function that connects the case managers to the patients. While education and self-care are necessary components that will be facilitated by information technology, clinical assessment of patients has to this point required that they either be at a medical facility or be attended to in their own homes by expensive labor, But a new type of technology is becoming available that will set off a revolution in remote care because it will provide the capacity for remote telemetry. The technology is the sensor, which converts analog, or real-life, signals into digital format, which computer systems can understand and therefore report on and react to.

The sensors that are being created for automobiles, video cameras, and all manner of other electronics will become cheap enough to drive their adoption in medical devices. Examples of how sensors may be used in remote telemetry include monitoring vital signs with wireless heart monitors; integrating digital signal creation by wireless or intermittently wired monitors, such as respiratory meters, blood pressure cuffs, or blood glucose monitors, with patient, plan, or provider information systems; and providing alerts from pharmaceutical dispensers that a needed pill hasn't been taken. At the back end of all these devices will be a link into the software for disease management or provider

Figure 9-4. Internet access is mostly for the wealthy and educated. (Percentage of U.S. households with access, by education and income,

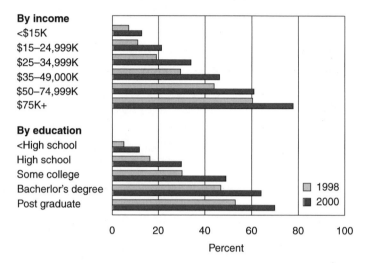

Source: IFTF; National Telecommunications and Information Administration.

Figure 9-5. Internet and computer penetration of the household will continue to increase. (Percentage of U.S. households with PCs and Internet connections)

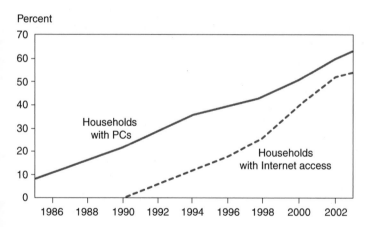

Source: NTIA and ESA, U.S. Department of Commerce, using U.S. Bureau of the Census Current Population Survey supplements; Forrester Research, 1999.

information organizations that will analyze, report, and react to abnormal results or the absence of them. This, in turn, should ensure appropriate follow-up, for instance a visit from a nurse, in more cases and better use of resources.

Inventing new ways of getting these technologies and the networks that support them into homes and smaller medical facilities will be an area of focus over the next 10 years, and these new approaches will draw on the experience of other industries, notably entertainment. In addition to monitoring the chronically ill, who tend to be high-end resource users, similar technologies will be used for patients' self-monitoring, including results reporting using a phone or computer—typically for those with less severe chronic conditions. For instance, lab testing will become increasingly decentralized. Advances in self-diagnosis with small, portable testing devices and immune assays will also be increasingly important. An example might be the "smart toilet," a very simple-to-use device that tests for problems in the digestive system. Results from these devices will be captured in computer systems and monitored in a similar way to the more active telemetry.

PROGRESSION OF INFORMATION TECHNOLOGY INTO HEALTH CARE

The four areas we've defined—process-management systems, clinical information interfaces, data analysis, and remote monitoring—are not the only aspects of information technology that will have an impact on health care,[6] although they are dominant themes that will encapsulate a great deal of the change that information technology will bring to health care. But it will not be an equal progression. The advent of electronic commerce will transform administrative processes in the next few years, and the new ways of administration will be ubiquitous by 2007. While great strides will have been made in other areas, the use of information systems by clinicians as an integral part of their work—the key vision of the EMR—will only develop in the latter part of the decade and will not be complete by 2010. However, the use of information systems will change the roles of the patient and the case manager intermediary in the next 10 years. Patients will become more informed and involved in their own care plans, and intermediaries responsible for medical management will use information technology extensively to assess cases in real time. Physicians will adapt their practice to adjust to this, but at a slow pace.

The adoption of technology will depend on the ability of health care organizations to set aside capital for investment and therefore depends on the ability of those organizations to become more like other types of corporations. While health care is moving in this direction (e.g., growth of physician groups), it will remain a fragmented industry that, as it consolidates, will struggle with the adoption and deployment of information technology. The use of that technology as an enabling driver to change health care will not really be felt until those consoli-

dated organizations are more stable, after 2005. By that time, the cost of the more complex clinical information systems will have fallen to the point that its widespread adoption need not be put off for economic reasons. After that, the vision of an information-intensive industry using information technology for consumer-friendly, high-quality, and low-cost patient care can become a real possibility.

Wild Cards

- With a new generation of software and hardware, diffusion of clinical information technology happens fully in the next 3 to 5 years. The EMR becomes commonplace, patients' records are standardized, and the clinical care process dramatically improves.

- Early large-scale implementation of information systems to support and case manage the chronically ill show no cost-benefit advantages compared to traditional lower-end technology care. Given the cost of system installation, the development of home monitoring and case management remains in its current embryonic state.

ENDNOTES

[1] Sheldon Dorenfest & Co.

[2] In its 1991 report, *The Computer-Based Patient Record,* the Institute of Medicine listed areas of technology that, when integrated, would make up a computer-based patient record (CPR). The technologies included databases and database management systems, workstations, data acquisition and retrieval, image processing and storage, data exchange and vocabulary standards, and system communications and network infrastructure.

[3] See Krall, M. A. Acceptance and performance by clinicians using an ambulatory electronic medical record in an HMO. *Proceedings of Annual Symposium of Computer Applications in Medical Care* 1995; 708–711 for a generally positive description of the implementation of the Epic EMR at Kaiser Northwest.

[4] See Bares, D. W., et al. Incidence of adverse drug events and potential adverse drug events: implications for prevention. *Journal of the American Medical Association* (July 5) 1995; 274(1):29–34. This describes the problems with drug interactions and other mistakes that Brigham and Womens Hospital more or less eliminated by switching to a computerized ordering system. See also Anderson, J. G., et al. Evaluating the potential effectiveness of using computerized information systems to prevent adverse drug events. *Proceedings of AMIA Annual Fall Symposium* 1997; 9:228–232.

[5] *Falling Through the Net: Defining the Digital Divide.* Washington, DC: National Telecommunications and Information Administration, July 1999. *Extreme Peaks Begin to Moderate as Adult On-line Usage Approaches 50%.* Interep Press Release, December 2000.

[6] For instance, telemedicine today is a fringe activity in which physician consults occur over dedicated videoconferencing facilities. This will stay a fringe activity, but some telemedicine will transmute into the use of groupware (computer communications) to share information between care teams and the use of online environments for collaboration between clinicians. In another example, the production of digital signals from imaging equipment will dramatically increase radiologists' ability to use computers to analyze and abstract information from X rays, MR images, and other imaging devices.

CHAPTER 10

Health Care Consumers

The Haves and the Have-Nots

We define "health care consumer" as anyone who receives or has the potential to receive health care services, regardless of whether or not that person pays for those services directly. Although employers and government, not health care consumers, are the most frequent purchasers of health insurance and thus pay for a great deal of the care provided, we discuss them in this chapter only in the context of their effects on individual consumers.

Consumers are more actively engaged in their own health care than in the past. Up until the mid-1980s, health care consumers in the United States generally had been passive recipients of care. Most patients submitted to whatever procedures a physician recommended, and most were happy to let the system take responsibility for decisions about their care. By and large, mainstream Americans revered doctors and trusted them—a culture sustained by the large information gap between highly educated doctors and the average patient. It was a gap further reinforced by doctors' political and economic power. Private physicians had a low awareness of the gap between their "customer service" and that of other services the public interact with, such as eye care or retailing.

Patients' impact on the organization of care was also slight because employers and government, not patients, were—as they still are—the purchasers of health care for a majority of working adults. Employers typically offered little choice among health insurance plans to their employees, making it difficult for patients to vote with their feet if they were dissatisfied with their coverage. Yet because traditional indemnity plans allowed free choice of provider, and because employers and government generally provided health care coverage as a defined benefit with low out-of-pocket costs, consumers' lack of plan choice did not seem to affect their care or their pocketbooks much, keeping dissatisfaction low among insured consumers. The uninsured have made do with limited coverage from safety-net funding streams and providers—a mix of public institutions and private charity—and have not had many advocates to speak for them. Although insured consumers and their advocates have had some impact on insurance legislation over the years, they have had little impact on the delivery of care. Their legislative voice has been muted in part because they haven't had many big issues to complain about.

As a consequence of these three factors— a culture of respect for physicians and their power sustained by an information gap, employer- and government-mediated purchasing, and defined benefits with free choice of providers—consumers have had relatively little effect on the organization of American health care. Until recently, providers (mostly hospitals and physicians in solo practice or small-group practice), health care plans, and purchasers (mostly employers and government) controlled how and where care was provided, who got it, and how much it cost the individual out-of-pocket in premiums, deductibles, and most recently, copayments. Individual consumers adapted to the system.

That picture is changing. As a new, more educated and informed generation of baby boomer consumers moves through the system and reaches the age where they use more health care services, a new culture of assertive skepticism is replac-

ing the old culture of passivity and respect. A rapidly growing group of consumers is trusting plans and providers less, demanding more information and choice from providers and plans, engaging in more self-care and self-management of disease, and showing more interest in sharing their health care decisions with providers. A study published in *Health Affairs* in 2000 showed that 55 percent of families had choices in their health coverage, and an improved likelihood of satisfaction because of these choices. Choice, self-care, and shared decision making are the key elements of consumer empowerment covered by our forecast.

Efforts by some payors to produce new "digital health plans" create an opportunity to provide health care and services without the inefficiencies of the old processes during the next decade. The resolution of the political struggle over the patient's rights to sue an HMO will potentially have a large impact on the economics of managed care during the next decade.

As baby boomers reach an age where they require doctor visits more frequently, employers are beginning to pass more health care costs on to employees, often by replacing defined benefits programs with defined contribution programs—thus potentially weakening employer mediation of consumption. The managed care revolution, triggered by escalating national health care costs has limited consumers' choice of providers and forced them to negotiate a thicket of primary care gatekeepers, access charges for specialists, and triage

The Three Modes of Empowerment

Informed Choice of Plans and Providers: The combination of employers' shifting to defined contribution programs and the increasing openness of provider networks available through plans will lead to a greater range of choices of providers and plans. Consumers will demand more sophisticated and comparative information about plans and providers to help them make these choices.

Self-Care and Self-Management: Increasing consumer access to medical information formerly known only to providers, combined with improved remote sensing technologies, will facilitate greater involvement of patients in their own health care, including preventive care (e.g., improving diet and lifestyle), treating acute episodes at home, and helping manage the course of their chronic diseases.

Shared Medical Decision Making: Improved medical record systems and increasingly sophisticated decision-support tools will facilitate patients' ability to understand complex medical decision-making processes and become more active in choosing treatments that match their preferences and values.

The Aging Baby Boomers

Baby boomers make up the generation born between 1945 and 1964. The first baby boomers will turn 65 in 2010. The percentage of the population that is over age 65 has been steadily increasing in this century, but the baby boomers will drive that percentage sharply higher (see Figure 10-1). Over the next 10 years, the baby boom cohort will begin to experience more chronic and severe illnesses. Those who are "new consumers" will be a particularly strong voice for change.

Figure 10-1. Population age 65 and older, 2000 to 2050

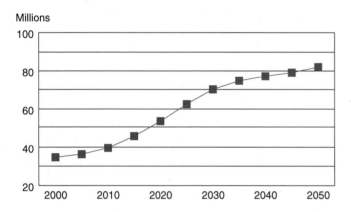

Source: U.S. Census Bureau, Statistical Abstract, 2000.

nurses on telephones in order to get the care they need. Combined with rising out-of-pocket costs, these limits have given the new, more informed and vocal consumers something to complain about. Change in the consumers' role is definitely in the wind.

Will the historically supply-driven health care market soon be forced to grapple with consumer demands? Will such changes be large and noticeable by 2010, or only incremental? To answer these questions, we need to know which consumers are likely to drive change the most, what changes they are likely to push most quickly, what forces will resist

them, and what impact the changes are likely to have on providers, purchasers, and plans. Will the overall impact on the system within the coming decade be striking, or a yawn?

To get at the answer, we first identify the three tiers of coverage into which consumers currently fall and the key issues facing each tier. We then forecast the changes most likely to occur in each tier and their implications for the system. We also take a look at some wild cards and identify a few emerging consumer needs that health care services may be able to fill in the future.

THREE TIERS OF HEALTH CARE CONSUMERS

Although legislators frequently hold up the ideal of a one-tier health care system, plans requiring major redistribution of resources have not been well received in Congress or by the public. The complexity of our existing system has created so many stakeholders that building consensus for a new one-tier single payer system has become a monumental task. In reality, three tiers exist.

The bottom tier is the rapidly growing group of Americans who lack access to the main system and are served largely by an increasingly tattered safety net because they are either uninsured or on Medicaid; currently, the number of uninsured is about 42 million when measured at a single point in time and about one-quarter of those are children.

The middle tier consists of those working Americans whose benefits are

Chapter 10: Health Care Consumers

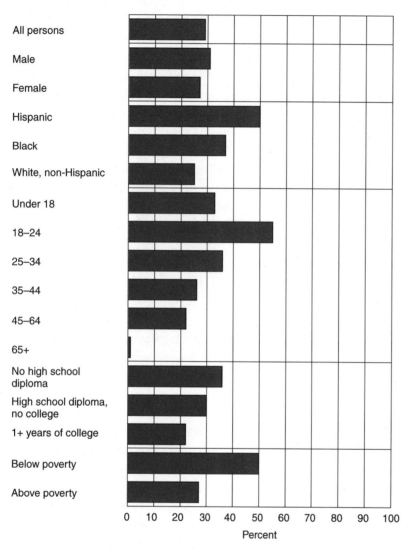

Figure 10-2. Benefits insecurity
(Percentage of group without health insurance for at least 1 month out of
36 months, 1993 to 1996)

All persons
Male
Female
Hispanic
Black
White, non-Hispanic
Under 18
18–24
25–34
35–44
45–64
65+
No high school
diploma
High school diploma,
no college
1+ years of college
Below poverty
Above poverty

0 10 20 30 40 50 60 70 80 90 100
Percent

Source: U.S. Census Bureau.

The top tier is made up of the very wealthy and the more securely employed, who have fewer restrictions on their care. The current system thus consists of a disenfranchised bottom tier (the excluded consumer), an insecurely enfranchised middle tier (the worried consumer), and a securely enfranchised top tier (the empowered consumer).

An alternative way to define the three tiers would be by the continuity of their insurance—to look at who is continuously insured, insured on and off, and continuously uninsured during a given period. If we examine the years between 1993 and 1996, we find that about 71 percent of Americans were continuously insured, 25 percent lacked coverage between 1 and 35 months, and 4 percent were continuously uninsured (see Figure 10-2). These three groups were further divided along ethnic lines: 50 percent of Hispanics lacked coverage for a month or more as compared to 37 percent of African Americans and 25 percent of whites.

The problem with using continuity of coverage as a means of defining the tiers is that many who are continuously insured are nonetheless worried about either the stability or the flexibility of their benefits. Furthermore, some of the insured have only very limited coverage, including those on Medicaid.

For those reasons, we have chosen to define the three tiers by the degree to which their benefits are adequate and perceived to be secure. Although we recognize that a fair amount of movement goes on between tiers, the three tiers themselves persist.

insecure because of threats to their jobs due to restructuring or ailing industries, low reemployability, employer benefits cuts, restrictions on providers and treatments, or potential inability to pay the insurance premiums passed on to them by their employers.

The New Consumers: Who Are They?

We define new consumers as people who have at least two of the following three characteristics:

1. Discretionary household income of $53,000 or more (in constant 1998 dollars)
2. At least 1 year of college education
3. Experience with information technology (e.g., owns a PC)

Figure 10-3. Description of new consumer attributes in 2005

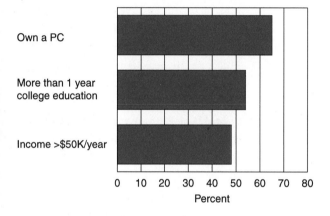

Source: IFTF; U.S. Department of Labor.

The consumers most likely to become empowered in the coming decade are the "new consumers" (see Figure 10-3). In contrast to traditional consumers, new consumers have at least two of the following three attributes: at least 1 year of college education, more than $50,000 in household income, and experience with information technology (e.g., computers). Because education, income, and experience with information technology are closely linked, most of the disenfranchised bottom tier consists of traditional consumers. Significant segments of the middle and upper tiers, however, are new consumers, including a large proportion of the baby boom generation.

In other sectors of the economy, such as retail and banking, the new consumers have already initiated a revolution in the way goods are purchased and customers are served. These consumers are also narrowing the patient–provider information gap. They are no longer in awe of physicians, and they will be the first to demand change from health care plans and providers as they interact with the system between now and 2010. In discussing the key issues facing each tier, we highlight the points at which the new consumers may have the most impact.

THE BOTTOM TIER: THE DISENFRANCHISED AND NEVER-ENFRANCHISED

The main issue for the disenfranchised, of course, is access to health care.[1] This tier consists of people under 65 who are uninsured, including a significant number of children, or who have very limited insurance—mostly through Medicaid, and a very small number on both Medicare and Medicaid. In 2000, 5 percent of the population in the United States comprised adults covered by Medicaid, 12 percent were uninsured adults, 5 percent were children on Medicaid, and 4 percent were uninsured children, for a total of 26 percent of the population in the bottom tier.

Access to care for this tier is severely limited because the safety net has become frayed. People in this tier depend utterly on the limited resources and strained generosity of safety-net funding streams and providers. Even those on Medicaid have limited choices. A significant proportion of people on Medicaid are mothers and children

Children: Patients and Beneficiaries, but Not Active Consumers

In 1998, children under age 18 made up roughly 27 percent of the United States population. Roughly one-third of this group, representing 9 percent of the total population, lacked coverage for at least 1 month in a 36-month period between 1993 and 1996.

Although we include children in our estimates of the percentage of the population falling into each tier—and the problem of uninsured children is a serious one—we do not discuss them further in this section because they are generally not active purchasers of or participants in their health care and will therefore exert little influence over it. See Chapter 13 for a discussion of children's health.

receiving AFDC. Their benefits depend on state budgets, where they compete for resources with prisons and schools.

Generally poor and lacking a college education, most people in the bottom tier will have serious trouble overcoming the information gap between providers and patients. Even the new consumers in this tier, the not-yet-insured recent college graduates who have not yet found stable jobs, will have trouble—but most quickly move up to the middle and top tiers.

THE MIDDLE TIER: THE INSECURELY ENFRANCHISED

The primary issue for the middle tier is benefits security. When unemployment is high, this tier is insecure about maintaining coverage. When unemployment is low, they are insecure about maintaining the flexibility and quality of coverage. Although at any one time most of this tier is insured, their benefits are not secure for a variety of reasons. Adults in the middle tier include (1) working people with unstable job security, including employees and owners of small or downsizing businesses, contract employees,

and employees of companies undergoing restructuring; and (2) early retirees (age 55 to 64 years) waiting for Medicare to kick in. We estimate that roughly 34 percent of the United States population falls into the middle tier.

The working group is worried because many of their employers are reducing or eliminating health care benefits or passing their costs on to employees, who may be unable to pay. Unstable job security and uncertain reemployability also put middle-tier members at risk for significant time periods without health insurance. The coverage this group does have tends increasingly to be in the form of HMO or PPO coverage, which limits to some extent both covered procedures and choice of providers.

Some early retirees are insecurely enfranchised because employers are increasingly cutting or restricting pension health benefits. Those benefits may include either managed care plans or traditional indemnity insurance. In 2001, 25 percent of employers offered health benefits to workers who retire after less than 5 years of company service compared to 90 percent in 1984.

Closely related to benefits security is the issue of value. As employers cut their premium contributions and reduce the scope of the benefits they offer, costs are increasingly passed on to the consumers in this tier and value—the amount of coverage per dollar spent—becomes more of an issue.

The new consumer segment of this tier—which is growing rapidly—will be the most informed about their choices and the most likely to demand good information to help them make those choices, taking a step in the direction of empowerment. As independent agencies and, increasingly, health plans have begun to generate "report cards" for employers on plans and providers, the information-savvy new consumer segment may take advantage of them. As middle-tier members increasingly gain access to PCs at home and at work, the Internet will be a rapidly growing and easily accessible source of plan and provider information.

In contrast, most of the traditional consumers in this tier have at most a high school education and thus tend to have lower incomes and less exposure to information technology. The patient–provider information gap will be hard for this segment of the tier to overcome, unless there is access to intermediaries from a disease management program.

THE TOP TIER: THE SECURELY ENFRANCHISED

The primary issue for the securely enfranchised tier will be empowerment. Although the changes that this tier drives in the system will be slow and incremental at first, they have the greatest ability to effect change. This tier consists mainly of consumers who are (1) securely employed or highly employable, (2) very wealthy and often self-insured, or (3) elderly and on Medicare, either with or without supplemental private insurance.

Many members of this tier are employed by large companies, many of which offer plans with generous benefits designs, pay the lion's share if not all of premiums,

and offer a choice of several different health insurance plans.

Medicare currently offers a rich benefits package, mostly FFS, although that is changing as Medicare HMOs become increasingly competitive.

Like the middle tier, the top tier consists of a mix of traditional and new consumers, with significant numbers in each category. Most of those over 65 in the top tier are traditional consumers. However, a large proportion of the group is made up of baby boomers who will turn 50 during the next decade. These new consumers will be interacting more and more with the system, and they will become a powerful force for change in the delivery of care.

People in the top tier are generally continuously insured in any given 2-year period. When they *do* lose their jobs, they are quickly reemployed thanks to their high level of education. In recent years, about 61 percent of the total United States population has been continuously insured by a plan other than Medicaid during any given 2-year period. Some are securely insured, some insecurely insured. About 13 percent of the population is covered by Medicare, usually supplemented by private insurance. We estimate that about 38 percent of the population constitute securely enfranchised consumers who thus fall into the top tier of coverage.

SUMMARY OF THE THREE TIERS

About one-third of the United States population currently falls into the middle tier of coverage, with a bit less than one-third occupying the bottom tier and a bit more than one-third the top tier (see Table 10-1). New consumers, who represent the largest potential for driving care delivery change in the next decade, are concentrated in the middle and upper tiers.

FORECAST AND ASSUMPTIONS

THE BOTTOM TIER: THE DISENFRANCHISED

Forecast

Because they largely lack a college education and have less access to information, and because their energy is focused on issues of access to care, this tier is unlikely to drive a consumer revolution or to be greatly affected by one. Although this group has many reasons to protest, it lacks voice and clout. Their advocates may push for legislation, particularly to cover children, but as a bloc these consumers have relatively little power over government or employers—their voter participation rates are lower than average, some are unemployed, their incomes are low, and a sizable group are minorities who face discrimination in many arenas. The (ab)use of emergency rooms by members of the bottom tier for basic primary care is currently a costly problem, although improved access to intermediaries or primary care during the next decade would reduce this cost. If the problem of access is to be solved for this tier, the solution will likely be driven by advocacy groups and members of the other two tiers. A factor that might motivate some action from the top two tiers would be the spread of drug-resistant

infectious diseases, exacerbated by lack of proper care, from the lower tier into the other two tiers.

Assumptions

- Lack of access to information and resources is a significant barrier to empowerment.

- Advocates for the bottom tier will be largely ineffective in changing legislation and the structure of care.

- Struggling for access prevents people from putting energy into other aspects of empowerment.

- The plight of the disenfranchised will not become so visibly horrible that it triggers the level of mass dissatisfaction with the health care system that would lead to comprehensive reform.

THE MIDDLE TIER: THE INSECURELY ENFRANCHISED

Forecast

The portion of new consumers in the middle tier and advocacy organizations representing them make up the first segment that will want the system to provide high-quality consumer-oriented information about performance. These middle-tier new consumers are a rapidly growing group—demographic factors are driving a steady transfer of people, about 2 percent a year, from the lower middle class into the new consumer group, and many of these are in the insecurely enfranchised middle tier.

Because benefits insecurity and worries about coverage and out-of-pocket costs are currently this group's major issues—especially during recessions—the first report cards have focused on the relative

Table 10-1. The tiers of coverage

	Traditional Consumers	New Consumers
The Securely Enfranchised (Roughly 38% of total U.S. population)	■ age 18 to 64, no college education, high-income workers (and spouses) with no PCs but high job security, with private managed care plans or fee-for-service insurance (paid by employers or self) ■ age 65+, no college education, moderate to high savings/resources, no PCs, Medicare only or Medicare and private insurance ■ children securely insured	■ age 18 to 64, college-educated, high-income workers (and spouses) with high job security, with private managed care plans or fee-for-service insurance (paid by employers or by self) ■ age 55 to 64, early retirees, college-educated, high savings/resources, private managed care plans or fee-for-service insurance (paid by generous former employers or by self) ■ age 65+, college-educated, moderate to high savings/resources, with PCs, Medicare + private insurance ■ children securely insured
The Insecurely Enfranchised (Roughly 34% of total U.S. population)	■ age 18 to 64, no college education, low- to moderate-income workers (and spouses) with low job security, in managed care plans (paid by employers or military) ■ age 55 to 64, early retirees, no college education, low to moderate incomes, in managed care plans (paid by former employers who are not reassuring about keeping retiree benefits, or have already tried to reduce them) ■ children securely insured	■ age 18 to 64, college-educated, middle-income workers (and spouses) with PCs and low job security, in managed care plans (paid by employers, by military, or by self) ■ age 55 to 64, early retirees, college-educated, high incomes, in managed care plans (paid by former employers who are not reassuring about keeping retiree benefits, or have already tried to reduce them) ■ age 18 to 54, no college education, high-income but low-job-security workers (and spouses), with PCs, in managed care plans (paid by employers) ■ children securely insured
The Disenfranchised (Roughly 28% of total U.S. population)	■ age 18 to 64, no college education, unemployed and/or very poor, uninsured or on Medicaid ■ children uninsured ■ children on Medicaid or other government assistance	■ age 18 to 34, temporarily uninsured, some college, with PCs, no full-time job yet or between early low-income jobs

Source: IFTF.

merits of health plans. Because many people in this tier work for small employers, however, many do not have a choice of plan. Thus employers initially will be the biggest market for this type of report card.

Report cards on plans are already stimulating demand for similar report cards on providers, to help both employers and their employees in this tier choose providers that offer the best value.

Because provider report cards are consistent with the cost-efficiency goals of plans, plans will continue to pursue their development both for hospitals and medical groups and eventually perhaps for individual physicians. Providers will object to such report cards, but they will be given little choice in the matter. Trusted intermediaries for processing such information will become more numerous during the next decade.

The older people in this tier, particularly the early retirees, are half new and half traditional consumers. Although the traditional consumers may complain more than they did in the past as American culture shifts from passivity to active skepticism, they will not have enough access to information to narrow the patient—provider information gap much, and thus will not be in the best position to demand change in the organization of their care. They will, however, be very experienced with the system and motivated to improve their care. They also vote. Increasing their access to information would help them have a greater impact.

Health consumers who have not yet retired may be able to put some pressure on their employers to keep their pension health benefits intact, but their numbers are too small for their complaints to stimulate major change. Employers are more concerned with pleasing young, educated employees. Older consumers will be heard primarily through their high voting rates and through advocacy groups like the American Association of Retired Persons (AARP). Although advocacy groups may change public policy, they may have less effect on provider behavior.

When the voices of the elderly traditional consumers in the middle tier are combined with those of the aging new consumers in the top two tiers, the elderly may be a major force for changes in the organization of care at both the provider and plan levels. As they get sicker, they will push for greater security of benefits and for greater flexibility, service, and coverage in managed care plans and from providers.

Assumptions
- Increased choice leads to increased need for information.
- Empowerment and access to information will be tightly linked.

THE TOP TIER: THE SECURELY ENFRANCHISED

Forecast

The aging upper-tier new consumers, though relatively small in numbers, now are growing rapidly as most of the baby boom generation turns 50 over the next decade. The growth of wealth occurring in society is still greatest in the older population, giving them access to information and health care. As these informed consumers begin to encounter the more chronic and severe illnesses that accompany advancing age, they will interact more frequently with providers and plans in demanding change. Indeed, they have already begun to drive a shift in the culture away from passive respect of providers and toward more active engagement in their care.

This segment will use all three major modes of empowerment: (1) choice of plans and providers; (2) ability to provide self-care and self-management of their chronic diseases; and (3) ability and desire to share medical decisions with their providers. By 2010, as the first of the baby boom cohort reaches 65, this group will have paved the way for a revolution in the organization of care—a revolution simultaneously being fomented in other sectors of the system, as noted in the other chapters of this report.

Because the new consumers in the top tier are information rich, and as health-related information sources like the Internet are growing rapidly, they are increasingly marshaling enough information to narrow the patient–provider information gap. They are not as preoccupied with benefits security as the new consumers in the middle tier are, so empowerment becomes their most pressing issue.

The youngest new consumers in this tier are not very sick and so many of them do not interact with providers with the frequency required to demand big changes. Some do, however, particularly women of childbearing age, who interact with providers both for OB/GYN care and on behalf of their children. Young men and

women will focus their demands on better customer service from plans and greater access to more open networks of providers.

Although continued employer mediation of health plan choices will limit new consumers' direct impact on plans to some extent, today's employers do tend to listen to the needs of their young employees. New consumers will encounter health plan customer service issues simply in the process of signing up for plans and choosing or switching primary care providers. They will encounter provider interaction issues when undergoing routine exams. They will affect plans by complaining to their employers and pressuring employers to complain to the plans or switch to more customer-friendly plans. Those new consumers who have a choice will simply switch. Because they are not sick enough to see very many providers very often, their effect on changing provider interactions and increasing shared decision making will be relatively small before 2010. Beyond 2010, these young new consumers will join the older group in driving a change toward patient-centered care.

In contrast to the young new consumers in this tier, the elderly are the sickest segment of the population, and they do interact frequently with providers. Most will purchase their care directly from providers and can take their Medicare money elsewhere if they don't like a particular provider. This gives them power in the health care market. Because the elderly are also a large voting bloc and have powerful lobbying organizations like the AARP, they are a potent force for both legislative and market change. Although we estimate that two-thirds of the elderly in the upper tier are traditional consumers whose impact on provider behavior will be greatly muted by their inability to bridge the information gap, even they will be influential in supporting legislation that protects their rights to privacy and dignity, especially in end-of-life medical decisions.

Both traditional and new elderly consumers in this tier will also be outlets for the voices of their adult children, many of whom are baby boomer new consumers. This baby boomer "sandwich generation"— especially the women— interacts with the health care system through both its children and its parents. These more assertive and informed baby boomers will attempt to intervene with providers as advocates for their parents, adding to the latter's impact. If large numbers of the traditional elderly consumers begin to switch providers or plans based on their children's advice, they will act as amplifiers of the voice of the new consumer. This amplified impact would be mostly in the direction of more patient-centered care and better service but to some degree, as some of the elderly have children in the middle tier, it might also push plans to address middle-tier issues by offering more coverage and better value.

Assumptions

- Health care legislation empowering patients will not be the primary force behind change in provider behavior and plans, although it may begin to have a larger effect as the baby boom generation ages and its voter participation increases.

- Most providers will not be motivated to bridge the patient–provider information gap, as that would reduce their power and status.

- Information technologies that would aid shared decision making (e.g., the EMR or smart databases) will be fairly slow to develop, limiting the development of the shared decision-making form of empowerment.

THREE LEVELS OF EMPOWERMENT WILL ARRIVE AT DIFFERENT TIMES

Of the three elements of consumer empowerment in health care, informed choice of providers and plans will develop first as middle- and upper-tier new consumers join forces with plans to create report cards. We estimate that roughly 10 percent to 15 percent of all people today have access to any information on plan quality. In some areas, such information is published in newspapers or on the Internet, but in most it is not yet available. We forecast that, by 2010, 50 percent of all consumers will have access to understandable comparative information on plan quality. Because networks will become increasingly more open, however, such information will become less and less useful over time. Provider report cards will be increasingly called for and are already being developed by some plans.

The other two elements of empowerment—self-care and shared decision making—depend more on the cooperation of providers, who right now are busy organizing themselves to resist the strictures being imposed on them by managed care. Of these two elements, self-care and self-management will be the next to emerge, in part because they will be assisted by pressures from plans to reduce costs. As the new consumers rapidly gain access to information, both online and through traditional media, they will narrow the patient–provider information gap and make effective self-care possible and desirable.

We forecast that, by 2010, 30 percent of health plan members will be able to identify the three most important threats to their health status, and a large proportion of these folks will be actively engaged in executing elements of their treatment plans. Right now, we estimate that only 5 to 10 percent of members engage in self-care or self-management. Medical technologies involving remote sensing of patients' vital signs will hasten this development.

Shared decision making will be the last element of consumer empowerment to take hold. Its tardy arrival is due partly to provider resistance to change and partly to the fact that many medical decisions are so complex that they require a sophisticated informational infrastructure to assist both patients and providers. This infrastructure will be slow to emerge. The issue of confidentiality of medical records may further slow the emergence of this infrastructure. The quality of medical information available on the Internet will also be a factor. We estimate that right now only 1 percent of consumers

share decision making with their providers. We forecast that by 2010, 10 percent of all consumers will be aware of the primary treatment choices implicit in the health risks they face and will share with their providers decisions about treatment paths, the providers helping them to pick paths in line with their personal preferences and values. Consumers with chronic illnesses are likely to be at the forefront of this shift. This element of empowerment also has the most potential to transform the system in the longer term and improve health status.

On the down side, shared decision making, if widely implemented, may exacerbate the widening gap in access and health status between the information-rich new consumers and the information-poor traditional consumers. Information access is key to effective shared decision making. Ultimately, beyond 2010, this could push us toward a two-tier system in which the information "haves" have secure access to high-value, patient-centered care whereas the information "have-nots" struggle for access, choice, and value.

All of these facets add up to a forecast for incremental consumer-driven change by 2010—not a full-blown consumer revolution. Nonetheless, consumer forces will build rapidly in the growing top tier by 2010, and this will shift the passive consumer culture significantly in the direction of active skepticism. The combination of this shift, the push toward self-care by cost-conscious plans, patients' rights legislation supported by the elderly, and slow but steady improvements in the information infrastructure will prepare the way for a major consumer revolution when the baby boomers begin to hit age 65 in 2010 and beyond.

WILD CARDS

- The "information poor" get "wired," gaining increased access to information, and thus become part of the force for change.

- The press and media discover a role for themselves in processing and repackaging health care information for the "un-wired information poor" in order to increase their readership/viewership.

- Employers switch en masse to a defined contribution system, making defined benefits obsolete and putting health care purchasing back in the hands of patients, thus converting health care to a demand-driven system well before 2010.

- Biosensors and other new medical technologies reduce costs dramatically, rather than increasing them, and lead to do-it-yourself home care improving access in the process.

- Spillover of infectious diseases from a rapidly growing uninsured population into the middle and top tiers leads to national legislation to fix the safety net, shrinking the bottom tier.

- Congress and the president join forces to push through legislation to reduce benefits insecurity, shrinking the middle tier.

- Congress and the president join forces to push Medicare entirely to HMOs or cut benefits drastically, shrinking the top tier—or igniting a revolution among the elderly.

ENDNOTE

[1] By "access to care" we do not mean convenience but rather ability to get even minimally adequate care when it is needed. This basic access is limited in this tier by inability to pay—either out of pocket, or for insurance —and by the poor quality and limited resources of the facilities available to those with limited ability to pay.

CHAPTER 11

Public Health Services

A Challenging Future

The goal of public health is to secure health and promote wellness, for both individuals and communities, by addressing the societal, environmental, and individual determinants of health. As defined by the WHO, health is "A state of complete well-being, physical, social, and mental, and not merely the absence of disease or infirmity."

Despite the merit of this intent, a lack of consensus on the public health mission, inadequate capacity in the field, disjointed decision making, hobbled leadership, and organizational fragmentation led the Institute of Medicine (IOM) in 1988 to liken public health to a "shattered vision." Almost 15 years later, has that assessment borne out? What does the future of public health look like today, and what will it look like by the end of the decade?

This chapter highlights some of the public health issues in the United States, reviewing briefly the development of the public health system and identifying broad social, political, and technological forces that will shape its future.

THE HISTORY OF PUBLIC HEALTH IN THE UNITED STATES

The IOM describes the history of the public health system in the United States as "a history of bringing knowledge and values together in the public arena to shape an approach to health problems." By understanding the history of today's public health system, we may forecast how public health might look tomorrow.

Before the 18th century, disease was widely believed to be associated primarily with a person's moral standing. During the 18th century, there evolved a sentiment that disease could be prevented, and an organized health infrastructure began to develop. Galvanized by industrial urbanization, by a realization that both rich and poor were vulnerable to disease, and by the "great sanitary awakening" of the early 19th century, the shape of public health changed profoundly as society developed a dynamic strategy to prevent disease through public action and environmental hygiene. By the second half of the 19th century, public health was dramatically altered again as evolution of the germ theory grounded public health in science. (See Table 11-1.)

Table 11-1. Stages of relations between public health and medicine

Period	Public Health	Medicine
Pre 20th century era of infectious disease: *Cooperation*	Focus on prevention: sanitary engineering, environmental hygiene, quarantine	Focus on treatment: direct patient care within comprehensive framework
Early 20th century era of bacteriology: *Professionalization*	Establishment of targeted disease control; Rockefeller Foundation report creates science-based schools of public health	Establishment of the biomedical model of disease, Flexner Report leading to standard science-based medical education
Post World War II era of biomedical paradigm: *Functional separation*	Focus on behavioral risk factors, development of publicly funded medical safety net (Medicaid/Medicare)	Pursuit of biological mechanisms of heart disease, cancer, and stroke, success with pharmacology, diagnostics, therapeutic procedures

Source: IFTF; Lasker, R., and the Committee on Medicine and Public Health of the New York Academy of Medicine. *Medicine and Public Health: The Power of Collaboration*. New York: NYAM, 1997.

Before the germ theory was propagated, public health's efforts at disease control aimed to improve living conditions through environmental hygiene, whereas medical efforts focused on individual treatment by private physicians. There was a great deal of interdependence between the two. With acceptance of the germ theory, the new domains of public health and private medicine could no longer be readily distinguished, as population health interventions—such as screening, immunization, and the treatment of communicable disease—were provided to individuals, usually in a physician's office. Problems deepened with the creation of the health care safety net that assigned to the public sector medical responsibility for patients unable to obtain care in the private sector. Whereas the public sector had traditionally addressed the health of the population, it was now to provide a mixture of population and personal health services.

With this change, the responsibility for public health progressively was placed in the hands of professional health experts, and programs were instituted that focused on specific disease transmission routes, established immunization programs and water sanitation as cornerstones of disease prevention, and expanded governmental participation in public health efforts.

The blurring of the distinction between population-based disease prevention and individual-based medical treatment extended into the 20th century. Roosevelt's New Deal in the 1930s and Johnson's Great Society programs in the 1960s served as bookends for the expansion of the federal role in health planning, promotion, education, and financing. With the Social Security Act and the Medicare and Medicaid programs, public health moved away from population-based approaches and became more involved in individual interventions. As health care costs increased and the resulting economic burden became unbearable, the social vision again changed as the focus turned to cost

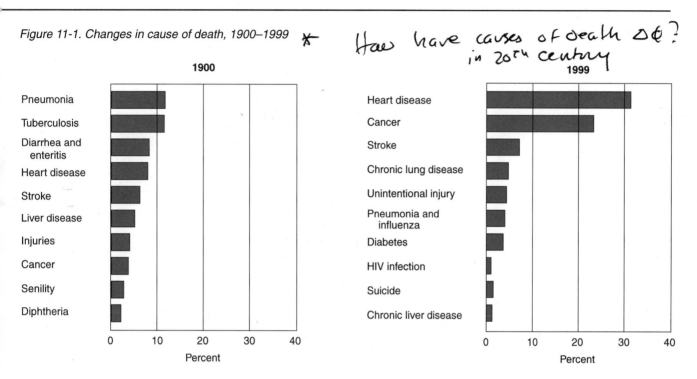

Figure 11-1. Changes in cause of death, 1900–1999

Handwritten note: How have causes of death ∆♦? in 20th century

Source: Centers for Disease Control and Prevention. Control of infectious diseases, 1900–1999. *Morbidity and Mortality Weekly Report* 1999; 48:621–629.

containment. The last decades of the 20th century ushered in the managed care system of health care delivery and further diminished support for a population-based public health infrastructure.

Table 11-2. Ten public health achievements, 1900–1999

Vaccination
Motor vehicle safety
Safer workplaces
Control of infectious diseases
Decline in deaths from coronary heart disease and stroke
Safer and healthier foods
Healthier mothers and babies
Family planning
Fluoridation of drinking water
Recognition of tobacco use as a health hazard

Source: Centers for Disease Control and Prevention. Ten great public health achievements—United States, 1900–1999. *Morbidity and Mortality Weekly Report* 1999; 48:241–243.

PUBLIC HEALTH ACHIEVEMENTS IN THE 20TH CENTURY

Over the course of the century, infectious diseases diminished as a major cause of morbidity and mortality while chronic disease and behavioral health risks grew. The 20th century brought Americans improved health and longevity, their life expectancy lengthening by 30 years since 1900.[1] According to the Centers for Disease Control and Prevention (CDC), 25 of those years can be attributed to advances in public health, which accomplished ten significant achievements during the 20th century (see Table 11-2).

There is much cause for celebration over the accomplishments of the 20th century, and yet much still needs to be done. (See Figure 11-1.)

PUBLIC HEALTH STRUCTURE AND FUNCTION TODAY

The mission of public health, as viewed by the IOM, is the use of knowledge to fulfill the public's interest in reducing human suffering and enhancing quality of life. The substance of this mission lies in organized community efforts that are aimed at the prevention of disease and the promotion of health. These efforts are guided by public health principles, which include a scientific basis for action, an orientation toward prevention of illness and promotion of wellness, a population-wide perspective, community-based participation and problem solving, and a respect for diversity. Ideally, these efforts and principles are applied within an organizational framework that encompasses governmental, private, voluntary, and individual activities.

The U.S. government is at the core of the public health system, acting as the primary source of leadership and accountability. The IOM delineates three functional pillars of public health that the government should guarantee: assessment, policy development, and assurance (see Figure 11-2).

Involvement of the federal government in public health efforts fluctuated during the 20th century. By the close of the century, federal intervention had been retracted, although the role of the federal government continued to be important because of its capacity to address interstate and international health issues, to develop overarching national health policy, and to coordinate national health data and research. State governments now have the greatest responsibility for the well-being of the state's residents, not only because of the reductions in federal intervention but also because of their constitutionally designated police powers. It is local government that is on the front line of public health action today, however. Local governments are critical to the public health system, providing an operational mechanism for public health action and serving as a liaison among professional experts, different governmental divisions, and the community.

Myriad other institutions contribute to public health practice, including private foundations, schools of public health, community-based organizations, private health care organizations, and community activist organizations. In this diversity of

---

Figure 11-2. The three pillars of public health

Assessment

The diagnosis of community health status and needs through epidemiology, surveillance, research, and evaluation of information about disease, behavioral, biological, environmental, and socioeconomic factors.

Policy Development

Planning and priority setting, based on scientific knowledge and under the leadership of the governmental agency, for the development of comprehensive public health policies and decision making.

Assurance

The securing of universal access to a set of essential personal and community-wide health services through delegation, regulation, or direct public provision of services.

Evaluation

Source: Institute of Medicine, Division of Health Care Services, 1988.

---

public health players lie both opportunity and challenge. Opportunity because public health problems tend to be complex and require integrated, multidisciplinary responses. Challenge because these various players can be uncoordinated and even competitive in their efforts.

KEY FACTORS AFFECTING PUBLIC HEALTH IN AMERICA TODAY

POLITICS: THE AMERICAN DREAM UNDER RECONSTRUCTION

The mid-20th century was a time of expansion of prosperity and the American dream, but the recessions of the 1970s and 1980s and government downsizing in the 1990s narrowed the government's social vision. Welfare and affirmative action receded. Government privatized the safety net, borrowed from Social Security, and embraced free trade. By 1999, government spending on infrastructure, education, and research had diminished from 24 percent of the federal budget to 14 percent.[2]

Yet, at the end of the 20th century, new health challenges emerged, such as AIDS infection and environmental contamination, that required strong centralized leadership and reintegration of population-based approaches to public health.

Two currents now flow through the mainstream, and one of them is likely to dominate in shaping the next social vision. One current is simultaneously populist, equitable, libertarian, pro-environment, fiscally conservative, and intrinsically supportive of effective public spending for social good. The other is fiscally conservative, characterized by market populism, and oriented toward increased privatization that would intrinsically limit government's involvement in health reforms.

The first political vision is fundamentally new, and the policies it would deliver are less certain. The second vision would definitely restrict government establishment of such policies as universal health coverage, a patient's bill of rights, and overall increases in social, health, and public health spending.

SOCIOECONOMIC AND POLITICAL FACTORS

Socioeconomic status is the number one predictor of poor health. The poor are more than three times as likely as the wealthy to die prematurely or have a disability from illness,[3] despite nearly two-thirds of the money for public health being directed to medical safety-net services. Socioeconomic status is a powerful factor among the determinants of intentional injury by homicide and suicide. The issue is clearly socioeconomic status and not ethnicity because when rates of household crowding are used as an index of socioeconomic status, Caucasians and African Americans living in comparable socioeconomic circumstances demonstrate similar rates of homicide.[4] The ill effects of poverty are particularly ominous in the light of an increasing economic gap between the rich and poor, which is independently associated with a worse health status for the bottom economic tiers of society.

Chapter 11: Public Health Services   169

Economic disparity in the United States has been increasing. From 1977 to 1999, the after-tax income for the richest 1 percent of the population increased 115 percent, whereas the after-tax income for the poorest 20 percent declined by 9 percent[5] (see Figure 11-3). Moreover, greater wealth is concentrated in a smaller segment of society today than has been the case at any time since the Great Depression. This disparity will have as large an effect on the future of public health as any other factors considered in this analysis.

GLOBAL FORCES DRIVING AND LIMITING PROGRESS

Global issues ultimately create the context for public health today and into the future. They are highly integrated economic, social, political, and technological forces that both drive and inhibit progress.

The world's economies are interconnected more than ever before, and the advent of free-trade agreements and expanded world travel are rapidly changing the context of public health in the United States. The main mechanism through which globalism is shaping public health is through the breakdown of natural and regulatory barriers to disease. Increased trade and travel are permitting diseases to spread to new populations that have no natural resistance and organisms to enter new environments with no natural controls.

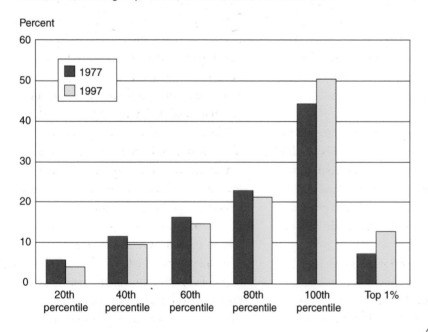

Figure 11-3. Changes in the share of national after-tax income held by various economic groups in the United States, 1977 and 1997

Percent

Legend:
- 1977
- 1997

(Bar chart categories: 20th percentile, 40th percentile, 60th percentile, 80th percentile, 100th percentile, Top 1%)

Source: IFTF; Shapiro, I., and Greenstein, R. *The Widening Income Gap.* Washington, DC: Center on Budget and Policy Priorities, 1999.

These forces of globalism are inevitably associated with health risks, including new infectious diseases, contaminated food, spread of emerging and drug-resistant disease, bioterrorism, and toxic substances, both legal and illegal. According to CDC, since 1995, nearly 50 percent of all cases of measles reported in the United States have been introduced from other countries,[6] as have been the influenza strains that affect the U.S. population every year. In 1997, 39 percent of all patients with tuberculosis reported in the United States, and 67 percent in California, were foreign born.[7] An increasing proportion of the foods Americans eat, including 40 percent of fruits and 60 percent of seafood, is produced abroad, where standards of pesticide use and sanitation can differ from the United States.[8]

International free trade is also challenging national and state health and safety regulations. The primary issue is how to maintain and advance U.S. health and environmental standards without violating trade accords and while remaining competitive. Reconciling this issue from a public health perspective will be like walking a tightrope, with liability and environmental and health risks all in the balance.

The next 10 years will see increasing international cooperation in vaccine preparation, disease control, and environmental and food safety. The reality and the perception of public health concerns and solutions in the United States by the end of the decade will be much more embedded in a global health and economic context. Policymakers and public health professionals will increasingly be called upon to protect the public and the environment in a way that both withstands the pressures and advances with the opportunities of global trade.

ENVIRONMENTAL FACTORS

A fragmentation of the infrastructure and information systems that supported environmental health until the last quarter of the 20th century has weakened the ability of public health agencies to protect the communities they serve. While there are ample data available, there is little usable information—a factor that has proved to be a serious barrier to public health agencies' ability to address emerging health problems, to educate decision makers and the public about specific environmental hazards, and to evaluate the effectiveness of interventions.[9]

The next 10 years will see public health professionals in the environmental health field creating multisectoral relationships like never before. Their success in creating links to government environmental agencies, environmental activist groups, human rights groups, labor unions, and technology agencies will be one of the primary determinants of the status of environmental health in the United States over the coming decade.

Three major areas will be of greatest importance: air quality, water quality, and food safety.

Air Quality

The good news is that Los Angeles no longer has the worst air quality in the nation. While California has broken new ground with air quality improvements, particularly in regard to motor vehicle emissions, other states have continued to pollute their air. The most important concerns in this area are the improvement of vehicular, diesel, industrial (especially power), and household product emissions.

The bad news is that failure to improve air quality has profound repercussions on health, including its relation to cancer, developmental problems, and asthma.

Asthma is one of the most common chronic diseases in the United States and is the ninth leading cause of hospitalization nationally. Despite medical advancements in its diagnosis and treatment, the prevalence rates linked to asthma are increasing nationally, and overall rates of death with asthma as the underlying cause—which decreased from 1962 through 1977—have gradually increased again in all race, sex, and

Chapter 11: Public Health Services   171

Figure 11-4. Trends in asthma prevalence by region and year, 1980–1994

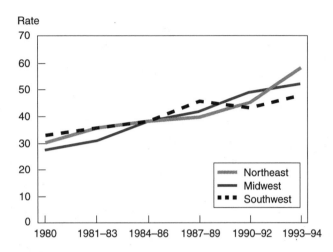

Source: Mannino, D. M., et al. Surveillance for asthma—United States, 1960–1995. *Morbidity and Mortality Weekly Report* 1998; 47 (SS-1):1–28.

Figure 11-5. Trends in asthma prevalence by year, 1980–1999

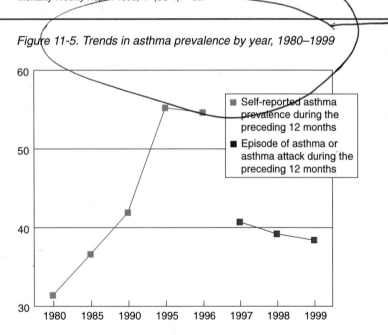

Source: Mannino, D. M., et al. Surveillance for asthma—United States, 1960–1995. *Morbidity and Mortality Weekly Report* 1998; 47 (SS-1):1–28.

Information Survey changed the measures of asthma prevalence. Now, two measures are used, both restricted to persons with a medical diagnosis of asthma. The first is referred to as lifetime asthma prevalence, which includes those respondents with a medical diagnosis of asthma at any time in their lives. In 1997, a total of 26.7 million persons reported a physician diagnosis of asthma during their lifetime, which is substantially higher than the 12-month prevalence measured before 1997. The second measure is a 12-month attack prevalence, which includes the number of persons with asthma who have had one or more attacks or episodes in the past 12 months. In 1997, the estimated prevalence of persons with asthma episodes or attacks was 11.1 million, lower than the 12-month prevalence estimated from the question wording used before 1997 (see Figure 11-5). A sufficient number of years with the new measures do not yet exist to determine whether the trends in ashtma are increasing or decreasing. Both 12-month prevalence (before 1997) and 12-month attack prevalence of asthma (since 1997) were higher among children aged 5–14 years, blacks compared with whites, and females. Neither 12-month prevalence nor episodes or attacks of asthma varied substantially among regions of the United States (data not indicated). The most substantial increases occurred among children from infancy to 14 years of age.[10,11] Allergic asthma costs an estimated $6.2 billion a year, according to the National Institute of Environmental Health Science.

Water Quality

Most attention to water quality has focused on drinking water, as public water systems are regulated under the

age strata. From 1980 to 1996, the prevalence of self-reported asthma in the United States increased 74 percent (see Figure 11-4). Beginning in 1997, the asthma questions on the National Health

Chapter 11: Public Health Services

Figure 11-6. Trends in waterborne disease outbreaks, 1971–1994

Number of outbreaks

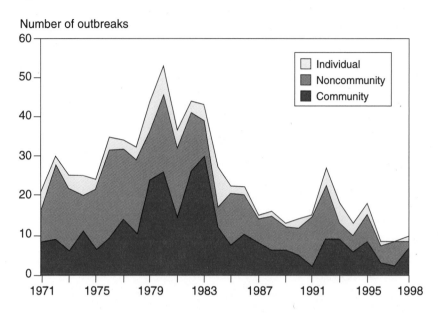

Source: Centers for Disease Control and Prevention. Surveillance for waterborne disease outbreaks—United States, 1993–1994. *Morbidity and Mortality Weekly Report* 1996; 45 (SS-1):1–33.

Two other sources of water contamination are also emerging areas for concern. According to the Environmental Protection Agency, farm animal waste produced at concentrated animal feeding operations has polluted 35,000 miles of rivers in 22 states and has contaminated groundwater in 17 states. Animal-factory pollution contributes to a range of physical and mental ailments in people, including headaches, nausea, depression, and even death. The practice of feeding animals large quantities of antibiotics also contributes to drug-resistant bacterial infections. Although the number of hog farms in the United States has dropped from 600,000 to 157,000 over the past 15 years, the total hog inventory for the United States has remained constant because of the increased animal concentration in large-scale farms. Securing water safety in the future will require structural, regulatory, or redesign interventions in this domain.

The second area of concern is increasing evidence of microcontaminants and pharmaceuticals in water supplies. Hormone-disrupting contaminants such as DDT-like compounds and waterborne perchlorate as well as other pesticides are of particular importance. An emerging issue is that greater than expected quantities of active pharmaceuticals are turning up in water, in large part excreted by humans who have not entirely metabolized the medicines that they take. In some cases, 50 to 90 percent of an administered drug may be excreted.[13] Drugs, however, are not traditionally considered pollutants and are regulated primarily by public health agencies that have little expertise in protecting natural ecosystems and water supplies. The full

[handwritten note: What challenges exist to keeping our water supply safe?]

federal Safe Drinking Water Act of 1974, as amended in 1986. Probably as a result of this regulation, the number of waterborne disease outbreaks reported annually has been similar for each year from 1987 through 1994, except for an increase in 1992[12] and has decreased since then (see Figures 11-6 and 11-7). Some outbreaks have disclosed the vulnerability of large metropolitan areas. However, the capacity to treat drinking water adequately in some metropolitan areas is being stretched to its limit, and the problem cannot necessarily be remedied by further regulation. As a consequence, municipalities increasingly will explore new technologies in water sanitation.

Chapter 11: Public Health Services

Figure 11-7. Patterns in waterborne disease outbreaks, 1997–1998

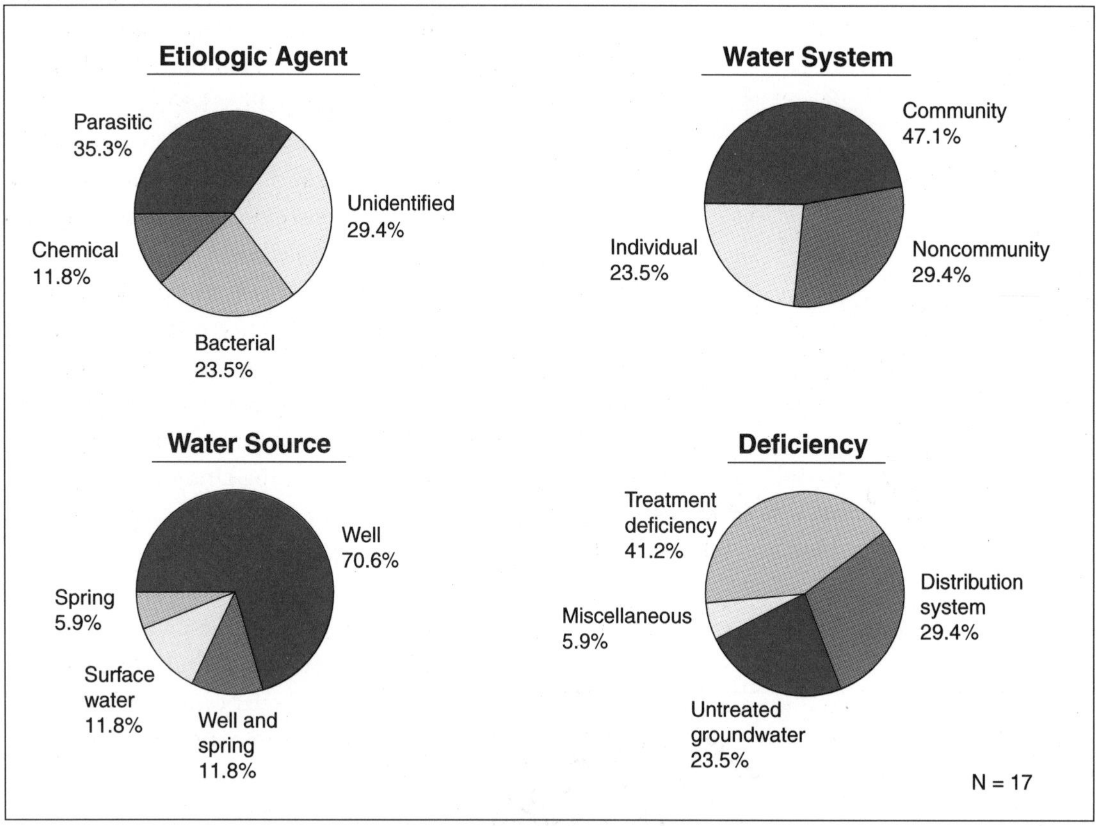

Source: Centers for Disease Control and Prevention. Surveillance for waterborne disease outbreaks—
United States, 1993–1994. *Morbidity and Mortality Weekly Report* 1996; 45 (SS-1):1–33.

impact of pharmaceuticals in the water supply is only beginning to emerge and may prompt new standards for drug approval and cross-sector collaboration in their control.

Food Safety

Two main areas of concern in food safety are outbreaks related to foodborne pathogens and pesticide use.

Each year, millions of people have a foodborne illness, but because only a fraction of them seek medical care and even fewer submit laboratory specimens, estimates of the magnitude of foodborne illness in the United States are imprecise. Since 1996, however, the Foodborne Diseases Active Surveillance Network (FoodNet) has collected data to monitor nine foodborne diseases at selected sites in the United States. As compared to the 1996 data, 2000 FoodNet data indicate a decline in several of the major bacterial and parasitic causes of foodborne illness.[14] These declines might in part reflect annual fluctuations, temporal variations in diagnostic practices, or implementation of disease prevention regulations. However, with the forces of increased international food trade and increased fast-food consumption, constant vigilance over this system is required to secure ongoing declines.

Pesticide use has implications for both food consumption and environmental or occupational exposure. Certain pesticides are known carcinogens, and others are under suspicion. Of particular concern is that these chemicals can be excreted in breast milk and that children consume the greatest concentration of pesticides. Mounting evidence shows that when children are exposed to ambient pesticides through proximity in or outside their home, their normal physical and intellectual development are profoundly affected. In adults, occupational exposure can be associated with bradycardia, diaphoresis, nausea, headache, eye irritation, or muscle weakness, as well as with a potential for more severe effects, including cancer, over the long term. Again, international differences in agricultural practices as well as trade agreements are major considerations in addressing these problems.

The Future of Air, Water, and Food Safety

In all cases of air, water, and food safety, it is children and developing fetuses who have the most adverse health consequences of environmental threats. Growing evidence to this effect has created an increasing momentum to change the way environmental health and safety standards are set. Within 10 years, the gold standard for setting levels for contaminants will be based on child health factors, with important implications for trade and industry. International accords will have as great a role in the setting of

environmental standards as will the work of national and state governments. The global context will require environmental health professionals to think in new ways and build alliances across environmental, labor, and technology sectors.

TECHNOLOGY

Technological advancements are so frequent and often dramatic now that change itself seems to be commonplace. Technology holds the greatest implications for public health in the areas of information, diagnostics, and genetic technologies. New information technologies are expanding public health's capacity to conduct epidemiology, disease surveillance, collaborative research, data-based policymaking, and advocacy. At the same time, tremendous struggles regarding privacy and data ownership, validity, and coordination have yet to be resolved.

Diagnostic technologies will continue to advance public health screening. New technologies include more sensitive mammograms, noninvasive screening with enzyme-linked immunoabsorbant assays and polymerase chain reaction tests, and computer-aided detection of abnormalities on pap smears and mammograms. These advances permit more and better screening, and also make it easier to screen in nontraditional settings, such as jails and community outreach sites, allowing access to otherwise hard-to-reach populations.

With progress in our understanding of genetic predispositions to disease, the implications for public health screening and epidemiology are impressive.

Chapter 11: Public Health Services   **175**

However, biotechnology also ushers in a new array of ethical struggles, as debate ignites issues of stem cell research, genetic screening, and international trials. Technology also helps drive the increase in resources expended on health care, further diminishing the funds available for public health services.

PUBLIC HEALTH FRAMEWORKS AND STRATEGIES: PROBLEMS OF PERCEPTION

PUBLIC HEALTH AS THE "ALSO RAN"

Ask most people on the street what public health means and they'll tell you, "welfare." Ask them what epidemiology means and they'll either blush or tell you it's the study of skin infections. Public health has an identity problem.

People often think of public health as publicly funded medical care for the poor. But while medicine and public health are inextricably entwined, they are also quite distinct. A physician's virtual black bag contains diagnostic tools, pharmaceuticals, treatments, and protocols. A public health professional's toolkit carries epidemiology and biostatistics, health education, program and policy development and evaluation, screening, and advocacy. Americans can see what doctors do any night of the week on television, but they have almost no exposure to what public health professionals do. This lack of understanding of public health can forestall reinvigoration of the public health system.

Furthermore, while people value the protections offered by public health, they do not know what it takes to achieve those protections. People value the *products* of public health, such as clean water, a clean environment, and control of communicable disease, but they do not as greatly value the *methods* of public health, such as disease surveillance and screening. The better public health's prevention strategies work, the more invisible they are to the public's eye. Ultimately, if the public does not value and support the means to the end, things will fall apart.

Two tendencies, one reactive and one active, indicate that improvements in public awareness are possible. Resurgence in public support for public health reforms does occur, but largely as reaction to a perceived crisis. It took 45,000 stray dogs and an epidemic of dog bites for Los Angeles County to reverse an 8-year trend of funding cuts to its animal control program. It has taken numerous mass shootings to galvanize the public and convince some politicians to take steps toward gun control. It may require a worsening of problems, such as drug-resistant tuberculosis or breaches in water-supply sanitation by microcontaminants, before the public becomes convinced that public health is not just for people on the outskirts of society, but rather is necessary for the well-being of the entire population. Public health professionals need to realize that embedded in these dilemmas are opportunities for heightening public awareness and support.

On a more positive note, another emerging trend—the rise of the "new consumer"—could put public health on the radar screen before disaster strikes. The new consumers not only are educated, they also have economic clout and are very well-informed about their health. With mounting exposure to public health information, the new consumers, if guided and organized, will serve as the opinion leaders necessary for enhancing the reputation and resources of public health. Moreover, these information-empowered consumers will become the majority of the adult population around 2005, and will bring with them a greater value for prevention (see Chapter 10).

ORGANIZATIONAL AND INSTITUTIONAL FORCES

Issues of public health leadership and professionalism, the organizational structure of public health, and public-private competition and accountability all influence the day-to-day functioning of the public health system. They also influence the potential for policy formation that could alter the course of public health in the future.

Public Health Professionalism: A Crisis of Leadership

Organizational factors that limit public health agencies' capacity to provide the leadership necessary to guarantee the three pillars of public health include uncompetitive wages, restrictive bureaucracies, and insufficient leadership training. Governmental public health officials' average wages are half those in medical and health services management and are less than one-third those of physicians.[15] Increasingly, public health practice relies on highly skilled professional staff, including epidemiologists, policy analysts, project directors, and information systems experts. Systemwide low salaries

impair public health agencies' ability to compete for talented personnel.

Compounding the problem is the administrative structure of public health agencies, which is not always well suited to a professional staff. Restrictive job classifications, restrictions on recruitment and hiring, out-of-date time management requirements, and outmoded or counterproductive administration of professional positions can make public health an uncompetitive field. Unlike the private sector, the public sector is also restricted in its ability to reward highly productive employees or lay off underachieving employees.

Show Me the Money

Inadequate funding is one of the greatest barriers to the completion of public health's mission and responsibilities. At all levels of government, but particularly the local level, officials are hamstrung by limited funding and are often forced to follow the money rather than address public health problems. Although states have been given considerable flexibility in their use of block grants, this restrictive funding mechanism has often compromised the ability of local agencies to meet the particular needs of their communities, especially as the grants are not discretionary.

Organizational Challenges to Public Health

The states have considerable latitude in fulfilling their public health mission. Partly because of that autonomy, the organizational structures of different states' public health agencies and their ties to related agencies vary widely.

Chapter 11: Public Health Services　**177**

Although greater uniformity is neither likely nor necessarily desirable, organizational variability can impede integration and coordination of health and social services.

A particular difficulty lies in creating functional organizational ties between public health and other agencies with overlapping missions, such as social services, environmental protection, environmental health, personal health care, and mental health agencies. When a new health problem emerges, health systems sometimes create organizational barriers, establishing a separate program for it rather than integrating that program into the existing infrastructure, as was the case with AIDS. The consequences of these barriers can include lack of coordination of program activities and policy priorities, inadequate and out-of-date data surveillance and information sharing, and competition for limited resources. The same problems exist between the government and private sectors, especially with the institution of managed care.

RECONCILING PUBLIC HEALTH AND PRIVATE MEDICINE

Perhaps the most significant example of an organizational threat to public health efficacy involves the interplay of the public and private sectors in the provision of personal health services. With the spectacular biomedical discoveries and their applications in the late 20th century has come expansion of the private medical sector, with concomitant further reductions in financial and public support of population-based public health

programs and training. To this day, although the interests of public health and medicine overlap, an adequate mechanism for coordinating activities between the two sectors is lacking.

The problems resulting from this arrangement continue to weaken the public health system and are fourfold.

First, the disproportionate allocation of public health resources to publicly funded medicine drains capacity and attention from community-wide public service, assessment, and policy development functions. At the state level, two-thirds of spending is for personal health services whereas spending for population-based health services is only 1.0 percent of total health care expenditures.[16] Of this, the largest amount (26 percent) is for enforcing laws and regulations that protect the health and ensure the safety of the public, whereas training (4 percent) and research (2 percent) received the smallest investments.[16]

Second, in both the public and private sectors, there is limited cooperation and coordination across public and personal health services for the provision of essential disease control functions. These services include screening, disease reporting, partner notification and treatment, treatment standardization, and diagnostic and treatment technology updates.

Third, opening of Medicaid and Medicare reimbursements to the private sector has reduced the resources available to state and local public health agencies. Initially, the public sector was able to support some of its infrastructure and provide care to the indigent through relatively high Medicaid reimbursements. Paradoxically, when private providers became eligible for those reimbursements, they successfully siphoned off the majority of reimbursement income and the healthiest patients, leaving the public sector with the burden of the indigent population but without the Medicaid/Medicare income. Moreover, private-sector involvement did not fundamentally increase health care coverage for the poor. As a result, the cash-strapped public health agencies are left providing medical care for the poor and provide little public health care for the overall population.

Fourth, as the government's public health agency became increasingly involved with the provision of medical care, the general public came to confuse public health with publicly funded medical services—with welfare. The consequence of the public's misunderstanding of the core functions of public health has diminished public support or sense of collective responsibility for public health actions. Some public health professionals even suggest that the public health field should change its name to population health to clarify things!

PRIVATIZATION: THE PROMISE OF PARTNERSHIPS

Market forces that affect the delivery of health care are significantly changing the financial base and functional role of public health agencies. With the emergence of managed care, the trend toward downsizing governmental agencies, and the overall reductions in public health funding, public health agencies have increasingly turned toward developing leaner, more efficient delivery systems. In par-

ticular, they have begun exploring "privatization" as a potential community-based approach for assuring delivery of necessary public health services. Table 11-3 reviews findings from a Public Health Foundation review of the privatization experience.[17]

However, when Medicaid and Medicare patients leave the public sector to enter private-sector care, public health loses control over some of the services it has traditionally assured its patients. For example, Medicaid recipients, as a medically vulnerable population, often require "wraparound" care that provides services, such as transportation or translation services, that help them gain access to or communicate with their medical provider. Currently, when patients leave the public sector to enter private managed care programs, essential wraparound services are not uniformly provided. The capacity of government agencies to assess the public's health status, expenditures, and disease control measures is significantly altered when patients enter the capitated world of private managed care.

The increasing delivery of health services in managed care environments is of particular concern for the poor, but is also of relevance to the general population. Between 1985 and 1998, the proportion of HMO members enrolled in investor-owned plans increased sharply from 26 percent to 62 percent. Between 1980 and 1998, the market share of group-model and staff-model plans decreased from 81 percent to 12 percent. A 1999 study analyzing differences between for-profit and not-for-profit health plans found that investor-owned HMOs deliver a lower quality of care than do

why did mgd care affect care for poor?

Table 11-3. Factors in the process of privatizing publicly funded public and personal health services

Measure	Finding
Reasons for privatization	Implementation of state Medicaid waivers
	Effort to achieve cost savings and address fiscal concerns
	Downsizing and reorganizing government
	Effort to improve quality and efficiency
Barriers	Personnel issues
	Philosophical differences
	Difficulty in finding able or willing partners in the private sector
Facilitators	Involved community
	Maintenance of the government's role in core functions of assessment, policy development, and assurance
	Public health agencies' savvy in corporate skills and collaboration
	History of partnering
	Strong local health department leadership
Outcomes	Public health agencies maintain service delivery components related to assurance and ultimate accountability
	Little impact on quality of services, except in the case of access, where access increases for clinical service and decreases for psychological services and health education
	Health departments evaluate and redirect revenues and expenditures regardless of privatization, although privatization allows them to focus on essential public health
	Privatization strengthens community relations, but occasionally can weaken them

Source: IFTF; *Privatization and Public Health: A Study of Initiatives and Early Lessons Learned.* Washington, DC: Public Health Foundation, September 1997. Research and writing supported by The Annie E. Casey Foundation, Baltimore, Maryland.

the not-for-profit plans. Compared with not-for-profit HMOs, investor-owned plans had lower rates for all 14 health plan employer data and information set (HEDIS) quality-of-care indicators. In particular, the investor-owned plans score lower in treatment of critical medical conditions and preventive health measures. Investor-owned plans had lower rates of immunization (63.9 versus 72.3 percent), mammography (69.4 versus 75.1 percent), Papanicolaou tests (69.2 versus 77.1 percent), and psychi-atric hospitalization (70.5 versus 77.1 percent). Staff-model and group-model HMOs had higher scores on virtually all quality-of-care indicators.[18]

Public health involvement in the reconciliation of these concerns has focused on increasing efforts to negotiate shared responsibilities either through government mandate or partnerships. Public-private partnerships are, to this date, the most prominent and perhaps most promising vehicle for guaranteeing

Chapter 11: Public Health Services

governmental assurance and assessment responsibilities and for transforming managed care settings into productive protagonists for public health. Through public-private partnerships, the local public health agency can engage the private sector and community representatives in building healthy communities.

Experimentation with several models is currently under way, including models serving the underinsured and the uninsured together with patients enrolled in Medicare and private programs. For example, Medicaid primary care case management interlaces managed care and FFS health services as an alternative to the traditional HMO model. Introduced in Texas in 1996, it quickly enrolled two-thirds of the state's eligible enrollees and may become the mainstream in other states as well. Such an arrangement fulfills the assurance function of the public health agency and streamlines the agency's assessment function as an added benefit to the community.

OTHER INSTITUTIONS: THE BREADTH OF PUBLIC HEALTH

Universities

University graduate schools of public health are, in a sense, the caretakers of the public health heritage. These schools train future public health professionals, provide technical support to government agencies, conduct basic research to further scientific understanding of health determinants, and provide leadership in public health ethics and health and human rights issues. In so doing, they are a force that can standardize and shape the skills, principles, capacity, and

knowledge of public health professionals at all levels.

Public health schools have an important role in shaping the future of public health. While there is a need for academics and researchers in public health, it is critical also to prepare future public health officials with skills in leadership, management, and negotiation. As a substantial proportion of current public health officials lack formal public health training and are resistant to efforts to further professionalize the field, more schools might follow the lead of schools that are developing distance education programs and creating nondegree certification programs.

Community-Based Organizations and Foundations

These organizations have the capacity to set political and program agendas through grassroots actions and financing of new initiatives. Community-based organizations are key members of any public-private partnership, as they are often among the strongest voices of constituency groups and can also provide services directly. Lack of funding consistently plagues community-based organizations, and innovative funding and public-private financing partnerships will have to be developed in the future. The potential for conflicts of interest resulting from new financing schemes will have to be evaluated. While community-based organizations seek funding, the foundations provide funding, and in so doing they play a leadership role in setting public health agendas and coordinating public health action.

THE FUTURE: SCENARIOS AND FORECASTS

OUTLOOK FOR PUBLIC-PRIVATE PARTNERSHIPS IN PERSONAL HEALTH CARE

There are three possible scenarios and three sets of key players whose leadership, management skills, and negotiation capabilities would predict the likelihood of particular scenario's occurrence. The three players determining the outlook for public-private relationships in personal health care include:

- public health agency directors

- private health care providers and organizations

- community-based organizations and leaders

Together, these players will lead their constituents through one of the following three scenarios.

Scenario One: Public-Private Community Partnerships

In this scenario, the medical services now provided by most government agencies are shifted to the private sector through a variety of public-private partnerships. The public health principles—especially those of prevention, shared standards and objectives, and community-based participation—potentiate this partnership. Public health agencies maintain a watchdog role to assure that vulnerable populations are served, but their focus returns primarily to assessment, policy development, and population-level interventions, such as health systems monitoring or monitoring of food and water sanitation systems.

Scenario Two: Dynamic Competition Rules

Local public health agencies continue to provide medical services, successfully competing with the private sector for both Medicaid and private pay patients. Competition is both dynamic and effective and is confined to the provision of medical services. In this area, the advances and achievements in each sector drive improvements in the other's services. For example, the public sector's success in providing wraparound services pushes the private sector to improve its own services in this area. Most of the larger public health functions are provided by the public sector, although the private sector does join in to some extent for the sake of positive public relations.

Scenario Three: Public Health in Tatters

Unable to compete directly with the private sector or to develop successful partnerships, local public health agencies retreat from the provision of medical services, leaving only a skeleton framework of services remaining in order to fulfill their minimum mandates. The private sector serves all of the insured population, leaving the government health care systems strapped for cash. Without the revenues generated from Medicaid reimbursements and with no additional funding, the public health functions of assessment, policy development, and assurance are in tatters. The "invisible" work of public health, such as water and food safety, becomes very visible as public health systems begin to fail and outbreaks and epidemics spread across the country. In some areas, community leaders begin to assist public health organizations through the private nonprofit sector.

FORECAST OF THE FUTURE: ORGANIZATIONAL ISSUES

The future of public health promises great struggle as public health leaders work to reinvigorate the infrastructure, approaches, and public attitudes that support a collective responsibility for society's well-being. It is not a question of whether there will be a future for public health—as long as people live together in society, public health will exist. Rather, the future asks the questions of how much, for how many, and how well?

Such questions are not easily answered at present. Money is short, organizing social vision is weak, and there predominates a sense that public health is relevant only to the poor. Our forecasts are based in this context. Nevertheless, there always exists the opportunity to challenge the future. We hope that, within these forecasts, public health professionals will see opportunities to shape a new era of public health that reaches its full potential to secure health for all.

During most of this decade, public health will continue to be underfunded and marginalized, and for the most part efforts to address the underlying problems will be incremental. Breaches in public health prevention systems will also become increasingly evident in the areas of food and water safety, air pollution, outbreaks of drug-resistant infections, and resurgence of sexually transmitted disease. As a result of these pressures, however, we think that government will begin to augment funding and pay attention to these systems.

Beyond the pressures of dysfunction, there are several key determinants of public health's future. These include the status of community health needs and community awareness, the relationship of the public health agency to the larger community, and the capacity of both the public and private sector to provide adequate personal health services to the community. Key public health actions will utilize policy, epidemiology, technology, public-private community coalitions, and information-empowered consumers. These are areas where focused energy will yield the greatest return.

IN PARTICULAR . . .

- *Community coalitions.* Coalitions establishing formal cooperative ties between community groups, private business, private health care agencies, community activists, and the government's health agency will become increasingly common. Ideally led by a public health official, these coalitions will be a powerful vehicle for building healthy communities. Their approach will be to develop collaborative initiatives that mutually benefit business and community. Their function for public health will be to monitor and assure access to basic personal and public health services, to verify their quality, and to provide some support to cash-strapped community-based organizations. It is possible that up to 45 percent of public health departments will be engaged in some type of public-private partnership by the year 2010.

- *Managed care.* While apparently destined to be the dominant Medicaid personal health care model for this

Chapter 11: Public Health Services   183

decade, up to 25 percent of public health agencies still will compete with the private marketplace to provide direct services to patients. Nevertheless, managed care will look different at the end of the decade than it does today. Competition and fiscal viability are continuing to drive innovation and experimentation. Patients' rights are going to be increasingly protected, which will also force managed care to either respond or fold. Think integration: of public and private partnerships, of insured and uninsured populations, and of managed care and FFS.

■ *Public health policy.* At the national level, public health policy will approach assurance functions primarily in a piecemeal fashion but will include development of a patient's bill of rights and experimentation with safety-net incentive strategies. At the state level, the states will be very active in developing protections for patients within HMOs and publicly funded personal health services systems that are fiscally viable. States will also address access to controversial services, such as family planning. By the end of the decade, it is likely that there will be enough momentum and shared experience at the state level to reinitiate federal-level comprehensive personal and public health care reforms. Along the way, another, more controversial, policy pathway increasingly will be taken: litigation. Following in the footsteps of the tobacco suits, there will be more court challenges to the public and personal health status quo. While this approach is provocative, in particular

in redirecting accountability to industry, it will take some time to evaluate its true value, as well as to expose its weaknesses.

■ *Epidemiology.* Epidemiology is the fundamental science of public health. As public health problems become more complex—both because of increased understanding of the problems and because of an increasingly integrated mix of stakeholders—public health will rely on the scientific foundation offered by epidemiology as one of its most useful guides and allies. Genetic epidemiology will help to introduce new strategies for health promotion and disease prevention— although these strategies will not replace basic public health prevention approaches. In the area of health services evaluation, information technology will enhance epidemiological research. Constantly changing management and payment structures will make access to consistent and informative data sets difficult, however, thereby presenting major challenges to solid epidemiological evaluation of health services.

■ *Universities.* Educational institutions will continue in their roles as researchers and advisors to policymakers and public health practitioners. Their role in training public health leaders will expand, especially through distance training programs and joint degree programs. Universities will also play a leadership role in studying and guiding ethical and human rights debates regarding emerging public health practices.

ENDNOTES

1 Centers for Disease Control and Prevention. Ten great public health achievements—United States, 1900–1999. *Morbidity and Mortality Weekly Report* 1999; 48:241–243.

2 Executive Office of the President, Office of Management and Budget, 1999.

3 Lantz, P., et al. Socioeconomic factors, health behaviors, and mortality. *Journal of the American Medical Association* 1998; 279:1703.

4 Centerwall, B. Race, socioeconomic status, and domestic homicide. *Journal of the American Medical Association* 1995; 273:1775.

5 Shapiro, I., and Greenstein, R. *The Widening Income Gap.* Washington, DC: Center on Budget and Policy Priorities, 1999.

6 Centers for Disease Control and Prevention. Measles—United States, 1997. *Morbidity and Mortality Weekly Report* 1998; 47:273–276.

7 *Reported Tuberculosis in the United States 1997.* Atlanta, GA: Centers for Disease Control and Prevention, July 1998.

8 Putnam, J. J., and Allshouse, J. E. Food consumption, prices, and expenditures, 1970–95. *Statistical Bulletin No. 939.* Washington, DC: Economic Research Service, U.S. Department of Agriculture, 1997.

9 Public Health Foundation. *Environmental Health Data Needs: An Action Plan for Federal Public Health Agencies.* Submitted to the Environmental Health Policy Committee Subcommittee on Data Needs. June 18, 1997.

10 Mannino, D. M., et al. Surveillance for asthma—United States, 1980–1999. *Morbidity and Mortality Weekly Report* 2002; 54 (SS01):1–13.

11 Centers for Disease Control and Prevention. Forecasted state-specific estimates of self-reported asthma prevalence—United States, 1998. *Morbidity and Mortality Weekly Report* 1998; 47:1022–1025.

12 Centers for Disease Control and Prevention. Surveillance for waterborne disease outbreaks—United States, 1997–1998. *Morbidity and Mortality Weekly Report* 2000; 49 (SS04):1–35.

13 Drugged waters: Does it matter that pharmaceuticals are turning up in water supplies? *Science News* (March 21) 1998; 153:187–189.

14 Centers for Disease Control and Prevention. Preliminary FoodNet data on the incidence of foodborne illnesses. *Morbidity and Mortality Weekly Report* 2002; 51(15): 325–329.

15 *Occupational Employment Statistics Survey by Occupation.* Washington, DC: U.S. Department of Labor, Bureau of Labor Statistics, 1997.

16 *Measuring Expenditures for Essential Public Health Services.* Prepared by Public Health Foundation for the Office of Disease Prevention and Health Promotion, Office of Public Health and Science, U.S. Department of Health and Human Services. November 1996, Washington DC.

17 *Privatization and Public Health: A Study of Initiatives and Early Lessons Learned.* Washington, DC: Public Health Foundation, September 1997. Research and writing supported by The Annie E. Casey Foundation, Baltimore, Maryland.

18 Himmelstein, D., et al. Quality of care in investor-owned vs. not-for-profit HMOs. *Journal of the American Medical Association* 1999; 282:159–163.

CHAPTER 12

Mental Health

The Hope of Science and Services

The mental health field is in transition. In the next ten years, a series of influential forces will emerge that could address problems that have plagued this field for a long time. Political support for parity—insurance coverage of mental illnesses that is comparable to that for more obviously physical disorders—combined with new frontiers in enhancing the scientific knowledge about mental illness, could provide a fortuitous climate for change. In many instances, these changes are inexorable and will demand new solutions to challenge the current status quo.

The main challenge for decision makers in mental health is the growing recognition that disability caused by mental disorders and serious mental illness is more significant than has previously been acknowledged. Shifting the focus from mortality rates to morbidity and disability issues, the WHO report on the *Global Burden of Disease* states that mental illness will replace cancer as the number two cause of disability in the next 10 years. In the United States, the Surgeon General's report on *Mental Health* has confirmed that in any one year, approximately 50 million Americans suffer from mental disorders, and that many do not seek help for their problem because of the stigma associated with this condition.

In spite of the many obstacles facing the mental health world at this time, there appear to be two forces for positive change in the next decade. The first basis for optimism derives from the hopes held out by biological and genetic research; the second is the implementation of parity for insurance coverage of mental illnesses at the same levels as "physical" illness. Neither of these forces will have all the answers for people with mental illness, and there will continue to be problems with the integration of policy and service systems. But there is every reason to believe that changes will incrementally improve the situation for people needing mental health services over the next 10 years.

CHALLENGES

Our forecast for mental health is affected by the many schisms that characterize society's responses to mental illness: The world of research holds out hope for better diagnostic and treatment modalities, but the care systems of treatment and rehabilitation, which are not integrated at present, may remain divided at the end of this decade. Although research is cautious about promising cures or cracking the genetic codes for major mental illnesses in the near future, emerging genetic and biological knowledge in concert with advances in imaging and computer technology will radically transform research methodology and generate useful information for clinical treatment and rational drug design. These will continue to grow rapidly in the near future and will contribute substantially to changing the face of mental health diagnosis and treatment.

A defining difference between mental and physical illness is the process by which mental illnesses are diagnosed. Historically, the diagnosis of mental illness has been dependent on clinical judgment, based on patient-reported symptoms and clinician assessment of behavior and symptoms. Treatment strategies to date have focused on symptom reduction (mainly through medications), and this emphasis has led to an ideological divide between those committed to pharmaceutical and technological solutions and those who see medications as only a partial (admittedly important) response to a "life crisis" condition. These two forces, although not necessarily mutually exclusive, could compete for funding if this schism persists.

Perhaps the most powerful force that keeps mental health systems anchored in their respective camps is the funding divide. The publicly funded mental health world currently bears the largest burden of responsibility for those with serious mental illness. This segregation between those in the public health system and those who are treated in the private sector will continue to stigmatize patients with severe mental illnesses; this divided system is not expected to materially change in 10 years.

Two additional national forces that will further affect the mental health world are anticipated demographic changes, and changes in provider partnerships that will challenge the status quo.

Mental health problems manifest themselves differently in different age groups and in the context of varied cultural norms. The aging of America, along with the anticipated increase of an ethnically mixed population will have major ramifications for the development of all health services, including mental health. Given the requirements for sensitivity in diagnosis and treatment of mental disorders, the need for age- and culturally sensitive solutions is being endorsed but will be difficult to implement across all systems of care.

Finally, the impending workforce "crisis" and its impact on services has been emerging as a concern in the provider world. At this time, there are strong calls to action to address the dwindling numbers of qualified clinicians. The clinical community has developed projections in every field that call for tremendous increases in professional groups. In many instances, these increases will not come to pass in 10 years unless extraordinary expenditures are undertaken immediately. This is unlikely to happen. What is more likely is that the traditional mix of services will change. The growth of self-help groups, and the eagerness with which these groups are inviting research to demonstrate their effectiveness, could challenge professional programs. If voluntary and self-help programs deliver on their objectives, and demonstrate to the payers that their interventions are effective, payers are increasingly going to prefer a self-care approach to treatment.

FACING THE PROBLEM AND THE FACTS

Mental illness generates fear in both those who experience it and those who come in contact with it. Historically, people with mental illness were hidden by their family members until the symptoms became too extreme to manage at home, when they were then admitted to and hidden in institutions. Suicide, then as now, was often a tragic outcome of this response. Societal fears and stigma colored and influenced funding levels for services as well as the types of services that were developed to respond to mental health needs.

Today, the hope for a more enlightened response to mental illness is being espoused by people recovering from mental illness, by their families, by mental health advocates, and by clinicians and scientists involved in discovering new knowledge about mental illness. The call for parity in access to services for mental illness is perhaps the most obvious sign of this new awareness.

Americans, however, are still not comfortable with mental illness. They spend up to $11 billion in out-of-pocket payments for mental health treatment, mostly to stop employers and insurance companies from finding out about their condition. When people with mental disorders seek help, they prefer to go to their primary care physician rather than a mental health specialist. The use of the Internet for self-help in mental health has been associated with patient preference for anonymity.

The impact that continued social denial about mental illness could have on the future of all knowledge-based economies has been highlighted in both the World Health Organization's *The Global Burden of Disease*, and *Mental Health: A Report of the Surgeon General*. Both reports bring mental illness into the forum of health issues in general, and link physical and mental illness in ways that express their similarities and not their differences.

The Surgeon General's report notes that in the United States about 20 percent of the adult population is estimated to be affected by mental disorders during any given year.[1] Mental health and mental illness cannot be ignored as conditions that do not affect "ordinary" people any more.

The WHO *Global Burden of Disease* report focuses on the loss of productivity in developed nations due to mental health problems, and issues a wake-up call for better management of these conditions. The most sobering fact emerging from this report is that unipolar depression will replace cancer as the second leading cause of morbidity in the next decade. The WHO report introduced an important concept in estimating the effects of both morbidity and mortality. This report noted that morbidity had far-reaching effects on a nation's economy. Psychological conditions contributed 1 percent to mortality, but comprised 11 percent of the disease burden worldwide. With this new yardstick, the WHO developed three potential scenarios for illness and disability in 2020 in developed regions of the world. In all scenarios (baseline, optimistic, and pessimistic), unipolar major depression,

Table 12-1. Projected future causes of disability

Baseline Scenario	Optimistic Scenario	Pessimistic Scenario
1. Iscemic heart disease	1. Iscemic heart disease	1. Iscemic heart disease
2. Cerebrovascular heart disease	2. *Unipolar major depression*	2. Cerebrovascular heart disease
3. *Unipolar major depression*	3. Cerebrovascular heart disease	3. *Unipolar major depression*
4. Trachea, bronchus and lung cancers	4. Trachea, bronchus and lung cancers	4. Trachea, bronchus and lung cancers
5. Road traffic accidents	5. Road traffic accidents	5. Road traffic accidents
6. *Alcohol use*	6. *Alcohol use*	6. *Alcohol use*
7. Osteoarthritis	7. Osteoarthritis	7. Osteoarthritis
8. *Dementia* and other degenerative and hereditary CNS disorders	8. *Dementia* and other degenerative and hereditary CNS disorders	8. *Dementia* and other degenerative and hereditary CNS disorders
9. Chronic obstructive pulmonary disease	9. Chronic obstructive pulmonary disease	9. Chronic obstructive pulmonary disease
10. Self Inflicted diseases	10. Self Inflicted diseases	10. Self Inflicted diseases

Source: Murray, Christopher, and Alan Lopez. *Global Health Statistics*. Harvard Center for Population and Development Studies, 1996.

alcohol use, and dementia rank in the top ten causes of disability, with unipolar major depression being in the top three causes among all three scenarios (Table 12-1). In addition, it is important to note that in many of the other conditions listed in these three scenarios (such as alcohol in road traffic accidents, and suicide attempts due to mental health problems), mental disorders often play a major role. Mental illness will be a growing cause of primary and secondary disability in the years to come.

THE PREVALENCE AND IMPACT OF MENTAL ILLNESS

In addition to providing detailed information about the depth and prevalence of mental illness in this country, the Surgeon General's report further notes that clinicians and others need to be aware of high rates of co-occurring disorders

within those who present with mental illness (about 3 percent). These people tend to have more chronic conditions and to be high users of health services (Table 12-2).

This report confirms that a huge number of people suffer from conditions related to their mental health, and that the magnitude of this impact is not yet fully understood by the general public, payers, providers, or public policymakers.

DETERMINING PRIORITIES FOR PUBLIC SPENDING

The Center for Mental Health Services, which provides states with block grants for mental health services, has developed policies to ensure that states allocate these grants to serving the needs of "the most seriously emotionally disturbed

Table 12-2. The most common mental health common disorders in the United States

Condition	Profile
Major Depression	Affects approximately 19 million adults (age 18–54) each year Affects nearly twice as many women as men Is treatable, but two out of three do not seek help Is often the side effect of major illness such as heart attack, stroke, diabetes, and cancer, and increases the risk of heart attack
Anxiety Disorders	Affect more than 16 million adults Include panic disorder, obsessive-compulsive disorder, post-traumatic stress disorder, social phobia, and generalized anxiety disorder Often complicated by depression, eating disorders, and substance abuse Often more than one disorder
Social Phobia	Affects 5.3 million adults Women twice as likely although men more likely to seek help Typically begins in childhood, rarely after age 25 Often accompanied by depression and may lead to alcohol and other substance abuse
Post-Traumatic Stress Disorder	Affects 5.2 million adults Women more at risk Can affect any age group Depression, anxiety disorder, substance abuse can accompany PTSD
Obsessive Compulsive Disorders	Affect 3.3 million adults Affect both sexes equally Social and economic losses resulting from OCDs total $8.4 billion a year
Bipolar Disorder	Affects more than 2.3 million adults 20 percent die by suicide Affects both sexes equally
Panic Disorders	Affect 2.4 million adults Usually young adulthood (before age 24) Women twice as likely Also likely to be depressed or with substance abuse problems
Schizophrenia	Affects 2 million adults In men usually appears in late teens or early twenties, in women in their late twenties to early thirties Affects both sexes with equal frequency Patients suffer chronically throughout their lives
Attention Deficit Hyperactivity Disorder (ADHD)	Affects 3 to 5 percent of youths age 9–17 in any 6-month period More boys (two to three times) than girls are affected Long-term impact on school work and social relationships Untreated disorder can lead to antisocial behavior, teenage pregnancy, drug abuse, injuries
Suicide	31,000 adults committed suicide in 1996 Almost all had a diagnosable mental disorder, most commonly depression or substance abuse Men more likely than women, with white men over age 85 most affected in United States In 1997, suicide was the third leading cause of death in 15- to 24-year-olds

Sources: *Mental Health: A Report of the Surgeon General,* 1999, and "The Numbers Count: Mental Disorders in America," NIH Publication No. 01-4584.

children and seriously mentally ill adults."[2] This latter category of serious mental illness includes persons diagnosed with schizophrenia, schizoaffective disorder, manic depressive disorder, autism, severe forms of major depression, panic disorder, or obsessive compulsive disorder. An additional criterion is the level of disability faced by these individuals, defined as significant impairment for the previous 12 months that precluded their participation in many of the acts of daily living (eating, bathing, dressing), instrumental living skills (maintaining a household, managing money, taking medications) and functioning in a social, family or vocational/ educational context. Children with diagnosable mental, behavioral, and emotional disorders are also covered by federal block grant funds. The definition also includes functional impairments, which interfere with their ability to function within their families, at school, or with their peers.

People with serious mental illnesses account for 5.4 percent of the population in most communities, while those with more severe and persistent illnesses account for 2.6 percent.

Many conditions, such as schizophrenia, exist in young adults who are no longer eligible for health insurance coverage through their parents' plans. Most private insurance coverage does not cover the life long needs of these patients, leaving patients dependent on either their families or their state and local services. Hence, the more severe the mental illness, the more likely it is that the patient will have to resort to the publicly funded care system. Although they are a very small proportion of the population,

these patients comprise the most severe cases and dominate public spending, often for the rest of their lives.

Mental health has a two-tiered payment system with illness and impairment-based inclusions and exclusions that are not, for the most part, paralleled in the physical health care system.

PUBLIC VERSUS PRIVATE SPENDING

Over the past decade, public payers (Medicare, Medicaid, state and local governments) have assumed a growing share of the mental health/substance abuse treatment costs. In fact, the public sector pays for almost two-thirds of substance abuse treatment and more than half of mental health treatment in America.

We forecast that public payers will continue to absorb a larger share of expenses for mental health care. Their share of costs will increase even more dramatically if the economy destabilizes, the percentage of uninsured Americans holds steady or increases over the next decade, and the number of individuals with serious mental illness increases in absolute numbers.

MENTAL HEALTH SPENDING GROWS SLOWER THAN SPENDING FOR ALL HEALTH CARE

Mental health and substance abuse spending growth averaged 6.8 percent a year between 1987 and 1997, while national health expenditures grew by 8.2 percent.[3] This slower rate of growth in mental health spending in comparison to general health spending is most likely the result of a trend to move patients out of hospitals and into community-based settings. The movement of patients out of hospitals and into community-based services is due to the devolution of the management of mental health services to the local and community levels, and, in part, to the advent of managed behavioral health care over the past 10 years.

CAVEATS

Current estimates of spending on mental illness are low in comparison with the need. The proportion of those with mental illness is expected to hover at around 20 percent by 2010. Given the overall population growth anticipated for the United States through 2010, the number of people needing care will outstrip growth in mental health spending. This serves as a warning that the gap is widening between addressing the needs of people with mental illness in comparison to those without mental illness.

It is important to note, however, that retail prescription drugs accounted for a growing share of mental health spending from 1987 to 1997, rising from 7.5 percent in 1987 to 12.3 percent in 1997. This cost will continue to climb, with hundreds of drugs for mental illness in the development pipeline.[4] Emerging technologies such as PET, SPECT, and MRI will add to the absolute costs spent on mental health care over the next decade.

There are some potential offsets that might affect some costs. If new drugs are effective and allow for effective rehabilitation of those in jails, prescription drugs and other new technologies may

serve to offset the costs associated with incarcerating individuals with mental illness. The costs of incarceration in state prisons per individual are estimated at an average of $20,000 per year.[5] This figure does not include the costs associated with the health and mental health treatment for these prisoners.

ECONOMIC AND SOCIAL COSTS OF MENTAL ILLNESS

In 1994, the total estimated economic cost to society of mental illness was $204.4 billion. About $91.7 billion (44.9 percent) of the total economic costs of mental illness were due to direct costs for medical care. Costs associated with loss of productivity due to illness were calculated at 43.2 percent and with premature death and lost productivity at 8.1 percent.[6]

Substantial health care costs for medical treatment and other services are associated with anxiety disorders, schizophrenia, and affective disorders. Affective disorders, such as depression, have greater mortality costs due to premature deaths (mainly suicides) than any of the other major mental health disorders. Anxiety disorders (such as panic disorders, phobias, and generalized anxiety disorders) have greater morbidity costs (such as reduced or lost productivity) than other major disorders.

Table 12-3 estimates the economic costs for the various key disorders. The impact of depression on workforce productivity (especially in a knowledge-based economy), and the loss of productivity ascribed to various mild to moderate mental health disorders are substantial.

Chapter 12: Mental Health

Table 12-3. Estimated economic costs of mental illness by type of disorder, 1994 (billions of dollars)[7]

Type of Cost	Anxiety Disorders	Schizophrenia	Affective Disorders	Other Disorders
Treatment/Health Care Service Costs	14.9	23.7	26.3	26.8
Mental Health Organizations	2.6	8.6	6.4	8.1
Short-Stay Hospitals	.5	3.4	6.1	7.5
Office-Based Physicians	.5	.5	1.5	2.2
Other Professional Services	.9	1.0	2.9	4.6
Nursing Homes	7.7	7.5	6.4	1.6
Drugs	1.5	.5	.5	.3
Support Costs	1.1	2.0	2.2	2.4
Morbidity Costs (Productivity loss due to illness)	47.8	15.0	3.1	22.4
Mortality Costs (Productivity loss due to premature death)	1.8	1.8	10.7	2.2
Other Related Costs	.5	4.4	1.9	1.3
Total	**79.8**	**68.4**	**68.0**	**79.4**

Source: SAMSHA Statistics Source Book.

CHANGE AGENTS IN RESEARCH

Biological research, specifically in the neurosciences, appears to hold the greatest potential for generating new knowledge about mental illnesses and for developing more effective tools for the prevention, diagnosis, and treatment of mental disorders. Although researchers are cautious about overstating the future, even small technological advances and incremental new knowledge about genetic risk and patterns of brain function are expected to generate useful, clinically relevant technologies or treatments. By the end of this decade, new directions will be forged from information generated by research in biological sciences.

The National Institute for Mental Health (NIMH) provides national leadership in determining research priorities for medical, neuroscientific, and behavioral research. The NIMH administers more than $170 million in grants for adult and geriatric research, child and adolescent treatment and prevention, and services research and clinical epidemiology.[8] To accelerate the pace of scientific discovery, the NIMH is advocating a strategy of shared knowledge, tools, and data. As the largest publicly funded research organization with a national mandate to develop new knowledge, the NIMH will influence major changes in the mental health world.

The NIMH's stated research goals shape both clinical and technical progress. The agency's three goals are

- to understand mental illness
- to understand how to treat and prevent mental illness
- to assure an adequate national capacity for research and dissemination

Two essential partners of the NIMH are the academic medical centers, which conduct most of the clinical research, and the pharmaceutical industry, which develops new medications, often in conjunction with the NIMH and the academic research community.

The academic research community is most often the generator of new knowledge, and the transfer of this knowledge to commercially viable treatment options links it to both the diagnostic and pharmaceutical industries. The academic community's role in clinical trials and in testing the efficacy and safety of new drugs makes it an integral partner with the pharmaceutical industry. The commercial objectives of the pharmaceutical companies and the large budgets involved, however, lead to consumer criticism that the scientific community is overly focused on pharmacological solutions.

Independent of the NIMH, the research-based pharmaceutical industry is establishing its own agenda in the private sector for the development of new drugs. With a collective $30 billion research budget in 2001 (up from $26.4 billion in 2000), pharmaceutical companies allocated $5.6 billion for products that

act on the central nervous system and sense organs, addressing diseases such as Alzheimer's, schizophrenia, depression, epilepsy, and Parkinson's. In the year 2000, there were at least 103 drugs in development for treating mental illnesses.[9]

These are not the only agencies involved in mental health research. Foundations, the Substance Abuse and Mental Health Services Administration (SAMHSA), University programs, and private grants fund a wide range of research projects. Some, like the private initiatives in genomic research, closely mirror the NIMH priorities and underscore the consensus around the importance of genomic research in general.

Since we think that the outcomes of neuroscience and technology are those likely to have a material impact on options for people with mental illnesses, we highlight these issues in the forecast. This is not to say that there is no research on other psychosocial issues. The need to understand the mind as well as the brain is a stated goal of the NIMH and other leaders in the field. But the reality of knowledge transfer continues to favor technological solutions; nontechnological developments are not easy to implement and therefore do not consistently affect service delivery, and in a field as fragmented and dispersed as this, we do not expect a major impact in the next decade. Within this context, we looked at the pace of change over the last two decades and concluded that the patterns of the past will persist: pharmaceuticals—aligned with two new partners, neuroscience research and computers—will continue to drive the system by providing more effective therapies than before. The mental health service world will continue to embrace technological opportunities faster than nontechnological interventions.

FORECAST

The following list highlights the major research outcomes that are forecast to occur in the next 10 years.

- Research in the neurosciences will create new information about the etiology and genetic basis of major mental illnesses.

- Research in molecular biology and genetics will provide greater diagnostic accuracy and better treatments in the mental health arena. By identifying *susceptibility genes* (the set of genes that create a predisposition to an illness), this research will also give rise to strategies to minimize the risk of onset, enhance patient resilience, and control environmental triggers.

- A new terminology for describing serious mental illnesses will begin to emerge and replace the current symptom-based approach.

- The overall research agenda will expand to include topics bearing on clinical practice, including relapse prevention and rehabilitation.

- New technologies (innovations in computer technology, drug-development methodologies, and diagnostic imaging) will enable the rapid development of new pharmaceuticals; in addition, new drug-

delivery systems will give clinicians and their patients more effective treatment options. The use of genetic data to target treatment responsiveness and to identify individuals likely to develop medication side effects is probable within the next 10 years. These innovations will have a significant impact on changing services to promote prevention and rehabilitation.

- New primary prevention strategies, including genetic testing and tracking of high-risk individuals, will prompt ethical debates and concerns about privacy and confidentiality.

- The Internet will emerge as a major tool not only in fostering collaboration among scientists but also in dispersing research findings to clinicians and, increasingly, the public.

- Social responses to these advances will manifest themselves in several ways. The first will be a widening schism between supporters of medication management and those who feel that there is an overemphasis on the use of technology to manage mental health. Second, there will be controversy over any proposals for genetic testing regarding susceptibility to disease. Finally, concerns over the confidentiality of mental health information, and over the consent required to be in a research trial will continue to challenge researchers and their agenda.

The following section details the direction this forecast could take in each of the areas identified above.

RESEARCH IN THE NEUROSCIENCES

In the field of neuroscience research, molecular biology (including genetics, pharmacology, and developmental research) and neuroimaging will provide pivotal information for understanding brain function, for diagnosing mental illness, and for developing treatment protocols. Rapid advances in computer technology will support this research.

The results of the Human Genome Project will create an unprecedented body of information about how the brain works. Key researchers warn against overstatement of the impact of this research, and note that it could be decades before all aspects of this research is concluded. Because 70 percent of genes are expressed in the brain and the central nervous system, genetic research will be the paramount preoccupation of major scientific research at the NIMH in the foreseeable future.[10]

In the next 10 years, researchers are likely to identify susceptibility genes, rather than a single genetic link, to most major mental illnesses. Susceptibility genes will be identified for schizophrenia, bipolar depression, and major depression. Susceptibility genes have already been identified for Alzheimer's disease and for many early childhood psychiatric and hereditary problems.[11]

Experts dismiss the development of any "gene therapy" (one that actually fixes defects in gene structure) in the next 10 years. However, if stem cell research develops and remains legal, the ability to clone and differentiate cells (possibly enabling the replacement of damaged brain cells) will open new treatment options, possibly including genetic manipulation. All in all, this research and the information it generates will provide greater diagnostic accuracy for all mental health problems in 10 years, and this in itself will contribute greatly towards defining proper treatment and service requirements for various conditions.

Identification of susceptibility genes is expected to trigger greater research in understanding (and perhaps controlling) environmental issues that trigger the onset of various diseases. This includes understanding factors that foster resilience (since not everyone who is susceptible or high risk is expected to progress to an onset of that disorder) or prevent the onset altogether. This is highly complex research, bringing together the worlds of social environment, stress management, coping strategies, and family engagement in ways that research is not currently designed to explore. This research is only just beginning (particularly in pediatrics), and will just be starting to explore its potential in 10 years.

The ability to diagnose mental disorders more accurately will lead to the need to adopt new terminology, based more on etiology and less on symptoms and resulting in material changes in the DSM IV.[12] While it is not expected that the DSM IV will be replaced in 10 years, we believe that it will begin to incorporate these tools into the development of diagnoses. Problems with diagnostic accuracy have presented challenges for clinicians, but the scientific evidence being developed that will

Chapter 12: Mental Health   **197**

improve diagnoses should diminish these problems in future.

RESEARCH IN PHARMACOLOGY

Medications have had a profound effect on service models in psychiatry, starting with drugs developed in the 1950s that enabled patients with schizophrenia to be treated in the community, rather than in state psychiatric hospitals. Pharmacology research entered a new era with the development of atypical antipsychotics about 10 years ago. In addition, the results of neuroscience research have led to new and revolutionary ways of evaluating drug effectiveness.

Over the coming decade, significant pharmacological innovation is expected in the following areas:

- The life cycle of new drug-development methodologies will shorten considerably and accelerate the speed at which drugs enter the marketplace. Science will enable pharmaceutical development to move away from time-consuming and costly trial-and-error drug development, and toward rational drug design. The ability to refine and improve drugs rapidly will be a major change from the past.

- More options to daily dosing, including patches, injections, and slow-release subcutaneous medications, will be available for more drugs. These options will increase therapeutic compliance for some and enable many to manage their symptoms with less disruption to their daily lives. New dosing options could also facilitate the shift of treatment into less acute settings, including primary care practices.

- Some drugs may be available to slow down or delay the onset of the more severe symptoms of some diseases (e.g., Alzheimer's disease).

- The use of genetic data to target treatment responsiveness and to identify individuals likely to develop medication side effects is probable within the next 10 years. The importance of this research is that it will target individual variations—incorporating age, gender, and any identified variations due to race and ethnic identity into the development of dosage and drug characteristics.

The important issue is that patients will have more choices. Not all patients will choose to use drugs, but for those who do use them, the fact that the drugs will have fewer side effects, could be more effective, and work in a shorter time frame is very good news. And this is likely to happen in the short space of 10 years.

RESEARCH IN NEUROIMAGING

Three imaging tools poised to expand their functionality in the mental health world are Positron Emission Technology (PET), Single Photon Emission Tomography (SPECT), and functional Magnetic Resonance Imaging (fMRI). SPECT and PET move studies of the brain from static views to continuous observations that enhance diagnosis and track the progress of treatment; functional imaging allows scientists to view brain function in real time. Rapid advances in these technologies will provide new information on:

- drug interactions

- signs of early onset of certain mental illnesses

- the effects of aging

- brain development processes in early childhood

- the development of brain disorders

- the impact of trauma

These technologies will build on developments now in use in cancer research and treatment.[13] As the cost of the technology decreases, neuroimaging will become clinically available in mental health. Among the first to benefit will be patients who have Alzheimer's disease or a serious mental illness.

RESEARCH IN COMPUTER TECHNOLOGY

Advances in computer technologies have greatly accelerated research in all areas of health, including mental illness. Computer technology has affected research in mental health in the following ways:

- harnessing immense and rapid data analyses

- modeling and analyzing drug responsiveness, leading to "rational" drug design

- facilitating the Internet as a tool for researchers, as well as supporting clinicians and consumers who are searching for current information

Computer technology's contributions to mental health research will derive from the capacity to store, interpret, model, and analyze large quantities of information. The development of data banks on early childhood development, and on highly complex multidisciplinary data sets for neuroscientific and biologic research, cannot happen without the power of computer technology.

Computer-aided drug design has become the norm. The ability to test compounds in high-throughput screening for binding to known neurotransmitter receptors will help to predict drug responses based on individual genetic variations. In 10 years, the ability to model human response to various drugs is very likely and will also allow safer clinical testing of new pharmaceuticals.

The Internet will be a huge asset to researchers, clinicians, and consumers. Its role in the Human Genome Project has already been demonstrated since the entire gene sequence is now available for researchers. The ability of clinicians to connect and share research on an international basis is just emerging, and the availability of large data banks makes the future world of research different from what we have known. In addition, the Internet facilitates interdisciplinary communication among research and clinical scientists. Clinicians' ability to access the latest study findings and to seek professional input into treatment plans for complex cases will be enhanced in 10 years. Finally, consumers and family members will be able to access the latest research news through the Internet, making them more educated and more aware of their options for treatment.

RESEARCH ON SOCIAL IMPLICATIONS

The role of medications in managing serious mental illnesses is unlikely to change over the next 10 years. However, public concern about the use of medications in mental health will continue to grow. Current controversies over the increase in the use of psychopharmaceuticals in children and the proliferation of such drugs as Prozac and other mood-disorder medications are a harbinger of things to come. The consumer movement is quite active in mental health areas and emphatically supports patient freedom of choice, especially in the area of drug treatment.

Pressure to demonstrate the effectiveness of nonmedication alternatives to treatment for mild to moderate mental health disorders will result in more treatment choices for patients, and more evidence about the effectiveness of combination therapies.

Social controversy over genetic testing will grow in the next decade. It is anticipated that there will be increasing challenges in the courts on the grounds of human and civil rights violations of people with mental illness. The impact of various genetic studies, the long-term effects of drug trials, and disease risk tracking in general will be controversial. In addition, advocacy groups will take up confidentiality issues posed by genetic testing. These groups will want regulations to govern the conditions under which genetic information can be used.

Confidentiality of mental health information will be addressed in 3 ways:

- Technological solutions will become more sophisticated and will include the encryption of data and increasing restriction of access to patient information.

- State, federal, or organizational regulations around privacy will be enacted and enforced, with appropriate penalties for violations.

- Protocols for patients' consent to participate in research trials will become more complex.[15]

Perhaps the greatest positive impact of the new research will be in the reduction of stigma. The ability to demonstrate biological evidence for mental illness will be a major factor in bringing both policymakers and the public to a new understanding of mental health disorders.

EMERGING RESEARCH TOPICS

As the Surgeon General's report notes, "No gene is equivalent to fate for mental illness." Biological research provides road maps and clues to mental illness— but the brain is not the mind and the need to understand such issues as factors that develop resilience to mental illness and that increase susceptibility to environmental stressors are of growing interest in research. Issues that affect the quality of life for people recovering from mental illness will also become a focus of research and treatment.

The following topics are being researched and could be future forces for creating improved mental health treatment programs:

- large-scale multicenter trials that organize, study, report, and develop implementation guidelines of best practice, including the use of pharmaceuticals

- clinical trials that include under-studied populations (e.g., children and older adults)

- epidemiologic and population-based studies on how different racial and ethnic groups interact with the formal mental health system

- multicenter trials in primary care centers where patients present a wide range of mental disorders

- studies of new tools (including self-screening tools) for screening depression in primary care

- studies to determine the effectiveness of self-help models and support groups in treating disorders, preventing relapse, and providing maintenance services

- studies of the role of families, especially those with a child affected by mental illness, in preventing relapse and avoiding recidivism

- studies of alternative therapies, including herbal remedies

Among the current roster of studies under way, those relating to the role of the primary care sector and to the role of rehabilitation after severe or acute mental illness are perhaps most likely to produce changes in the mental health system. In both cases, new participants with new skills appear ready to formalize their role in managing mental illness.

TRANSFERRING RESEARCH TO PRACTICE

The NIMH has acknowledged that transferring knowledge from research to practice has been slow, sporadic, and not always related to clinical practice. In response, the NIMH's National Advisory Mental Health Council has established an ambitious agenda.[16] It aims to provide a more inclusive tone, to reflect clinical and consumer input, to look at whether the review process hinders or dictates methodologies that are not appropriate for all research, and to develop new sampling and methodological approaches.

MENTAL HEALTH SERVICES CHANGES IN THE NEXT DECADE

Mental health care services are delivered through two systems—one publicly funded and the other privately sponsored. While this structure mirrors the overall health system, mental health's "two tiered" system results in people with serious and disabling mental illnesses being at greater risk of defaulting to the public system. There are two reasons for this. First, some serious mental illnesses have their onset in late adolescence, when young people are no longer covered by their parents' health insurance but have not yet established adequate employment bases to qualify for their own insurance. Second, given the discrepancies in current coverage for mental illness, those who do have insurance soon exhaust their coverage for acute mental health benefits. Their recourse at this point is either to pay for these services out of pocket or to qualify for public services. Such a shift does not occur as often with serious physical illnesses. The movement to achieve parity between physical and mental health insurance coverage is expected to bring access to mental health services on a par with access to all other health services, but its impact on changing this two-tiered system will be evident only minimally in the next 10 years.

SERVICE UTILIZATION

The publicly funded mental health system is the social safety net and provides a substantial portion of care for people affected by serious mental illnesses: schizophrenia, schizoaffective disorder, manic depressive disorder, autism, severe forms of major depression, panic disorder, and obsessive-compulsive disorder. Many of these people require multiple social services (low-cost housing, transportation, education, vocational assistance, etc.), rely on county emergency departments for care, and have high rates of relapse. A small number need hospitalization in an acute setting. Those whose illnesses fit the criteria of serious mental illness often depend on the public system to provide lifetime care.

The public system also provides mental health services through community mental health and substance-abuse treatment centers and in hospitals. Children receive mental health services through multiple agencies at their schools and within the community. Juvenile and correctional services provide mental health diagnosis and treatment (funded separately from the health system) for inmates with mental health needs. In addition, the publicly funded system is responsible for the mental health needs of people who are homeless or uninsured or who cannot afford private mental health care.

According to a survey conducted by the researchers with the National Comorbidity Survey (NCS), 28.1 percent of the U.S. population was affected by a diagnosable mental or addictive disorder.[17] The prevalence of mental disorders, excluding substance abuse, is estimated at around 20 percent for adults in the United States. NCS research data further illustrated that people access a wide range of services, from highly specialized mental health services to care provided by the "volunteer sector," including family, friends, spiritual leaders, churches, and self-help groups. The percentage of the adult U.S. population using mental or addictive disorder services in one year was reported as follows:

- 6.4 percent used their general medical health system.

- 5.9 percent used specialty mental/addictive health services.

- 3.0 percent sought services from other human services professionals.

- 4.1 percent turned to the volunteer services sector.

The most important finding of this study is that when overlaps and duplications of services were accounted for, barely half (14.7 percent) of the 28.1 percent of the population with a mental health need actually reported using the health system. Making services more accessible, and helping people find services will be a major challenge for the mental health system in the near future.

When patients do seek mental health services, there are a myriad of entry points through which they can obtain help. Each entry point has its own philosophy and criteria for managing the same condition. A patient with depression will receive very different services in the voluntary services network, in the paid service sector (psychologists, psychiatrists, other therapists), in the community mental health system, and in emergency departments.

This fragmentation of the mental health system is a well-documented problem. Although mental health services are available, and in some settings are organized to facilitate links among services, such coordination is not the norm. The consistency with which referrals occur depends first on the patient's ability to pay for services and then on the system's referral services and relationships. People who are recovering from severe mental illnesses require regular and frequent contact with medical services to organize their medication management. If the care of these patients isn't coordinated, they often appear in hospital emergency rooms—a regular source of care for people who are both mentally ill and homeless.

The system is particularly fragmented when patients present with co-occurring conditions (e.g., mental health disorders and substance abuse problems). Clinicians and researchers have demonstrated the need to address multiple co-morbidi-ties simultaneously, but few programs are organized to provide these services in a coordinated way.

FORECAST

The following list summarizes the major changes anticipated in the mental health service system during the next decade. A detailed discussion of each issue follows.

- Unless the current service system changes dramatically, growth and change in population demographics will overwhelm it in 10 years. The aging of the population and the rapid growth in the number of children and adolescents of diverse ethnic and racial groups will significantly challenge current systems.

- Fragmentation and a lack of coordination within service delivery systems will continue to impede implementation of service models that have demonstrated good outcomes.

- Technological advances will be a two-edged sword. New technologies, especially pharmaceuticals, will be very expensive and yet will be adopted rapidly within both the public and private mental health service systems. While new drugs may enable more compliance with medications and potentially ensure better outcomes, they will compete with all other mental health services for scarce financial resources.

- The Internet will emerge as a major resource for consumers and service providers.

- The growing self-help movement will take root alongside traditional service models.

- Employers will expand Employee Assistance Programs (EAPs) to provide greater access to services earlier in the onset of mental health problems.

- The workforce mix will change as will the roles of traditional service providers in mental health. The role of psychiatry will become more focused on providing highly specialized medical interventions for people with very complex mental illnesses; primary care physicians will assume a greater role in providing general mental health services; and nontraditional care providers will assist the traditional service system to meet expanding needs.

THE IMPACT OF DEMOGRAPHIC CHANGE

The population of the United States will increase from 273 million in 1999 to over 300 million in 2010, or by roughly 10 percent in this decade. With experts estimating that 20 percent of all Americans experience some form of mental disorder each year, mental health care providers must prepare for a significant increase in the demand for services. The rate of population growth will be higher among groups that have special needs and tend to have greater difficulty accessing mental health services. These vulnerable groups include older people, children, and people of different ethnic and racial backgrounds whose mental health needs are generally unmet. Their utilization of services varies dramatically in comparison to the general population, and their mental health outcomes are affected by the cultural context of services provided. The potential for creative solutions using shared resources, telecommunications, and alternative settings for service is great, but these improvements are unlikely to be funded and implemented before demographic changes increase the demand on clinical services.

SYSTEM FRAGMENTATION

Pockets of excellence exist within the public mental health care system, and these organizations have often led the way in integrating services (such as Systems of Care initiatives for children). Regrettably, integrated programs are few and far between, and most parts of the current mental health system will remain fragmented in the future. Public health leaders have called for a "mainstreaming" of mental health services, underscoring the need to address mental health needs in the same way that we plan and fund other health programs. Such a change will require massive restructuring of government agencies, funding, and organizational policies, and is unlikely to be accomplished in the next 10 years. However, there is no doubt that these calls will increase as mental health's links to all other health conditions are highlighted by scientific advances, and the barriers between the mental health profession and other health professions will disappear over time.

THE IMPACT OF TECHNOLOGICAL ADVANCES

Medications and new diagnostic technologies will allow for quicker, more effective management of various mental

Service Coordination for People with Mental Illness and Substance Abuse

Three percent of adults have both mental health and substance-abuse disorders. The Surgeon General's report notes that these individuals are likely to use more health services. In addition, they have high rates of co-morbidity, which affects the service mix they need. In 1997, the Substance Abuse and Mental Health Services Administration (SAMHSA) reported that most treatment models for substance abuse were outpatient-based and that clients of these treatment facilities were primarily young, with Caucasians representing 57–61 percent of the client load and African Americans making up 21–25 percent. Less than half of the facilities reviewed by SAMHSA offered programs for those who were diagnosed with both disorders. Only 38 percent provided programs for adolescents. Although more effective pharmaceuticals will become available to manage substance abuse, the coordination of these medications with those for mental illness will require considerable expertise.[18] Consequently, this cohort of people with both mental illness and substance abuse problems will continue to have limited access to effective, coordinated treatment programs.

However, self-help programs such as Alcoholics Anonymous (AA) have fueled a growing self-help movement for patients with both mental illness and substance abuse diagnoses.[19] Given the growing use of medication treatment for the two disorders, these groups have developed alternative 12-step programs for their unique needs. Preliminary studies indicate that self-help groups can be successful with co-morbid patients. Long-term studies are pending, but self-help programs for this group are expected to grow in future.

illnesses and will increase the number of candidates for recovery programs. New medications will continue to reduce the number of patients who require hospitalization and will shorten the length of those hospitalizations.[20] The number of psychiatric beds in hospitals will continue to decline as inpatient admissions decrease, and the remaining beds will be primarily for the small numbers of patients who have acute crises. The elimination of daily dosing, better-defined dosage levels, and fewer side effects should continue to improve symptom management and patient compliance and allow more patients to utilize services in community-based settings.

The number of psychiatric acute beds (in both specialized and general hospitals) declined throughout the 1980s and 1990s, and this reduction is expected to continue for the next decade even though more private psychiatric hospitals are now offering overnight services.[21] Inpatient days dropped from 475 per 1000 patients in 1988 to 275 per 1000 in 1997.[22] State mental health hospitals are excluded from accessing federal community mental health service block grants awarded to states, and this adds to the pressure on states to reduce the use of inpatient services. Some experts argue that state mental hospitals should be phased out entirely, but this is unlikely to happen in the next 10 years.

As genetic links to mental illness are discovered they will raise the issue of opportunities for prevention. Currently, there are few effective strategies for preventing the onset of mental illnesses. When scientists identify susceptibility genes for serious mental illnesses, testing individuals for risk could be the next step. Without the availability of any real prevention programs to offer these individuals, the value of identifying risk will provoke heated ethical debates about patient consent, privacy, and the legitimate use of genetic data. Hence the real value of genetic screening will be limited until there are effective prevention services.

THE INTERNET

The Internet is growing as a particularly useful tool for people with mental disorders because of the anonymity it affords. It has become a major source of information about, and communication among, people with mental health needs. In addition, the growing self-help movement and Internet use are mutually reinforcing. At present there are over 200 websites related to mental health, ranging from those of government agencies to advocacy organizations and support groups. The website of the National Mental Health Self-Help Clearinghouse provides technical training, advice on establishing self-help groups, information about local organizations, and data about mental health policies.

As more patients seek the greater flexibility allowed by electronic communications, a growing cadre of clinicians will turn to the Internet as a means of providing clinical care.[23] Although telemedicine is unlikely to replace the initial development of a clinician-consumer relationship, follow-up will be done on the Internet if the patient prefers. Some health plans already provide Internet-based behavioral health services for their enrollees (e.g., Epotec On-Line Behavioral Health).

The pace of these changes will accelerate as the following barriers are overcome:

- Concerns about patient privacy are addressed.

- User-friendly, inexpensive Internet access becomes available, making Internet access as simple as a phone call is today.

- Licensure issues for the provision of support and clinical services across states are resolved.

- Guidelines for telemedicine and clinical practice are developed.

The impact of Internet technology on mental health care is just beginning to be understood, and it is hard to predict how much material change in the service delivery system will occur due to this technology. Wireless transmission, systems of access that do not require computers, and a technology that is ubiquitous will offer opportunities that we cannot now envision. Already, technology makes it possible for clinicians to process prescriptions, manage appointments, and receive results using the Internet. Given the stresses forecast for the mental health system, the Internet could provide major support to both clinicians and patients.

THE EMPOWERED CONSUMER AND THE GROWING SELF-HELP MOVEMENT

The new consumer movement in mental health is expected to spearhead many changes within the service sector.[24] The main contribution of this movement is to change the profile of the mental health consumer from a passive recipient of services to an active participant in decision making about care. This recovery model emphasizes post-illness rehabilitation and independence. As medical treatment outcomes improve and patients can be returned to functional independence, rehabilitation will assume a greater treatment role both for the chronically ill and for those with moderate to mild disorders.

The recovery model reflects the belief that medical and pharmaceutical management is only part of the treatment for mental health disorders. Individuals with chronic mental illnesses also need

Self-Help Within a Managed Care Plan

Value Options, currently the third-largest managed behavioral care company in the United States, covers 3.8 million Medicaid recipients in six states under 18 separate contracts. It has implemented a successful self-care program to rehabilitate patients with serious mental illnesses within state mental health programs. The goals are to help these individuals maintain an optimal state of recovery between episodes, to provide them with support, and to teach them to recognize potential signs of relapse and take appropriate action to prevent relapses.

Value Options uses a multi-system treatment model, which provides training and the support required to set up self-help groups. Within four years of implementing a self-help model, the numbers of groups within its service area grew to 45 in 1998. Using a Quality of Life Interview Data questionnaire they were able to demonstrate statistically significant improvement in social functioning. They were also able to demonstrate higher levels of service penetration to serve a more seriously ill population than anticipated.

An important variable identified by Value Options in engendering success was the support of their professional clinical service providers. Without this support, such programs not only do not come to the attention of their patients, but also affect patient confidence in participation.

help rebuilding and maintaining family, social, and work relationships and skills that will allow them to regain as much functional independence as possible. While most patients and advocates agree that medications are essential in many cases, they emphasize the need for adjunct services that help prevent future episodes and re-establish patient self-esteem.

Self-help and peer support groups have evolved from the consumer movement and teach participants to overcome the "learned helplessness" that is brought on by dependence and social isolation. The stigma attached to their disease exacerbates these feelings.[25] Self-help groups provide services using trained peer leaders and professionals and are based on the premise that "people with a shared condition who come together can help themselves and each other to cope,"[26] but philosophy, structure, and approach vary. Approximately 3 percent of Americans who have a mental disorder or illness participated in some form of self-help group at any one time.

Self-help consumers are among the most intrepid users of online information and resources,[27] and self-help services will continue to proliferate on the Internet. America Online, for example, hosts more than 400 live self-help groups each month.[28] Studies have shown that participation in self-help groups can result in decreased perception of isolation, increased practical knowledge of an illness, increased awareness of available options, and increased ability to cope with an illness overall. In the long term, these benefits can lead to reduced rates of hospitalization, to better health, and to an increased sense of well-being.

Rehabilitation of patients affected by schizophrenia, severe depression, and other more serious illnesses is a major new trend. Successful rehabilitation and recovery of all patients will relieve pressure on the mental health system.[29] However, rehabilitating people with chronic conditions will require additional resources and infrastructure since these are new services, not currently in widespread use. Current programs, such as the Assertive Community Treatment (ACT) program or Intensive Case Management (ICM) developed originally through the Patient Outcomes Research Team (PORTS) efforts of the NIMH are widely adopted and endorsed by state mental health departments. Another popular model is the Clubhouse model, which is widely implemented. Both of these models will find that their clients and client needs will change in 10 years since they will be using better medications, and that they will need a different mix of services than are provided today. Self-help models may have preempted the more organized professional groups in anticipating the future needs of their community.

As more research is conducted to assess the efficacy of self-help interventions, self-help is likely to prove extremely cost-effective and to become a component of both public and private care.

EMPLOYERS AND LOST PRODUCTIVITY

Large employers are expected to emerge as the real leaders in the area of mental health system reform in the next decade. Employer interest in maintaining the health of the workforce is a key ingredient in health system reform. In addition to the costs of treatment, depression is estimated to cost employers $11.7 billion annually in absenteeism from work, and $12.1 billion in lost productivity.[30] Coupled with the impact of substance abuse on employee productivity, these facts could prompt employers to look at issues that they feel the health services sector is not handling in a timely manner. The real change in this instance will be not in service delivery, but in including a variety of mental health services within EAPs.

Some major corporations have already enhanced their EAPs to provide information, screening, and support for disease prevention and mental health–

maintaining behaviors.[31] In time, more large employers will act to make sure that such services are available to their employees. The cost of lost productivity will provide the economic motive, but employers and employees must also overcome the stigma attached to mental disorders.

THE CHANGING WORKFORCE

Primary Care. Primary care physicians have always been the first point of health care contact for patients. Historically there has been evidence that mental disorders were not diagnosed and treated properly in a general medical setting. Researchers in the field of general medicine feel that this is changing, and that patient willingness to address mental health problems with their primary care physicians is the first step in this direction.

Patients' personal preferences and fear of the stigma of seeing mental health specialists will continue to lead them to seek help from their primary care doctor. A survey of five primary care practices reported that when patients were identified as having "emotional distress," 60 percent wanted counseling through their primary care services, 33 percent wanted medication, and only 5 percent wanted a referral to a mental health specialist.[32]

The number of practicing psychiatrists is expected to decline due to reductions in the numbers of medical students electing to enter this specialty. Primary care physicians will have little choice but to continue to manage their patients' mental health needs.

Primary care will continue to develop partnerships with psychiatrists and other mental health clinicians, allowing more patients to be treated in the primary care setting. There are a number of multi-center trials testing new diagnostic tools that will facilitate the screening of at-risk patients in the primary care setting.[33] Furthermore, new medications will make it easier for primary care doctors to manage the treatment of most mild to moderate mental illness on an ambulatory basis. These doctors will refer to psychiatrists only those patients whose needs are severe or complex.

The Role of the Psychiatrist. Just at a time when there are greater efforts to reduce the stigma associated with seeking mental health care, the numbers of mental health specialists are shrinking. Fewer medical students are selecting psychiatry as a specialty, although the numbers of available residencies have remained steady. Within the sub-specialists, shortages of psychiatrists with interests in gerontological psychiatry, childrens' mental health, and child development could create major access problems in the future. Concurrently, resources to provide culturally competent services that mirror the needs caused by growing racial and ethnic diversity in the population will not meet the needs of the population.

Leaders in the field have identified the need for a new role for psychiatrists. In the coming decade, psychiatrists will provide specialist services that address the needs of patients who do not respond to standard treatment protocols and will also manage medication therapy

for a wide range of patients. This is inevitable, given the continued reductions in the psychiatry workforce forecast for this decade.

CHANGES IN THE WORKFORCE MIX

The following changes are forecast in the workforce mix as a response to new therapies, innovative post-acute recovery programs, new technologies, and the limited availability of psychiatrists in the future:

- Counselors, psychologists, and social workers will assume more significant roles in both the public and private mental health systems. Managed care already uses these clinicians to reduce the costs of care, and the future shortage of psychiatrists will generate more demand for these professionals.

- New diagnostic and treatment models—especially the development of more effective drugs—will allow psychiatrists to manage more patients than in the past. In addition, the ability of primary care physicians to manage more patients with better medications will allow psychiatrists to manage those with more complex medication needs.

- More foreign-trained physicians will take psychiatric residencies and will provide some relief to the public mental health system in the next decade.

- General practitioners will create new partnerships with mental health professionals.

Complementary and Alternative Medicine (CAM)

If traditional providers cannot meet the growing demand for mental health care, there is every indication that other alternatives will emerge to augment, and even challenge, their roles.

The use of Complementary and Alternative Medicines (CAM) is on the rise in the United States. In 1998, the Congress established the National Center for Complementary and Alternative medicine (NCCAM) at the National Institutes of Health to "stimulate, develop, and support research on CAM for the bene-fit of the public."[34] This reflects the fact that about one-third to one-half of Americans admit to using alternative therapies, and are expected to spend close to $27 billion a year on complementary therapies (an increase of almost 46 percent compared to expenditures in 1990), most of it paid for out of pocket.[35] This spending exceeds out-of-pocket spending for all U.S. hospitalizations. In one survey, almost all patients were seeing a physician, but 72 percent did not tell their doctors they were using nontraditional medicines as well, prompting one researcher to advise mental health clinicians to ask their patients about any other treatments they were receiving in order to manage drug interactions and to address conflicting advice.[36] Almost two-thirds of U.S. medical schools offer courses in alternative medicine and 47 percent of doctors in one study admitted to using alternative therapies themselves.

Alternative medicine practitioners use herbs and vitamins, acupuncture, spiritual healing, massage, guided imagery, hypnosis, and stress release for patients who have anxiety and other mental health needs. Most people who use alternative medicine do so to maintain good health and prevent disease, to "boost" their immune system, and to fight infections. Interest in alternative treatments has prompted pharmaceutical companies to add natural and herbal supplements to their commercial lines.

Some health insurance companies cover acupuncture and chiropractic care, but most alternative care is paid for directly by patients. A Milbank Memorial Fund report lists a wide range of health plans that recently have begun providing some coverage for alternative medicine. The use of CAM will grow in the next 10 years, and traditional medicine will need to acknowledge that these practices appeal to people who perceive that there is a lack of interest within traditional medicine in holistic, integrated, mind/body care.

POLICY AND LEGISLATION

Policymaking for mental health care is, and will continue to be, broadly distributed among all three branches at the federal, state, county, and municipal levels of government. Upcoming policy debates will be dominated by the issues of parity, the role of managed care in the public and private health care systems, and the expansion of the civil rights of people affected by mental illnesses. Progress in the effort to remove the stigma of mental illness will in part determine the tenor of these discussions.

FORECAST

- The U.S. Congress will follow the lead of the states and enact federal parity requirements in mental health and substance abuse.

- Eligibility for Medicaid will expand, but the portion of Medicaid funding allocated to mental health services will grow more slowly than funding for general health services.

- States will continue to shift responsibility for mental health care to the counties, and state and county agencies will subcontract out specialized services.

- In the private sector, managed behavioral health care will thrive.

PARITY IN FEDERAL LEGISLATION

The Mental Health Parity Act of 1996 imposed federal standards on mental health coverage offered under most employer-sponsored group health plans. That law prohibits employer plans from imposing annual or lifetime dollar limits on mental health coverage that are more restrictive than those imposed on medical and surgical coverage. Three types of insurance coverage are exempt, however:

- plans sponsored by an employer with 50 or fewer employees

- group plans that experience an increase in claims costs of at least 1 percent because of compliance

- coverage sold in the individual (non-group) market

Scientific evidence for the biological basis of mental illness, the gradual removal of mental illness stigmas, and the lobbying efforts of better-organized consumers favor the expansion of parity. Before 2010, Congress will enact legislation to mandate more comprehensive coverage for mental health benefits and ban the imposition of higher co-payments or deductibles for mental health care.

THE FEDERAL EMPLOYEE HEALTH BENEFITS PROGRAM

The Federal Employees Health Benefits (FEHB) program is required to provide parity in mental health coverage for its 9 million federal employees and their dependents. This program often serves as a benchmark for private sector benefit plans. Because of the FEHB requirement, parity likely will be offered in the private sector for all DSM IV illnesses by 2010, especially if initial studies of the cost-effectiveness of parity in the FEHB program are encouraging.

A unique feature of the FEHB program is that beneficiaries choose from an extensive menu of health plan options; they may elect to pay a minimum amount for a basic, "no-frills" package or to pay more for a plan with more benefits. This element of choice, combined with out-of-pocket expenses for increased coverage, serves as a template for a hybrid model of purchasing health

insurance in the private sector. Under this model, employees would have the option to choose a health plan (either in the open market or from a menu of plans laid out by an employer) that offers basic or substantial mental health benefits. With federal parity enacted by 2010, all plans would be required to provide at least a minimal level of mental health coverage, thus reducing the threat of adverse risk selection.

PARITY IN STATE LEGISLATION

Many states have parity laws that exceed the basic standards set by the federal statute. Some states require coverage only for a set of biologically based mental illnesses, whereas others are more generous and include coverage for substance abuse. Studies show an increase in insurance premiums from 1 to 4 percent in states that require full parity. The cost increase to employers offering coverage depends upon the level of the benefits offered to employees before parity was enacted. Employers who formerly offered very limited or no benefits see a higher range of premium costs. Employers with more generous prior benefits and who use managed care approaches to mental health see little or no difference or perhaps a decline in premium costs.

THE UNINSURED

Efforts to expand parity will not affect the uninsured and the underinsured, and no serious momentum is driving lawmakers to find a way to provide mental health coverage for these populations. In 2010, only 56 percent of Americans will receive health insurance from their employers or through the individual market. Public health programs (Medicare and Medicaid) will insure 29 percent, and 15 percent will have no insurance, with the ranks of the uninsured increasing by 500,000 per year through 2010.

We forecast that the gulf will widen between the "haves" and the "have nots." Parity will mean nothing to the uninsured, and people affected by chronic or severe mental illness will continue to be at risk for homelessness, incarceration, and premature death.

FUNDING AND THE ROLE OF MANAGED CARE

The public sector funds 53 percent of mental health care. Public sector services are directly operated by government agencies and include state and county mental hospitals as well as services financed through Medicaid and Medicare. Both state Medicaid and private insurers depend heavily on managed health care to provide mental health services.

The federal government plays a smaller role in financing care for mental illness than in financing general health care, generally about 35 percent of care, as opposed to 46 percent. Federal programs include block grants for adults and children with serious mental illnesses and disorders, as well as safety-net services for individuals who have severe mental illnesses or who are indigent. In relative spending terms, however, these grants are small in comparison to other grant dollars for health care and they are less important to mental health than they are to substance-abuse prevention and treatment.

While federal funding for mental health is increasing in absolute dollars, it is decreasing as a percentage of the federal health care budget. The Substance Abuse and Mental Health Services Administration reports that expenditures for mental health and substance-abuse treatment represented 7.8 percent of all U.S. health care expenditures in 1997, down from 8.8 percent in 1987. This trend will continue over the next 10 years.

STATE AND LOCAL SPENDING

By and large, the states play a larger role than the federal government does in financing mental health care. State- and county-funded mental health services are a catchall for people unable to obtain private health insurance. These services are part of a complex web of social services that include health, social welfare, housing, criminal justice, and education. States distribute their funding for mental health services in three ways: In 5 states, the state mental health agency runs local health centers and agencies; in 25 states, the state distributes money to county governments, which fund local agencies; and in 20 states, the state mental health agency directly contracts with local agencies.

Most states rely on a discounted fee-for-service system for mental health services. If the federal government continues to allow the states greater flexibility in funding allocations for mental health services, more states will privatize their mental health systems through contracts with corporations. With costs and administrative pressures increasing, states—especially the larger states—will continue to shift mental health care costs onto local entities, which will develop county-based systems. The 750 local and county mental health systems in the United States will assume an increasing share of the cost of caring for the mentally ill.

Local systems with financial resources, determination, and skills can often provide high-quality mental health care. But many local governments—especially those in rural counties, many of which currently provide no mental health services at all—are shifting the risk to community mental health organizations. To improve efficiency and reduce costs, we believe that local and state systems will become better integrated. As the states continue to devolve mental health services to the local level, local agencies will create integrated mental health programs funded through a single source.

Medicaid is the primary payer of public mental health services, and states rely heavily on Medicaid funding for community mental health services. Roughly 25 percent of individuals under age 65 who qualify for Medicaid by disability status have a severe mental disorder. In all, Medicaid represents 19 percent of total mental health expenditures by payer.

Despite the exodus of the "welfare-to-work" population from the Medicaid program, we forecast that the total pool of people in Medicaid will increase over the next 10 years. These people will require more general health services (particularly given the fact that many individuals covered completely by Medicaid are the Supplemental Security Income (SSI) population, most of whom are disabled and require extensive gen-

eral health care services). Consequently, a smaller proportion of Medicaid funds will be available for mental health services over the coming decade.

MEDICAID MANAGED CARE

Relationships between the states and managed care organizations are tenuous, with local forces in each community shaping the experience. Many states contract with private managed behavioral health organizations (MBHOs), which have the information systems management and financial management skills needed to administer programs for large populations. But other states have ended their contracts with MBHOs because the MBHOs have failed to provide care for certain populations or have been inaccurate or late in making provider payments. Furthermore, MBHOs have complained that payment levels from states are inadequate and, consequently, are reducing their partnership with the Medicaid market.

We forecast that states and counties will retain control of their mental health systems but, despite the contentious issues surrounding Medicaid managed care, will continue to contract with private managed care organizations (MBHOs) for niche services, such as information systems management, utilization review, and outcomes monitoring. This is also the preference of many MBHOs, which have found statewide comprehensive care management contracts unprofitable and thus prefer to provide specialized managed care services. Contracting out database management and data analysis will remain cost-effective for state and local governments, which lack the hardware, software, and technical staff needed to conduct data-intensive outcomes and performance analyses.

PRIVATE SECTOR FUNDING

The affordability and access provided by MBHOs will allow managed care organizations to retain a strong share of the mental health care market in the private sector as well. Indeed, the economic viability of parity will largely depend on the ability of managed care organizations to control costs for mental health services through MBHOs.

As parity mandates are strengthened, employers' demands for efficiency in purchasing will lead managed care organizations to offer integrated coverage packages. The provision of mental health services in the private sector will thus be linked to, but not fully integrated with, general medical services. Although researchers will discover more about the biological nature of mental illness, treatment of serious mental illness will remain a specialized field and will not be integrated by insurers into general medical care coverage.

CIVIL RIGHTS

The burgeoning consumer advocacy movement will lobby successfully for federal and state legislation to provide greater rights for people affected by mental illnesses. At stake are issues such as guardianship, custody, family versus individual rights, and employment and housing rights. The courts will also extend the principles of equal opportunity and nondiscrimination to the mentally ill. These legal and judicial actions,

combined with better care and treatment, will serve to "normalize" the lives of those with mental illness. Specific issues will include:

- *The Americans with Disabilities Act.* The courts have been hostile to mental health claims under the Americans with Disabilities Act (ADA), holding that Congress did not intend to include mental illness claims as a disability issue. Legal analysts believe that laws patterned after the ADA will be enacted to guarantee nondiscrimination in housing and employment to people affected by mental illness, however, and to ensure equality in insurance coverage for those with disabilities caused by mental illness.

- *Confidentiality.* Concerns about confidentiality, especially in the context of employer-sponsored mental health care coverage, may impede the integration of services. Without strongly enforced federal regulations to safeguard patient privacy, mental health care providers will hesitate to share patient information with general medical organizations. Most likely, however, privacy rights will be expanded in the coming years.

- *Medical necessity.* As MBHOs shift their attention from case management of the provider–patient relationship to systemic outcomes issues, the definition of "medical necessity" will become less contentious. Insurers use the standard of "medical necessity" to approve or deny treatment. In the past, individuals with severe mental illness who did not warrant institutionalization have been denied extended treatment by insurers who judged the treatment as not being medically necessary. For those cases that reach the courts, judges are expected to apply a more pro-patient interpretation of "medical necessity."

■ *Outpatient civil commitment.* The debate over state laws allowing for outpatient civil commitment (court-ordered outpatient treatment for people whose voluntary compliance with treatment is poor) peaked in recent years and will wane by the end of the decade.

THE UNFINISHED AGENDA

Political will is always unpredictable, but it is the catalyst to fostering change in all national systems, mental health included. The political agenda of the executive, legislative, and judicial branches could speed or delay the pace of progress toward mental health parity, an integrated care agenda, and mental health care reform. Public opinion and public response to various events either fires up political will or defeats it. With mental health, public opinion

and stigma continue to be a drag on progress.

It seems unlikely—but not impossible—that the United States will develop and implement universal health coverage during the next decade. It also seems unlikely that the nation will adopt a public health approach to mental health care, one that values prevention (both primary and secondary) as much as it values diagnosis and treatment. Without a national mandate, health plans do not have the incentive to fund treatments that could prevent chronic diseases from developing in adolescents or in older adults. Until that happens, it will be up to each health plan and the government to include programs that add value to society as an essential part of their coverage.

The realization of an integrated, coordinated mental health system where programs are funded according to best-practice principles and outcomes, and where mental health is an integral part of all health services, is unlikely to be realized within the next ten years.

ENDNOTES

[1] Fundamentals of Mental Health and Mental Illness. *Mental Health: A Report of the Surgeon General*. 1999.

[2] Federal Register. 58, no. 96. Thursday May 20, 1993. Notice 29423.

[3] Mark, T., et. al. Spending on mental health and substance abuse treatment, 1987–1997. *Health Affairs* 19(4):108.

[4] PhRMA. 2000 Survey, New Medicines in Development for Mental Illness. www.phrma.org/charts/archive/2000/mental_00.html.

[5] U.S. Department of Justice. State Prison Expenditures, 1996. Bureau of Justice Statistics.

[6] SAMHSA Sources: Rice, D. P. Costs of Mental Illness. Unpublished Data. 1997. The 1994 estimates are projections from basic conceptual and analytic work done under contract with the Alcohol, Drug Abuse and Mental Health Administration and presented in: Rice, D. P., S. Kelman, L. S. Miller, and S. Dunmeyer. *The Economic Costs of Alcohol and Drug Abuse, and Mental Illness: 1985*. DHHS Publication No. (ADM) 90-1964. 1990. The 1994 costs were based on socioeconomic indexes applied to the 1985 cost estimates by Dorothy Rice.

[7] NIMH. *Bridging Science and Service: A Report by the National Advisory Mental Health Council's Clinical Treatment and Services Research Group*. NIH Publication No. 99-4353. 1999.

[8] R&D The Key to Innovation. *Pharmaceutical Industry Profile 2000*. www.phrma.org.

[9] NIMH. *Genetics and Mental Disorders: Report of the National Institute of Mental Health's Genetics Workgroup*. September 1997. CMHS. 1998:7–10

[10] State, Mathew W., et. al. The genetics of childhood psychiatric disorders: A decade of progress. *American Academy of Child and Adolescent Psychiatry* (August)2000; 39(8):946–962.

[11] Ibid, p. 14. See also: Pincus, Harold. Test your futurist skills: What Will Be the Future of Psychiatric Diagnosis. Pre-Meeting Briefing Papers, The Future of Mental Health Services. CMHS. 1998:7–10.

[12] Meltzet, Carolyn Cidis, et al. Serotinin in aging, late-life depression, and Alzheimer's disease: The emerging role of funcitonal imaging. *Neuropsychopharmacology* 1998; 18(6):407–430. See also: Schuckit, M. A., et al. Difficult differential diagnoses in psychiatry: The clinical use of SPECT. *Journal of Clinical Psychiatry* 1995; (56):539–546. See also: Longworth, Catherine, G. Honey, and T. Sharma. Functional imaging tomography in neuropsychiatry: Clinical review: Science medicine and the future. *British Medical Journal* (11 December) 1999; 318(7224): 1551–1554.

[13] Michels, Robert. Are research ethics bad for our mental health. *The New England Journal of Medicine* (May) 1999; 340(18).

[14] NIMH. *Bridging Science and Service: A Report by the National Advisory Mental Health Council's Clinical Treatment and Services Research Group*. NIH Publication No. 99-4353. 1999.

[15] Regier, D. A., et al. The de facto US mental and addictive disorders service system. *Arch of Gen Psychiatry* (February) 1993; 50:85–94.

[16] Ustun, Bedirhan T. The global burden of mental disorders. *American Journal of Public Health* (September) 1999; 89:1315–1318.

[17] California Health Care Foundation. The State of Behavioral Health in California. 2000.

[18] Vogel, Howard, E. Knight, et. al. double trouble in recovery: Self-help for people with dual diagnosis. *Psychiatric Rehabilitation Journal* (Spring) 1998; 21(4).

[19] The only exception to this will be in the needs for the elderly who will be entering the health system in larger numbers in the future. Their needs for nursing and hospital services for multiple problems, of which mental illness will be one, will be quite significant and is discussed in Chapter 14.

[20] Witkin, Michael J., et. al. Highlights of Organized Mental Health Services in 1994

and Major National and State Trends. *Mental Health, United States 1998*. CMHS, USDHS. See also: Mechanic, David. Emerging trends in mental health policy and practice. *Health Affairs* 1998; 17(6):82–98.

[21] Saphir, Ann. Fiscally challenged: Psychiatric industry's hope is in consolidation, focusing Services. *Modern Healthcare*. March 27, 2000.

[22] Nichelson, D. W. Telehealth and the evolving health care system: Strategic opportunities for professional psychology. *Professional Psychology: Research and Practice* 1998; (29):527–535. One example of an entrepreneur in the area of telehealth is the "Dr. Bobs" website. Dr. Bob Hsuing, a Chicago psychiatrist and founder of this website posts links to a wide variety of resources, and also claims that he does not hesitate to use e-mail for communicating with his established patients. Also see www.mentalhealth.com, which lists a wide variety of information for consumers, including lists of common medications, and organizations that consumers might wish to use.

[23] Van Tosh, Laura, Ruth O. Ralph, and Jean Campbell. The Rise of Consumerism, A Contribution to the Surgeon General's Report, 1999, provided by the author.

[24] Forquer, Sandy. Self Help and Recovery— Quality Improvement Activity. Unpublished report. Colorado Health Hetworks, 1999.

[25] www.medhelp.org/forums/MentalHealth/index.htm

[26] AMA Cultural Competence Compendium. Section VII: Patient Support Materials, including Self-help Group Resources. pp. 285–308.

[27] Madera, Edward J. The Mutual-Aid Self-help Online Revolution. www.cmhc.com/perspectives/articles/art03987.htm. March 27, 1998.

[28] Kane, John. Mental Health Treatments: What Approaches Will We Be Using in Ten Years. Pre-Meeting Briefing Papers, The Future of Mental Health Services. CMHS. 1998:11–12

[29] Center for the Advancement of Health. Depression Outlook Lifts with Ongoing Management and Care. Special Series: Collaborative Management of Chronic Conditions. November 1999. 4(8).

[30] Alliance for Health Reform. Managed Care and Vulnerable Americans—Mental Health Care Coverage. February 1998.

[31] Brody, D. S. et. al. Patients' perspectives on the management of emotional distress in primary care settings. *Journal of Internal Medicine* (July) 1997; 12(7):403–406.

[32] Katzelnick, David J., Gregory E. Simon, et al. Randomized trial of a depression management program in high utilizers of medical care. *Archives of Family Medicine* (2000); 9:345–351. See also: Spitzer, Robert L., et al. Validation and utility of a self-report version of prime-MD. *JAMA*. (November 10) 1999; 282(18):1737–1744.

[33] Sierles, F. S., and M. A. Taylor. Decline of U.S. medical student career choice of psychiatry and what to do about it. *American Journal of Psychiatry* 1995; 152:1416–1426.

[34] National Institutes of Health. General Information about CAM and the NCAM. Publication M-42. NCCAM Clearinghouse. June, 2000.

[35] El Feki, Shereen. *Dr Nature's Surgery—The World in 2000*. The Economist Publications.

[36] Yager, Joel. Use of Alternative Remedies by Psychiatric Patients: Illustrative Vignettes and a Discussion of the Issues. *American Journal of Psychiatry* (September) 1999; 156:1432–1438.

[37] Milbank Memorial Fund. Enhancing the Accountability of Alternative Medicine. January 1998.

CHAPTER 13

Children's Health

A Good Investment

Children are among the healthiest populations in the United States. On average, those under age 18 account for 26 percent of the population and only 18 percent of inpatient hospital stays.[1] Yet there's been a public move in recent years to improve the health care of children. Indeed, after the Clinton administration's universal health care reform was defeated, the administration opted for a more incremental approach and focused on getting children health insurance. President Bush's 2001 budget proposal, "A Blueprint for New Beginnings," didn't stray from this course but included a focus on education, plus tax credits as priorities that will improve the well-being of America's children. If children are so healthy, then what's all the fuss? Why should a health care system already pushed to its limits put scarce resources toward caring for a population that's rarely very sick?

The short answer is, to keep them healthy and to improve their health status where we can. The longer answer is both philosophical and practical.

Philosophically, we should insist on the best possible health care for our children for the same reason we bore them—they are our future. They are our legacy and should be cared for because they aren't able to protect themselves, either physically or politically. When children's needs, such as preschool programs, are discussed in policy circles, kids often lose out for simple lack of representation.

Practically, we should work to improve child health because child health today is a determinant of adult health tomorrow.[2] Morbidity in childhood is correlated with morbidity and mortality in adulthood. Children are inexpensive to care for and offer a huge return on investment. Preventing childhood diseases with immunizations and other forms of preventive medicine such as well-child care saves the system the later costs of treating these diseases.[3] A health care system that's trying to slow the growth of costs overall can't afford *not* to embark on this critical strategy of child health promotion and disease prevention, one that is often the first to be cut in any conflict of resources.

To ensure the future health of United States children, while at the same time keeping down costs of the health care system as a whole, policymakers must ask themselves these questions:

- What keeps children healthy?
- How well are we doing?
- What's in store in the future?

WHAT KEEPS KIDS HEALTHY? ACCESS AND ENVIRONMENT

Two significant impacts on children's health are their access to health care and their environment. Studies such as those led by Paul Newacheck of the Institute for Health Policy Studies at the University of California, San Francisco, have shown that access to health services is associated with improved health, and that access to some form of health insurance or health care funding is the best proxy for access to services.[4,5]

In 2000, 88.4 percent of children had health insurance coverage, reflecting a decline from 9.1 million to 8.5 million uninsured children since 1999. The percentage of children covered by some form of health insurance has fluctuated somewhat over the past decade, but between 85 and 87 percent of children have had health insurance since 1987.[6,7]

Even if children have health insurance, they don't necessarily get the care they need. There aren't enough pediatricians and other children's health care providers to go around, especially in geographic and socioeconomic areas traditionally short of adequate health care services— rural and inner-city areas.[8] And these are precisely the areas most susceptible to the negative effects of another important determinant of children's health—their environment. Health insurance and health care are not enough to keep children healthy; a relatively clean, safe environment is also important.[9] How and where children grow up have very specific effects on their health, with implications for public policy beyond the realm of health care.

ACCESS TO HEALTH INSURANCE OR OTHER FINANCING

"Simply put, health insurance is a powerful predictor of children's degree of access to and use of primary care. . . . The effect of insurance remained substantial and statistically significant even after we controlled for several potentially confounding variables, such as family income and children's health status."[10]

PRIVATE HEALTH INSURANCE

With the booming economy of the late 1990s, employment-based coverage for children increased from 58.1 percent in 1994 to 61.5 percent in 1999.[11] (See Chaper 4.) This increase happened because the percentage of children with a working parent increased, the percentage of children in families with incomes below the poverty level decreased, and more children had a working parent employed in a large firm. The increase in employment-based coverage can, in part, be attributed to a combination of welfare reform and the strong economy, both of which resulted in fewer adult women on welfare and more adult women working. During these years of an extremely robust economy and tight labor market, profitable companies were inclined to offer health insurance to attract and keep good employees.

Though the recent increases in covered children are heartening, their link to the health of the economy means fluctuations in the unemployment rate will determine the number of children covered in the future. Now and in the near future as the economy faces the "R" word—recession—companies are likely to cut costs. They'll ask employees to foot more of their own health care premiums by no longer insuring dependents, or by eliminating health insurance altogether where they can. While the average monthly worker contribution for single coverage has fluctuated up and down since 1993, family coverage has become increasingly expensive to the worker. This cost shifting and cost sharing will be increasingly common as firms hire more part-time employees, as expected in the next 10 years.[12] Also, low-income workers that make too much money to qualify for Medicaid are likely to decline health insurance if co-pays become too great of a financial burden.[13] And what about those children without health insurance?

The majority of those working without health insurance benefits are in service sector jobs, which are traditionally less likely to offer insurance at any time.[14] Also, almost 10 percent of the current American workforce is temporary, part-time, or contract workers. Such workers are much less likely to receive benefits, and buying private health insurance is prohibitively expensive for them. The number of working Americans in service sector jobs is expected to increase by 20 percent in the next 10 years; and just over 70 percent of businesses will use part-time or temporary workers by then. (Since 1970, most job growth has been in the service-producing sector, a trend expected to continue as nonhousehold service-producing jobs are projected to increase by 17.6 million between 1996 and 2006.) These changes could result in a decrease in the proportion of children covered by their parents' employers, with a corresponding drop in the number of children receiving basic care.

MEDICAID PICKS UP SOME SLACK

With an estimated 8.5 million children without health insurance in 2000, the government has made a concerted effort to provide insurance and health services to as many uninsured children as possible.[15] In 1965, Title XIX of the Social Security Act established Medicaid, a public health financing program for low-income families and individuals. In 2000, Medicaid insured 21 million children. For most families covered through Medicaid, private health insurance is unavailable or unaffordable; with Medicaid, they gain access to medical, dental, vision, and behavioral health services, including preventive care, acute care, and LTC, with little or no cost sharing.[16] Although Medicaid is not specifically designed to serve children, the number of children who rely on Medicaid for coverage has grown in recent years.

More than half a million children have joined the Medicaid rolls each year since the late 1980s. The number of children enrolled in Medicaid increased substantially, from 9.8 million children in 1985 to 21 million children in 1998. This is due primarily to the deliberate expansion of Medicaid to cover children above the poverty line, in compliance with the Omnibus Budget Reconciliation Acts (OBRAs) of the late 1980s. This broadening program scope for low-income families is reflected in trends in enrollment and spending.

As a result of these increases, 58.5 percent of those eligible for Medicaid are children; Medicaid covers 25 percent of America's youth. In metropolitan areas, the percentage of children on Medicaid is higher. Medicaid pays for more than 50 percent of births in New York City, for example; and in the United States as a whole, Medicaid covers 39 percent of all births.[17] Medicaid pays for a broad range of other services for children, including well-child care, immunizations, prescription drugs, doctor visits, and hospitalizations, as well as long-term care for disabled children.[18]

The value of Medicaid is underscored by the contrast in outcomes between the poor with Medicaid and the uninsured poor. Studies consistently show that the uninsured fall well behind those with Medicaid with respect to access to services, while those with Medicaid fare favorably compared to the privately insured.[19] Children with Medicaid are only slightly less likely than privately insured, nonpoor children to have a regular source of care and reasonable access to care, but poor uninsured children face significant deficits.[20] Also, few differences have been found in access to, use of, or satisfaction with health care services for children under Medicaid managed care relative to Medicaid fee-for-service.[21] Though covered by Medicaid, groups at risk of less-than-optimal access to health care are chronically ill and disabled children in poor families. While numerous state and federal programs provide services and cash assistance for them, recent changes in Supplemental Security Income (SSI) and Medicaid have fundamentally altered the financing of services for this population. In 1995, President Clinton announced cuts in SSI to disabled children as a part of his welfare reform pack-

age. Although disability benefits to more than 135,000 children were cut, their health care needs were met through their Medicaid eligibility.[22]

Partly as a result of this influx of eligible children into Medicaid, many states are moving children with special health care needs into managed care by means of Medicaid health maintenance organizations (HMOs). Managed care promises, among other things, disease-state management programs that have had mixed success in treating the chronically ill at lower cost. In reality, the rapid expansion of managed care has unknown consequences for children with chronic illnesses and disabilities. Since Medicaid reimbursements are lower than Medicare and private insurance reimbursements, some HMOs are opting out of the Medicaid market.[23]

The bulk of Medicaid spending does not go to care for adults and children in low-income families. In 1998, the Health Care Financing Administration estimated the average annual cost of Medicaid coverage per child to be $1,225, as opposed to the average Medicaid cost per disabled person of $9,558 and per elderly adult of $11,235.[24] Adults and children in low-income families make up 73 percent of enrollees, but account for only 25 percent of Medicaid expenditures, a fact that underscores the importance of early preventive care in keeping total system costs down.[25]

Ultimately, even though Medicaid is picking up much of the slack left by decreasing private health insurance, the quality of care may not be as high.

Incremental Medicaid Expansion Is Nothing New

During the 1980s, Medicaid rapidly expanded beyond its AFDC base to cover increasing numbers of low-income children and their mothers. The following expansions occurred:

- *Deficit Reduction Act of 1984*   mandated coverage of all AFDC-eligible children born after September 30, 1983, and extended coverage to AFDC-eligible first-time pregnant women and two-parent families.

- *Consolidated Omnibus Budget Reconciliation Act of 1984*   extended coverage to all remaining AFDC-eligible pregnant women.

- *Omnibus Reconciliation Act of 1986 (OBRA)*   allowed coverage of pregnant women and children under age 1 up to 100 percent of the federal poverty level (FPL).

- *OBRA 1987*   permitted coverage of pregnant women and children under age 1 up to 185 percent of the FPL

- *Medicare Catastrophic Coverage Act of 1988*   required coverage of all pregnant women and children under age 1 up to 100 percent of the FPL, and allowed states the option to extend coverage to families with incomes higher than 185 percent of the FPL.

- *OBRA 1989*   raised the minimum eligibility requirement to 133 percent of the FPL for pregnant women and children up to age 6.

- *OBRA 1990*   mandated coverage for children born after September 30, 1983, with family incomes below 100 percent of the FPL.[26]

Medicaid's early and periodic screening, diagnostic, and treatment (EPSDT) services represent the single most important source of financing and programmatic guidance for children's public health programs. EPSDT requires states to periodically screen Medicaid-eligible children under 22 years old for illnesses, abnormalities, or treatable conditions, and refer them for definitive treatment.

As a result of these policies, by 1999 Medicaid was the major insurer of children, covering 25 percent of children under 18 and 27 percent of children under age 6.[27] Nationwide, the number of children covered by Medicaid grew in response to the expanded eligibility policy, particularly among those not receiving cash assistance, rising from 11.5 million in 1990 to more than 21 million in 2001.

THEIR SCHIP CAME IN . . .

With the continued enactment legislation, lawmakers have done considerably more than expand Medicaid eligibility. In what *The New York Times* called the largest expansion of government-paid health insurance since the formation of Medicaid 32 years before, the Balanced Budget Act of 1997 (BBA) created Title XXI of the Social Security Act. This act set aside more than $24 billion through 2002 in the form of the State Children's Health Insurance Program (SCHIP). The goal was to provide health insurance coverage for 5 million of those uninsured, low-income children.

These funds became available to states on October 1, 1997, and states were required to develop federally approved plans by the end of FY 1998 to receive funding. Since then, many states have substantially expanded eligibility for children's health insurance. States are required to provide matching funds equal to 30 percent of their current Medicaid state-matching rate. The legislation allocated an additional $4 billion over 5 years for, among other things, those states choosing to provide Medicaid coverage to children for a continuous 12-month period or states adopting presumptive eligibility (allowing children likely to be eligible for Medicaid to receive coverage while awaiting final determination). In 1999, 94 percent of children whose families earned up to 200 percent of the FPL qualified for Medicaid or SCHIP. As of July 2000, 50 states, the District of Columbia, and five U.S. Territories have implemented SCHIP, covering over 2 million children.[28]

Of these approved plans, 15 states have created a separate child health program, 23 states have expanded Medicaid, and 18 states have developed a combination of a separate state and Medicaid expansion program. Prior to SCHIP, only 4 states covered children with family incomes up to at least 200 percent of the federal poverty level. In 2000, 30 states had plans approved to cover children with incomes up to at least this level.

. . . BUT IT MAY BE LEAKY

Though SCHIP is a windfall for uninsured children in the short run, in the long run there may be problems with the legislation.

- Some critics were concerned that after passing the SCHIP legislation, federal and state legislators would rest on their laurels and no longer be motivated to take significant action on behalf of the remaining uninsured children for the next 5 to 10 years. There are currently several minor measures before Congress that would help state agencies ease administrative barriers and improve enrollment processes so low-income families could more easily enroll their children. In praising what he considered the early success of SCHIP, President Clinton sponsored enrollment initiatives through school lunch programs and child care centers. These measures affect only children eligible for public support; they don't touch the remaining uninsured children in families above 200 percent of the poverty line. Many states have had a difficult time spending the SCHIP funds that Congress set aside, with only 10 states successfully doing so by the end of 2000.

- SCHIP decreased Disproportionate Share Hospital (DSH) funding, which has traditionally reimbursed safety-net providers for charity care, resulting in a squeeze on provision of services to children who remained uninsured despite SCHIP. Under SCHIP, a nominal amount of DSH funding was returned to states with hospitals that report treating a disproportionate share of low-income individuals.

- One popular option for implementing SCHIP was by expanding Medicaid, but many children eligible for Medicaid do not enroll. Indeed, in his 1998 State of the Union address, President Clinton encouraged increasing the enrollment of 3 million Medicaid-eligible-but-not-enrolled children. In 1999, 63 percent of uninsured children with family incomes below 200 percent of the poverty line were eligible for Medicaid or SCHIP but were not enrolled. Aside from the stigma associated with public assistance programs, other reasons eligible children are not enrolled include fluctuating eligibility requirements, plus complex and lengthy applications—up to 12 pages long in some states. Before SCHIP made provision for presumptive eligibility for a year from application, up to 4 percent of children on Medicaid lost eligibility every month.

As a result of these stumbling blocks, there are many different estimates of the true number of previously uninsured children for whom SCHIP will provide health insurance. The Congressional Budget Office estimated in 1997 that the final BBA will cover a net gain of only 1.5 to 1.6 million of the 10 million uninsured children, and will result in a 3.4 million gross gain in coverage.[29] Even with more generous estimates of 20 percent coverage of uninsured chil-

Q most new cared by SCHP?
(F)

dren, SCHIP's impact will be significant but not dramatic or sufficient.

UNINSURED CHILDREN WILL BE WITH US STILL

Though the BBA makes strides toward providing for uninsured children, many children will remain without either health insurance or a consistent source of health care. In 1999, approximately 3.5 million uninsured children were in families that earned more than 200 percent of federal poverty level. These children will remain without health insurance even under SCHIP. This is a problem. A recent study published in the *Journal of the American Medical Association* found that the uninsured are four times more likely to report an episode of needing care but not getting it than those who are insured. Research shows that uninsured children are less likely than insured kids to have a regular doctor or receive routine preventive and dental care. Studies indicate that lack of coverage negatively affects access to care among low-income children—41 percent of parents of eligible uninsured children postponed seeking medical care for their child because they could not afford it.

In Chapter 1's middle scenario titled "The Long and Winding Road," we forecast that 47 million Americans or 16 percent of the population will be uninsured in 2010. Of that uninsured group, 11.6 million will be children. The SCHIP has been implemented in all states, but the amount of money allocated to the program is preset and not enough to provide access to care for the children in need. There will not be much

new activity beyond the efforts already undertaken by each state.

ACCESS TO HEALTH SERVICES: ENOUGH PROVIDERS?

The financial side of the healthy child equation is not all that needs attention. Even if we assume that in the near future children who need health insurance or some other form of financing get it, there's still a long way to go to ensure that children receive actual care by qualified pediatric providers. Like other clinical specialists, pediatricians and other ancillary providers with pediatric training are not distributed evenly throughout the U.S. population, sometimes making it difficult for the patients who most need health care services to attain them.

NOT ENOUGH PEDIATRICIANS TO GO AROUND

Pediatricians monitor and treat the physical, emotional, and social health of children from birth to young adulthood. Thus, pediatric care encompasses a broad spectrum of health services ranging from preventive health care to the diagnosis and treatment of acute and chronic diseases. Pediatricians also increasingly provide guidance and therapeutic interventions for a large number of behavioral problems, school difficulties, risk-taking behaviors, and environmental threats to the well-being of children. Not all health care providers are capable of this range of activities.

In the United States, there are over 55,000 pediatricians, accounting for more than 7 percent of the physician population. Pediatrics is the third largest specialty after internal medicine and family practice. Pediatricians are given the specialty training necessary to care for seriously sick children. The main activity of more than 90 percent of pediatricians is the provision of patient care in office-based and hospital-based settings. They provide approximately 50 percent of all office-based visits for children and youth from birth to age 19 in the United States, and pediatricians and family practitioners combined provide 90 percent of kids' office-based visits. This proportion has increased steadily for all age groups, from 39 percent in 1976–77 to 50 percent in the 1990s.[30] That average is a little deceptive, however. Pediatricians provided 72 percent of all office-based visits for U.S. children from birth to 2 years of age, but only 24 percent of all office-based visits for those aged 10 to 19 years.

Most pediatricians practice in metropolitan areas: Few serve rural or inner-city communities.[31] Even when health care coverage for poor children increases with SCHIP, if a community has a limited number of health care providers, access to care remains limited.

Community health clinics play an important role in filling the need for pediatric care. Studies have shown that poor children, even those with Medicaid, are much less likely than other children to receive routine care in a physician's office and more likely to receive care in community and hospital clinics. Though better than no care at all, the routine care children receive in community clinics is likely to lack continuity, which results in parents using emergency departments as their children's usual source of sick care. These alternatives are neither high quality nor cost-effective.[32]

Whether in an office or a clinic, family practitioners, international medical graduates (IMGs), and pediatric nurse practitioners provide primary care services to the majority of children who do not receive them from pediatricians. There are many caring and skilled individuals in these groups, with more general, less specialized training.

The most specifically trained of these caregivers are family practice physicians, who learn to care for children as a part of the family unit. Family practice grew out of general practice in the 1960s. Since then, the number of general practice physicians has decreased significantly as medical students have chosen to become family practitioners instead. There is an inequitable distribution of physicians throughout the United States, with less than 11 percent of physicians living in rural areas where 20 percent of the population lives. However, 54 percent of the physicians in rural areas are in primary care versus 38 percent in metropolitan areas.

In 1999, there were 191,418 international medical graduates (IMGs), or medical students from other countries who are studying in the United States.[33] They serve as an important part of the physician workforce, making up 25 percent of medical school graduates.[34] Moreover, a disproportionate number train in residency programs that provide ambulatory and inpatient services for the urban poor and uninsured. After they graduate, many remain in these underserved communities as a vital source of pediatric care. Over the past 5 years,

Chapter 13: Children's Health

policies addressing the oversupply of physicians in America, such as the Balanced Budget Act of 1997, have targeted IMGs' residency opportunities for cuts, decreasing this source of providers for poor children.[35]

A much less expensive option for providing health care to children is the pediatric nurse practitioner. Approximately 10,000 pediatric nurse practitioners are active in the United States today, the majority of whom are involved in the delivery of primary care services.[36] More than 60 percent of the members of the National Association of Pediatric Nurse Associates and Practitioners work in urban areas with populations of more than 100,000, increasing access for many poor, underserved families. There will likely be an increasing reliance on these mid-level providers in the future, as they have shown they can meet the majority of children's primary care needs.

The quality of children's individual health services will change, driven by the continuation of existing trends toward cost containment, medical and technological advances, and the pressure of managed care. These changes will occur as insurers, businesses, and governments attempt to contain costs in a generally healthy and cheap-to-care-for population, and medical schools and pediatric training programs compete for funding under competitive financial pressures.

THE IMPACT OF ENVIRONMENT

Access to health insurance and adequate care doesn't tell the whole story of kids' health. Studies have found that environ-

ment—broadly construed to include socioeconomic status, the behavior of surrounding adults, the level of violence in the community, pollution in the physical environment, and so on—is as important if not more so.[37] In particular, the following environmental risk factors increase the likelihood of illness for certain children:

- Having poor or single parents

- Exposure to toxic physical environments such as substandard housing, air pollution, increased violence, and so on.

SOCIOECONOMIC ENVIRONMENT

Children's access to health care and education, as well as the overall level of violence and safety in their neighborhoods, is directly linked to their socioeconomic status.[38] Children's socioeconomic status comprises more than just their parents' income bracket. The parents' level of poverty, their education, their employment status, and their household composition combine to determine the individual and community-based resources available for maintaining good health and treating the health problems that do occur, although access to resources is only a small part of the effect of socioeconomic status on health.

CHILDREN LIVING IN POVERTY

National data show that the poverty rate among children under age 18 increased from 19 percent in 1989 to 22 percent in 1993 before declining again to 16.2 percent (11.6 million children) in 2000, the lowest it has been since 1979.[39]

As you might expect, poverty rates are not evenly distributed among ethnic groups. In 1999, the poverty rates among Hispanic children (30 percent) and African American children (33 percent) were almost twice those for white children (9 percent).[40] And let's be clear—by families in poverty, we don't mean only those who are unemployed and on welfare. The U.S. Census Bureau reported that the number of poor families with children, headed by someone who worked during the year, reached 3.8 million in 1999, higher than any year since 1975. Of all poor children, 78 percent lived in a family where someone (not always the head of the household) worked in 1999, also a record high and up from 61 percent in 1993.

Education, ethnicity, and age are factors that strongly affect hourly wages and labor force activity and, hence, adult earnings. Children who live with poorly educated, relatively young, or Hispanic or African American adults are more likely to be poor than are children who do not live in such families. By extension, these are the families that are the least likely to be covered by adequate health insurance and services.[41] The children who live in these families are most at risk of living in poverty and with little or no access to regular health care.

INCREASING ETHNIC DIVERSITY

Ethnic and racial diversity has grown dramatically in the United States in the past three decades. This diversity is projected to increase even more in the decades to come. As a result, ethnically diverse children are a rapidly growing sector of society.

In 2000, 64 percent of American children were white, non-Hispanic;

15 percent were African American, non-Hispanic; 16 percent were Hispanic; 4.2 percent were Asian or Pacific Islander; and 1 percent were American Indian or Alaskan Native. The percentage of children who are classified as minorities increased from 26 percent in 1980 to 36 percent in 2000 (see Figure 13-1).

The Hispanic population has grown more rapidly than other ethnic groups, increasing from 9 percent of the child population in 1980 to 16 percent in 1999. In the decade from 1995 to 2005, the number of Hispanic children is projected to increase by 30 percent, and by 2020, it is projected that more than one in five children in the United States will be Hispanic. Although the base is smaller, the percentage of children who are Asian or Pacific Islanders has also increased quickly, doubling from 2 to 4.2 percent of all children between 1980 and 2000. This population segment is expected to grow to 6 percent of all children by 2010. Between 1995 and 2005, the number of Asian or Pacific Islander children will increase by 39 percent.

This increasing diversity will affect the delivery of health care for children. Ethnic groups sometimes differ in cultural attitudes toward health, in health needs, and in how they access services.[42,43] For example, in some Hispanic cultures it is considered impolite to complain of pain, and thus someone in dire need of treatment may remain undiagnosed.

Increasing diversity will also affect other aspects of the environment, especially education. As more children who speak English as a second language enroll in

Figure 13-1. *U.S. ethnic diversity increasing at accelerating rate*

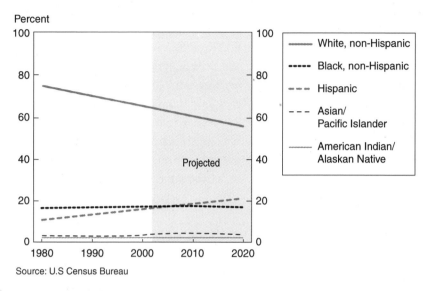

Percent

Source: U.S Census Bureau

Figure 13-2. *Children 5–17 years old who speak a language other than English at home*

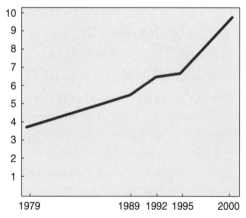

Number of children in millions

Source: U.S Census, 2000 Census summary file 3: Age by language spoken at home by ability to speak English for the population 5 years and older.

schools, for example, there will be an increased need for multilingual teachers and resources (see Figure 13-2). Indeed, more teachers of all stripes will be needed. A recent Department of Education report predicted a teacher shortage

of 150,000 since high school enrollment, which added 1.1 million students in the past decade, will climb by another 1.9 million or 13 percent between 1997 and 2007. This enrollment surge will be most dramatic in California, where the ranks of high school students are expected to jump by approximately 35 percent. Since level of education is linked to health status, those students who receive substandard education due to resource shortages will not be as healthy as those who receive a better education.

HOUSEHOLD COMPOSITION

Another much-discussed factor associated with an increase in child poverty in recent years is the increase in single-parent, mother-only families. In recent decades, the delay of marriage and having children, more couples living longer, a high divorce rate, and a growing out-of-wedlock birthrate have contributed to a decline in the number of adults per child per family.[44] With fewer adults, a family's earning potential is reduced, increasing the likelihood that children in these families will be poor and thus at risk for inadequate health care.

It is estimated that children in mother-only families are five times more likely to be poor than are children of two-parent families.[45] In 2000, 27.9 percent of children living in female households were living in poverty and nearly 69.8 percent of children living only with their nonworking mothers were living in poverty. Research indicates that poverty, in turn, increases the risk that a child will experience significant health difficulties. Children of unmarried mothers are at higher risk for adverse birth outcomes because their mothers are less likely to have received adequate prenatal care, less likely to have gained adequate weight during pregnancy, and more likely to have smoked during pregnancy. This applies even when differences in age and educational level are taken into account. Studies have shown that 8 to 12 years after birth, a child born to an unmarried, teenage high school dropout is 10 times as likely to be living in poverty as a child born to a mother with none of these three characteristics.[46]

In 2000, 69 percent of American children lived with two parents, down from 78 percent in 1970. Also in 2000, 22 percent of children lived with only their mothers; 4 percent lived with only their fathers; and 4 percent lived with neither parent. The number of female-parent households is projected to increase by 12 percent (from 6.4 to 7.2 million) between 1995 and 2010. The percentage of children living with two parents is declining among all major ethnic groups. By 2010, household composition will have changed, with only one in five households comprised of a mother, father, and children under 18, compared with one in four currently. White children are much more likely than Hispanic children and somewhat more likely than African American children to live with two parents. In 1999, 77 percent of white children lived with two parents, compared to 35 percent of African American children and 63 percent of Hispanic children.

Among the factors contributing to the increased percentage of children living with just one parent is the sharp rise in births to unmarried mothers: from 18 percent in 1980 to 33 percent in 1999. This increase is linked to a decline in the proportion of women of childbearing age who are married (from 71 percent in 1960 to 53 percent in 1995), a decline in births to married women (from 4 million in 1960 to 2.6 million in 1995), and a decline in the birthrate for married women (from 157 per thousand in 1960 to 84 per thousand in 1995). Some of the decline in marriages reflects increases in cohabitation; 20 to 25 percent of unmarried women aged 25 to 44 were in cohabiting relationships from 1992 to 1994.

Increases in households that are most likely to be below the poverty line and thus more likely to encounter greater health difficulties will put even more stresses on a health care system that can ill afford them.

PHYSICAL ENVIRONMENT AND INCREASING CHRONIC ILLNESS

A more obvious connection can be drawn between children's physical environment and their health status. Air pollution has been linked with an increased incidence of asthma, for example, and studies have shown associations between pesticide use in the home and increased incidence of childhood cancers.[47] Other aspects of physical environment such as stress and violence have been linked to neuropsychiatric illnesses in children, such as post-traumatic stress disorder.[48]

ASTHMA

Asthma in children has increased at approximately 5 percent per year since 1980 and is perhaps the best example of a disease with a strong link to environmental factors. According to the American Lung Association, of the 26 million Americans who have been diagnosed with asthma, 8.6 million are under the age of 18. 3.8 million of these youth have had an asthma episode in the past 12 months.[49] Asthma affects 7 percent of children. The number of cases has risen nearly 80 percent in the past 15 years and the death rate for children 18 years and younger increased by 78 percent since 1982.[50] The reason isn't entirely clear, but an increased prevalence of asthma is correlated with social and environmental factors such as poverty, maternal smoking, family size, home size, birth weight, and maternal education. In 1990, asthma in children was estimated to cost $6.2 billion per year. In 2000, the cost was estimated to double to $14.5 billion.[51]

Environmental causes of asthma are associated with an increased incidence in metropolitan areas and the prevalence of the condition among inner-city children is three times higher than national estimates. The highest prevalence of asthma continues to be among African American inner-city children. Since more urban African Americans than whites tend to be poor, sociodemographic factors have been suggested as the reason for this disparity. These factors include poorer environment (exposure to industrial effluents, air pollution, and potential allergens like dust mites and cockroaches) and reduced access to or inadequate use of primary care. Other studies associate race with genetic predisposition to asthma. African American children are particularly vulnerable to the disease. In fact, asthma is 26 percent

more prevalent in black children than in white children.[52]

Asthmatics are profoundly influenced by pollution. As an inflammatory disease, asthma's severity is directly affected by the number of particulates in the air.[53] And though recent efforts to lower air pollution nationwide have met with some success, national air pollution standards are based on exposure limits for protecting the average person. But a child is not the average person. Children's respiratory systems are more vulnerable to lower levels of toxins than adults', and children spend considerably more time out of doors—at play and at school—where they are more likely to breathe airborne pollutants. Recently, the Environmental Protection Agency announced new, tighter air pollution standards, but even these standards may be inadequate to protect children.[54]

CANCER

Another group of chronically ill children profoundly affected by their environment is those diagnosed with cancer. Cancer follows unintentional injuries and homicide as the third leading cause of death in children between 1 and 19 years of age, and an estimated 2,300 children died from cancer in 2000.[55] The numbers of children getting a particular cancer are so small, however, that recent increases in incidence may not be statistically significant.

Factors contributing to the increase in cancer are unknown, as is the cause of most cancers. Some argue that the rates of childhood cancer have risen only because detection methods are more discriminating, while other studies point to increased exposure to environmental pollutants, such as home pesticides.[56]

Overall childhood cancer incidence increased by 10 percent between 1973 and 1991, then leveled off and declined slightly through 1996. Mortality has decreased steadily for all cancer sites combined and most sites have decreased by more than 50 percent. This decrease in mortality is evident in substantial increases in 5-year survival rates, from less than 30 percent in the early 1990s to almost 75 percent in 1999. Decreased mortality from childhood cancers is due in part to technological and pharmaceutical advances in treatment. It also is likely due to technological advances in the state-of-the-art medical care given to most children with cancer. Seventy percent of children with cancer are enrolled in clinical cancer trials and are given access to the latest therapies and breakthrough technologies.

The National Cancer Institute predicts that cancer trends in children will remain flat or decline through the year 2010. These predictions incorporate the potential positive impact of technological advances in gene and vaccine therapy and rational drug design.

NEUROPSYCHIATRIC CONDITIONS

Some neuropsychiatric conditions in children, such as depression and attention deficit hyperactivity disorder (ADHD), can be linked to environmental factors such as stress and violence and are becoming more prevalent. Whether such prevalence indicates a true increase in major depression in children or better detection methods remains open to further study. Nonetheless, the number of prescriptions for drugs such as Prozac and Ritalin has increased tremendously. Between 1990 and 1995, the number of prescriptions for Ritalin among school-aged children increased 260 percent. In a given year, major depression affects an estimated 5 percent of 5- to 12-year-olds and 10 percent of adolescents (the same rate as adults). The condition is a major factor in the growing tragedy of teen suicide—rates have tripled since the 1950s—and a common cause of school failures and dropouts. Another neuropsychiatric condition, ADHD, is estimated to affect 4 percent of youth aged 9 to 17—perhaps as many as 2 million children.[57]

Both depression and ADHD are linked to factors in a child's home environment, according to a study by A. Leung and W. Robson.[58] Those problems are also linked to low birth weight and the amount of alcohol and drugs a mother uses while pregnant.

With diseases as varied as childhood asthma and teen suicide attributed to environmental effects, some health care policymakers are launching a two-pronged attack. First, they are supporting further studies of the perceived link between pollution and asthma, for example, or daily violence and teen suicide. Second, they are taking a holistic approach, working with policymakers outside the realm of health care to create better, healthier environments for children; for example, working to improve housing standards, lessen air pollution, or eliminate violence from neighborhoods by means of gun control.

HOW ARE WE DOING?

Currently, the United States health care system is not doing a bad job of caring for children. Most kids (88 percent in 2000) have access to health insurance and, by extension, health services.

By the same token, approximately 70 percent of children can be considered to be generally healthy.[59] These children require little medical attention other than treatment of minor acute illnesses, preventive checkups, and regular immunizations. They are estimated to incur less than 10 percent of all medical expenditures for children (see Figure 13-3).

Another 20 percent of children have minor chronic problems such as persistent ear infections, asthma, or allergies. The annual expenditures for these chil-

dren are double or triple the expenditures for the average healthy child, but these costs can be contained by consistent, state-of-the-art care for those with access to health insurance. Those without access are not as well served by the system, and can use help in the form of a better-integrated and more comprehensive community clinic system.

The remaining 10 percent of children use the largest proportion of medical services. These children have one or more severe chronic illnesses that limit their activity and ability to function. Within this subpopulation, illnesses range in severity from correctable birth defects such as congenital heart disease to ailments for which treatment may be futile (such as pulmonary failure). Again, those with health insurance are likely to get the care they need, and severely disabled children may be covered by Medicaid, depending on state requirements.

The number of children with chronic conditions today is three times the number in the 1960s. This may be

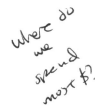
where do we spend most $?

Figure 13-3. Most kids are well covered—and are well.

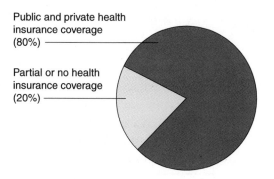

Public and private health insurance coverage (80%)

Partial or no health insurance coverage (20%)

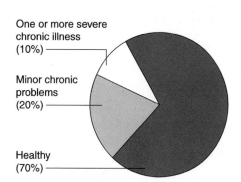

One or more severe chronic illness (10%)

Minor chronic problems (20%)

Healthy (70%)

Source: Newacheck et al.,1998, IFTF.

because data collection methods have become more comprehensive and inclusive, and some illnesses have been newly defined (e.g., ADHD is a relatively new diagnosis). It may also be that clinical innovations allow more children with disabilities to survive longer, or that the change is due to some combination of all of these factors.

In 1998, 7 percent of children ages 5 to 17 years old were limited in their normal activity by one or more chronic health conditions. This is significantly higher than the 3 percent of children under 5 years old with limited activity, possibly because some developmental and learning disabilities are not diagnosed until children enter school.

While children with moderate to severe chronic illnesses and disabilities in the aggregate may represent up to 10 percent of the childhood population, individually each diagnosis is infrequent to rare. The most common chronic illness in childhood is asthma, which has an age-adjusted prevalence rate of approximately 53 per 1,000.[60] Congenital heart disease has a prevalence of about 3 per 1,000 under age 18, but the diagnosis includes many different anomalies. Most other chronic illnesses have prevalences below 3 per 1,000. Epilepsy, cerebral palsy, diabetes, and Down's syndrome have prevalences of between 1 and 2.7 per 1,000. Conditions such as acute leukemia, neural tube defects, cystic fibrosis, muscular dystrophy, hemophilia, and hereditary metabolic disorders have prevalences that are considerably less than one per 1,000.

In the future, some incidence of chronic conditions may increase as a result of technological innovations that now are saving the lives of increasing numbers of premature and low-birth-weight babies. A recent study of extremely low-birth-weight babies (less than 1 kg) of higher socioeconomic status found that 20 percent had significant disabilities, including cerebral palsy, mental retardation, autism, and low intelligence with severe learning problems.[61] As more of these babies enter the population, the costs of caring for them will be higher, and more of them will slip through the cracks.

Who Are Children with Special Health Care Needs?

Differences in the definition of children with special health care needs produce varying estimates of the size of this population. The CDC estimates that approximately 17 percent of children less than 18 years old have developmental disabilities.[62] These are a diverse group of physical, cognitive, psychological, sensory, and speech impairments that may begin any time during development, up to 18 years of age.

Different states and programs define the population differently and target their medical care services to specific subsets of the population, resulting in overlapping services in some areas and no services in others. This lack of standard definitions blurs the lines between the mildly and severely disabled. As a result, many states do not know how to fairly allocate the small share of their health care dollar intended for disabled children.

CHILDREN'S CURRENT HEALTH STATUS INDICATORS

One way of measuring the health care system's success in caring for children is by using changes in global health indicators as rough estimates of children's overall health. While many measures can be used to assess the health status of America's children, we have chosen those indicators for which trends are changing. Generally, the changes have been positive and child health has improved, but some positive trends overall hide negative trends in sub-populations.

PRENATAL CARE

The Department of Health and Human Service's 1990 goals for improving child health by the year 2000 included improving maternal and child health outcomes measured by early prenatal care, infant mortality, and low birth weight.[63] In 1999, 83.2 percent of babies were born to mothers who had begun prenatal care in the first trimester of pregnancy, compared with 75.8 percent in 1990. By contrast, the rate of early prenatal care had fallen between 1980 and 1990 (see Table 13-1).

INFANT MORTALITY

The infant mortality rate has declined steadily for the past 50 years, from 47.0 deaths per 1,000 live births in 1940 to a low of 7.2 deaths per 1,000 live births in 1998. However, a comparison of health indicators in industrialized countries found that in 1998 the United States ranked 24th out of 29 in infant mortality even though it spends the most of all industrial nations on health care as a percentage of gross domestic product.

One explanation is that large disparities can still be observed in infant mortality rates across racial/ethnic subgroups in America. A recent study found that the infant mortality rate for children born into poor families (13.5 deaths per 1,000 live births) was more than 50 percent higher than that for children born into families with incomes above the poverty line (8.3 deaths per 1,000 live births).[64] The link between poverty and infant mortality helps explain why the infant mortality rate of African Americans, who have higher poverty rates, remains more than twice that of whites (13.9 compared to 5.8 deaths per 1,000 live births in 1998). The current system is failing this population.

Table 13-1. Healthy People 2000 goals for maternal and child health

Indicator	Race	1991 Rate	1994 Rate	2000 Goal	Estimated 2000 Rate	Projected Year Goal Reached
Early prenatal care	Overall	76.2% of all births	80.2%	90%	88.2%	2002
	Black	61%	68.3%	90%	81.1%	2005
	Hispanic	61%	68.9%	90%	84.7%	2002
Low birth weight	Overall	7.1% of all births	7.3%	5%	7.7%	Never
	Black	13.6%	13.2%	9%	12.4%	2026
Infant mortality	Overall	8.9 infant deaths per 1,000 live births	8.0	7.0	6.2	1998
	Black	17.6	15.8	11.0	12.2	2002

Source: Healthy People 2000. Maternal and Infant Health Indicator Review, May 2–4, 1999.
Website http://www.cdc.gov/nchs/about/otheract/hp2000/childhlt/mchb&w.pdf

Low-Birth-Weight Infants

Technological advances have increased the likelihood that smaller and more premature babies will survive to their first birthday and resulted in a decrease in infant mortality. Though these life-saving advances are awesome, there now are relatively more preterm deliveries and low-birth-weight babies—a population with long-term, expensive health care needs.

Nationally, 301,183 babies were born in 1999 weighing less than 2,500 grams (about 5.5 pounds).[65] The percentage of low-birth-weight infants increased from a low of 6.8 percent in 1985 to 7.6 percent in 1999 and is projected to continue to increase. Babies born to African American mothers are almost twice as likely to be of low birth weight as white babies. The Institute of Medicine identifies a mother's low level of education as a prominent risk factor for having a low-birth-weight baby, though education may be a proxy for socioeconomic status.[66] And since African American women are more likely to have lower levels of education, they're more at risk for low-birth-weight babies.

Immunizations

Fully immunizing 90 percent of children by age 2 was another Department of Health and Human Services goal for maternal and child health for the year 2000.[67] In 1999, 78 percent of children 19–35 months of age were fully immunized, up from 69 percent in 1994 and 55 percent in 1992. Childhood immunizations help prevent serious illnesses, such as polio, tetanus, whooping cough, mumps, measles, and meningitis. To create immunization registries and track the entire child population within a state, local and state public health agencies have increased collaboration efforts with private physicians. In 1998, only 100 cases of measles were reported, down from 28,000 cases in 1990, providing impressive evidence of how successful vaccination has been in increasing the population's immunity to measles.

The Children's Defense Fund estimates that providing immunizations yields a ten-to-one economic return on investments to reduce medical expenditures. This part of the system seems to be working. If we hit the goal of 90 percent immunization, then the system will be taking an important step toward keeping children healthy and long-term medical costs down.

As with other measures, there is a problem getting inner-city and rural children immunized. In one study of Los Angeles County, an 83.2 percent immunization rate in the overall population fell to 57 percent for the inner-city subpopulation. Though some studies have proven case management effective in increasing immunizations among inner-city populations, case management is costly because it is so labor intensive. The biggest problem appears to be with late-cycle immunizations, perhaps because parents with lower education don't understand the importance of going through the whole cycle, or because the lack of a consistent and single place to go for medical care creates gaps in coverage. Creating consistent services will go a long way toward getting all children immunized regardless of socioeconomic status, which may in the long run keep down the costs of caring for this population.

TEEN PREGNANCY

After decades of declining birthrates among U.S. teens ages 15 to 19, they spiked during the late 1980s and early 1990s, increasing from 50.2 births per 1,000 females in 1986 to 56.8 in 1995. Teen birthrates have decreased recently, to 49.6 in 1999, the lowest rate in 60 years. The drop was more pronounced among young teens, ages 15–17, who registered a decline of 6 percent between 1998 and 1999 (see Figure 13-4). The number of births to unmarried teenagers was 2 percent lower in 1999 than in 1998. In addition, the number of births for the youngest teenage group, ages 10–14, dropped by 4 percent to the lowest level in 30 years. However, it is important to recognize that "out-of-wedlock" births among teens continue to increase even as the overall teen birthrate has fallen. This means that fewer people are marrying in their teens and having babies, and that more teens who are having babies are not married.

As mentioned earlier, children of one-parent families are more apt to live in poverty, which means they are also more likely to have health problems. The health care system can help in at least two ways: by working to prevent births to unmarried teens and by targeting the children of unmarried teens for extra medical attention and follow-up.

Many teen pregnancy experts attribute the drop of teen births overall to the growing effectiveness of teen pregnancy education and prevention campaigns. Experts believe the teen birthrate is falling, in part, because more teens are choosing to delay sexual activity and those who are sexually active are more likely to use contraceptives.

If childbearing prevention programs focus solely on female teenagers, however, they may be missing an important segment of participants in this problem. Of sexually active 15- to 17-year-olds,

---

Figure 13-4. Unmarried, with children

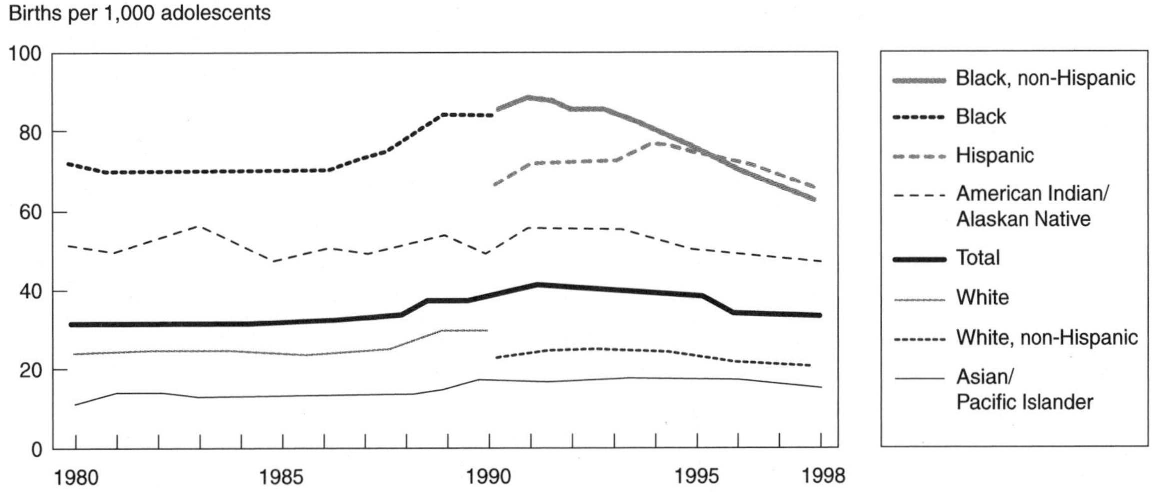

Births per 1,000 adolescents

Source: America's Children: Key National Indicator of Well-Being, Federal Interagency Forum on Child and Family Statistics, 2000.

29 percent have sexual partners who are 3–5 years older, and 7 percent have partners who are 6 or more years older.[68,69] Furthermore, while data are still scattered and preliminary, there seems to be growing evidence that the births experienced by many young teens may be the result of coerced sex.[70] Young adult men in high-risk communities should be targeted for education programs and held accountable for the children they father.

SMOKING AND DRUG USE

In 2000, the National Institute on Drug Abuse reported good news with the results of its annual national survey of illicit drug use among 8th, 10th, and 12th graders.[71] Use of illicit drugs in the preceding month among 12- to 17-year-olds remained stable for the fourth year in a row. Since 1996 or 1997, there have been decreases in the use of inhalants, hallucinogens such as LSD, and smoked methamphetamine. The few recent statistically significant increases were in the use of Ecstasy, anabolic-androgenic steroids among 10th graders, and heroin use among 12th graders.

Alcohol use among teens also peaked in 1997 and has been declining since then, as surveys taken in 2000 indicate, with 50 percent of 12th graders, 41 percent of 10th graders, and 22 percent of 8th graders reporting alcohol use in the preceding month. Cigarette use among teens has also decreased, with 31 percent of 12th graders, 24 percent of 10th graders, and 15 percent of 8th graders reporting use in the preceding month in 2000. Recent attacks on the tobacco industry by federal and state governments and public health programs may have resulted in significant efforts by both to decrease teen smoking.

The long-term detrimental effects of teen drinking and smoking are obvious. Increased alcohol use results in increased risk of accidents, violence, and high-risk sexual behavior. At the same time, smokers who start in their teens are less likely to be able to quit.[72] Though the recent trend is heartening, any increases in these behaviors will result in higher health care costs for the system in the future.

VIOLENCE AND CRIME

The problem of violence shows itself in two ways—violence perpetrated against children and violence perpetrated by children. The number of youth victims of crime increased steadily between 1980 and 1994 when it peaked and started declining (see Figure 13-5).

One form of violence against children, child abuse and neglect, has declined from just over 900,000 children in 1998 to an estimated 826,000 victims of maltreatment in 1999 nationwide. The incidence rate of children victimized by maltreatment also declined to 11.8 per 1,000 children, a decrease from the 1998 rate of 12.6 per 1,000.[73]

In a trend that began in 1994, the number of victimized children has decreased approximately 19.2 percent from a record of 1,018,692 in 1993. Parents continue to be the main perpetrators of child maltreatment. More than 87 percent of all victims were maltreated by at least one parent. The most common pattern of

Figure 13-5. Youthful victims of violence: Rate of serious violent crime victimization of youth, ages 12–17 by gender

Per 1,000 youths, ages 12–17

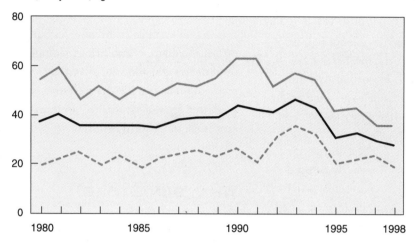

Source: America's Children: Key National Indicator of Well-Being, Federal Interagency Forum on Child and Family Statistics, 2000.

Figure 13-6. Serious violent crime offending rate

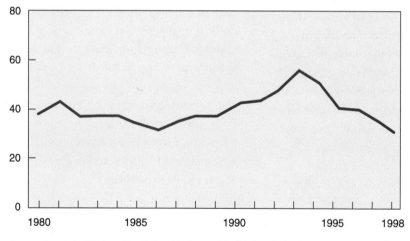

Source: America's Children: Key National Indicator of Well-Being, Federal Interagency Forum on Child and Family Statistics, 2000.

maltreatment (44.7%) was a child victimized by a female parent acting alone. Female parents were identified as the perpetrators of neglect and physical abuse for the highest percentage of child vic-

tims. In contrast, male parents were identified as the perpetrators of sexual abuse for the highest percentage of victims.

As for violence by children, the Department of Justice reported that as the adult arrest rate for murder fell 7 percent from 1978 to 1993, the juvenile murder rate surged by 177 percent, peaked in 1993, and has been declining since then. At the same time, the arrest rate of teens for all violent crimes (involving use of force) climbed 79 percent, almost three times the rise in the adult rate. Nationally, the juvenile violent crime arrest rate increased from 305 per 100,000 youths ages 10 to 17 in 1985 to peak at 517 in 1994.

In response to this perception of an onslaught by a "wave of superpredators," pressure was put on Congress to treat juvenile violent offenders like adults by locking them up with adult inmates. Such a tactic doesn't do much for the health of the juvenile offenders, however. Juveniles in adult jails commit suicide eight times as often as other prisoners, are five times as likely to be sexually assaulted, and are twice as likely to be beaten by staff.

Since 1995, juvenile arrests for violent crimes—murder, rape, robbery, and aggravated assault—have declined and in 1998 the juvenile violent crime arrest rate was at its lowest point in 10 years (Figure 13-6). Young people under age 15 accounted for more than half of the decline of these arrests, suggesting that, despite perceptions from the media, perhaps there was no wave of violent youth crime. In fact, most (19 out of 20) juvenile arrests were for nonviolent crimes.[74]

Chapter 13: Children's Health

ADOLESCENT DEATHS

Deaths from injuries—accidents, homicides, and suicides—accounted for 75 percent of all adolescent deaths among 10- to 19-year-olds in 1998. While perceptions of increasing violence in our country highlight the implications of this indicator, it is important to note that accidents continue to account for far more teen deaths than any other source.

Nonetheless, since 1985, a decline in fatal teen accidents (primarily automobile accidents) has been offset by a doubling in the number of homicides. The number of teen deaths due to accidents reduced from 8,202 in 1985 to 6,565 in 1994, while the number of teen homicides ballooned from 1,602 to 3,569 during the same period. The number of teen suicides increased slightly during the period (from 1,849 to 1,948). It is important to note that rates of teen death vary greatly by geographic region, urbanization level, and state gun laws. In general, motor vehicle death rates are higher in less densely populated settings and firearm homicide is higher in more densely populated settings.[75]

Despite some good news about decreasing violence, the fact is that many children live with increasing anxiety induced by expectations of violence and even death. Moreover, children are not oblivious to what's happening around them. In a recent study by Kaiser Family Foundation and Children Now, children aged 7 to 17, regardless of age, religion, or demographic group, said they were "gripped by fears of violence and early death because of physical, sexual, and drug abuse." Of those aged 7 to 10 years old, 63 percent said they were worried they would die young, while 70 percent were afraid of getting shot or stabbed at home or in school or feared they would be hit by an adult.[76] This anxiety affects children's health in many ways, causing a higher incidence of conditions ranging from depression and suicide to the common cold. Until these circumstances are addressed by society at large, attempts to keep children healthy will remain incomplete.

WHAT'S IN STORE?

Balancing the positive trends of most indicators of children's health against continuing discrepancies by social status (poverty, race/ethnicity, etc.) and our poor performance when compared with other countries around the world, we have to say the system appears to be doing a mediocre job of keeping U.S. children healthy. But what's in store for the future?

The apparent success of the current health care system for children is somewhat a lucky accident—a precarious balancing act of public and private resources. But the balance isn't likely to hold for long.

For one thing, children are not a monolithic, homogeneous group. The health care needs of children vary dramatically by age group. For example, prenatal care and immunizations have the greatest impact for 1- to 3-year-olds, whereas adolescent health care focuses more on social and behavioral concerns such as substance abuse and pregnancy prevention. This wide range of diverse needs, combined with poorly integrated public and private care, has created what Madlyn Morreale, of Johns Hopkins University School of Hygiene and Public Health, described as a "non-system" of health care services for children.[77]

Neither public- nor private-sector efforts have been sufficient to address the broad spectrum of child and adolescent health care needs. Private efforts consist of individually focused primary health care that is removed from—and not coordinated with—population-based care. Public sector programs are extremely complex and lack coordination.

For example, federally legislated child health programs implemented today represent a mix of income-based entitlement programs (Medicaid and EPSDT), quasi-entitlement programs (Women, Infants and Children), categorical population or disease-specific programs (immunization, pediatric AIDS, lead poisoning, health care for the homeless, and family planning programs), and age-specific entitlement programs (early intervention services for infants and toddlers with disabilities). "Gap-filling" grant-funded programs (Title V prenatal and child health services) and categorical grants to localities for community and migrant health centers are also included. Health services, too, are embedded in entitlement and categorical programs for education (special education and school health services) and social services (Head Start and family preservation programs).

The system as a whole is a threadbare, patchwork net ready to snap if too much more weight is added. Policymakers face significant challenges in strengthening that net to develop a coordinated and integrated system of care for this population, in that the categorical funding streams often prevent consolidation of these overlapping or related services. A family trying to access services has no central place to go and must apply to each agency separately. This takes the kind of resources and time that much of the underserved population just doesn't have. An obvious solution, then, is to create a health care system for children that has as close to "one-stop shopping" as possible, given the different levels of government and private institutions involved. With the trend toward increased public funding of children's health insurance, opportunities exist for the creation of public-private partnerships that consolidate and link vital services.

Meanwhile, it seems that the population of children that makes the most demands on the system—the chronically ill—is likely to increase in the next 10 years. Though tempered by advances in technology, the number of children born with significant disabilities is growing. Increasingly younger and smaller premature babies are being born and are surviving, thanks to amazing and expensive neonatal technology. As more premature babies of low birth weight survive into childhood, the numbers of younger disabled are expected to increase. Technological advances also will increase the number of children who survive disabling accidents.

Of the 500,000 children in need of long-term care, 330,000 are unable to play or attend school because of conditions such as epilepsy, asthma, and cystic fibrosis. The remaining 170,000 are severely disabled with cerebral palsy or mental retardation.[78]

Most children with chronic illnesses requiring long-term care are cared for by their families at home.[79] Children under 18 make up only 3 percent of the total long-term care population. These children have disabling physical and/or cognitive conditions that leave them unable to engage in age-appropriate activities or school. The definition of this population is problematic, as traditional measures of function and disability for adults do not apply to children (that is, dressing and feeding themselves). As more children move into the population that needs long-term care, the system will be stretched even further.

CHILDREN ARE MEANT TO BE SEEN AND NOT HEARD

In any debate about allocating scarce resources, it always comes down to: Who has the political clout to get things done their way? The issue of children's health care may ultimately come down to a battle between children and senior citizens since together they make up the nation's "dependent population," or those persons whose age makes them less likely to be employed than others.

This is a battle children have no chance of winning.

Though children represent a smaller percentage of the population today than in 1960, they are nevertheless a stable and substantial portion and will remain so into the next century. In contrast, senior citizens have increased from 8 to 13 percent of the total population since 1950. In 1960, children made up 79 percent of the dependent population; by 2000, they made up approximately 65 percent. That percentage is expected to continue decreasing through 2020.

Not only are children a shrinking portion of the whole, but they have no voice—they cannot speak for themselves. They don't vote, and for many of the underserved, neither do their parents. The tendency to vote is tied to education level. Thus the majority voice of the voter is an older, more affluent voice that probably doesn't recognize the needs of children's health issues, especially for underserved populations. Voting is just one way that interest groups influence policy. As children become a smaller share of the "dependent population," and the elderly share of the U.S. population grows, there may be less intergenerational equity, and school bond initiatives and children's health measures will give way to expanding Medicare.

How much should we be concerned about this silent population? As noted previously, most kids are in pretty good shape. Most have health insurance and access to some form of health care services. And even though these services are fragmented, uncoordinated, and geographically patchy, the fact that, increasingly, one payer for those services—the government—picks up the tab means there are opportunities for stakeholders to collaborate in each local community.

But a substantial proportion of children—about 20 percent—do not have access to insurance and have only difficult access to services. This is a large and significant group. These children are not well served by the system, as it is; they need some help! Medicaid expansion and SCHIP have targeted these kids, but the two programs are likely to serve only a net gain of 1.6 million of the total of 11.6 million children who are likely to be uninsured in 10 years. And with the possible decrease in employer-based health insurance in a worldwide economic slowdown, the number of uninsured is likely to increase even more (though experts are on the fence about the extent of the likely decline in employer-based health insurance). It will be important to watch the local initiatives for children and the makeup of employee benefit packages to see what the future of health care holds for America's children.

IMPLICATIONS OF CURRENT TRENDS FOR CHILDREN'S FUTURE HEALTH

The current system of health care for children is holding its own, but is unlikely to be able to handle additional stresses. These stresses are coming, however, in the form of decreasing private health insurance, the likely inability of public financing to continue taking up the slack, a maldistribution of adequate pediatric health care providers, and environmental factors that are getting worse instead of better.

These trends have important implications for children's health in the future:

- *Catch them early.* Children are relatively inexpensive to care for and offer a huge return on investment. Preventing childhood disease with immuniza-

tions and other forms of preventive medicine saves the system the later costs of treating these diseases by tenfold, according to some estimates. A health care system that's trying to slow the overall growth of costs can't afford not to take this strategy seriously.

- *Don't expect Medicaid to do it all.* As the wave of reform was implemented through the Balanced Budget Act of 1997, the channel for replacing private health insurance reductions with some form of public financing—Medicaid and SCHIP—has been effectively narrowed. Policymakers will have to find other ways to make sure children get access to health care. Possibilities include school-based health programs that will teach children healthy behavior and make health care available to them on a daily basis.

- *Plan for decreases in private insurance coverage.* More employers will increase employees' share of their health insurance premiums and decrease dependent coverage, and more employees will forgo coverage to save money, especially now that the world economy seems to be heading for recession. Since health insurance is a good proxy for health care services, fewer children will receive adequate health care under this scenario unless the booming economy rebounds quickly from a slowdown, and the labor shortage compels companies to offer full benefits, including health insurance for dependents, to attract strong employees.

- *Make pediatric care available across the board.* Pediatricians are not adequately distributed across the United States, with most in metropolitan areas and few in rural or inner-city communities. Although community health clinics play an important role in these areas, children who receive routine care in community clinics instead of physicians' offices are likely to lack continuity of care and to use emergency facilities as their usual source of sick care. This is both expensive and self-defeating.

- *Forge creative partnerships beyond health care.* With diseases as varied as childhood asthma and teen suicide attributed to environmental effects, health care policymakers must work with policymakers outside of health care to create better, healthier environments for children. Health care policymakers can work with environmentalists, for example, to decrease air pollution in crowded urban areas, or with gun control lobbyists to limit the violence to which children are often exposed.

- *Prepare to serve a growing chronically ill population.* Because of new technologies, more of the chronically ill will live longer, and more and earlier preterm and low-birth-weight babies—a proportion of which are chronically ill—will live past their first year. The system must be prepared to care for the surge in these populations.

- *Create a system with one-stop shopping,* especially for the chronically ill. Categorical funding streams prevent consolidation of overlapping or related services. A family trying to access services has no central place to go for care and must apply to each agency separately. Health care stakeholders

must attempt to provide one-stop shopping for such families.

- *Agree on a universal definition of "special needs."* Different states and programs define the population differently and target services to specific subsets, resulting in overlapping services in some areas and no services in others. For the system to best serve the people who need help the most, it must define these populations consistently and act on these definitions.

- *Pay attention to cross-cultural differences.* Since many poor people belong to nonwhite ethnic groups, caregivers must try to reach these groups in new ways. Better translation services are a start, while cross-cultural health education programs are also important. Programs that pay attention to the needs of diverse communities must be created, expanded, and financed for the long run.

- *Work to decrease teen pregnancy.* Although teen pregnancy as a whole is decreasing, out-of-wedlock teen pregnancy continues to increase. The children of these unwed mothers are often born with low birth weights and their attendant (and expensive) health problems. These same babies will be most at risk for inadequate early health care and more expensive interventions later on. School-based programs targeting these at-risk teen populations need to continue, with an increased focus on the role and responsibilities of young men.

- *Work the environmental issues.* For certain populations, such as urban, inner-city children exposed to air pollution and the contaminants associated with substandard housing (lead paint, cockroaches, dust mites), and rural children exposed to pesticides, the environment seems to be a significant enemy of good health. The powerful health care lobbies—those for doctors and insurance companies—can use their clout to influence local, regional, and federal legislatures to do the right thing in reducing these environmental dangers.

WILDCARDS

- The recession of the beginning of the new millennium grows deep and sustained, adding to the rolls of the uninsured and Medicaid-eligible. Medicaid reimbursements will not be able to cover the increasing costs of care, leaving millions with nowhere to turn for services.

- Converging forces, such as the decentralization of responsibility to local communities and the privatization of public health services, lead to the widespread collapse of health care safety nets, triggering major infusions of federal and state funds. This collapse will divert funds intended for other health purposes and most likely will be too little, too late.

- Legislation sinks managed care. Concomitantly, the American public's appetite for new technology, including drugs, drives the nation's health care bill through the ceiling. A legislative backlash strikes the most vulnerable.

- Not satisfied with the relatively small net gain in health insurance coverage that SCHIP and Medicaid provide for children, federal and state legislators expand Medicaid to include children above 200 percent of FPL (with some familial contribution), reaching some of the 3.5 million uninsured children in that income bracket.

ENDNOTES

[1] Elixhauser, A., K. Yu, C. Steiner, and A. S. Bierman. *Hospitalization in the United States, 1997.* Rockville, MD: Agency for Healthcare Research and Quality, 2000. Health Care Utilization Project (HCUP) Fact Book No. 1. Agency for Healthcare Research and Quality (AHRQ) Publication No. 00-0031.

[2] Barker D.J.P., C. Osmond, P. D. Winter, B. Margetts, and S. J. Simmonds. Weight in infancy and death from ischaemic heart disease *Lancet* 1989; 2: 577–580 and Guo, S.S., A. F. Roche, W. C. Chumlea, J. D. Gardner, and R. M. Siervogel. The predictive value of childhood body mass index values for overweight at age 35 y. *Am J Clin Nutr* 1994; 59: 810–819 and Nieto, F. J., M. Szklo, G. W. Comstock. Childhood weight and growth rate as predictors of adult mortality. *Am J Epidemiol* 1992; 136: 201–213

[3] Children's Defense Fund, *Immunizations*, http://www.childrensdefense.org/hs_tp_imm uniz.php.

[4] Newacheck, P. W., M. Pearl, D. C. Hughes, and N. Halfon. The role of Medicaid in ensuring children's access to care. *Journal of the American Medical Association* 1998; 280:1789–1793.

[5] Newacheck, P. W,. et al. Health insurance and access to primary care for children. *New England Journal of Medicine* 1998; 338:513–519.

[6] U.S. Census Bureau. *Health Insurance Coverage: 2000.* Current Population Reports. 2001.

[7] Federal Interagency Forum on Child and Family Statistics. *America's Children: Key National Indicators of Well-Being, 2001.* Federal Interagency Forum on Child and Family Statistics. Washington, DC: U.S. Government Printing Office.

[8] DeAngelis, C., et al. Final Report of the FOPE II Pediatric Workforce Group. *Pediatrics* 2000; 106(5):1245–1255.

[9] Shogren, J. Children and the environment: valuing indirect effects on a child's life chances. *Contemporary Economic Policy* (October) 2001; 19(4):382–396.

[10] Newacheck, P. W., J. J. Stoddard, D. C. Hughes, and M. Pearl. Health insurance and access to primary care for children. *New England Journal of Medicine* (February 19) 1998; 338(8):513–519.

[11] Fronstin, P. *Employment-Based Health Benefits: Trends and Outlook.* Employee Benefit Research Institute. May 2001.

[12] Department of Labor. *Futurework: Trends and Challenges for Work in the Twenty-First Century 1999.* www.dol.gov/dol/asp/public/futurework/report/chapter4/main.htm#4b.

[13] Duchon, L., et. al. *Listening to Workers: Challenges for Employer-Sponsored Coverage in the 21st Century.* New York: The Commonwealth Fund, Taskforce for the Future of Health Insurance for Working Americans. January 2000.

[14] Salisbury, D. *EBRI Research Highlights: Retirement and Health Data.* Employee Benefit Research Institute. January 2001.

[15] U.S. Census Bureau. *Health Insurance Coverage: 2000.* Current Population Reports. 2001.

[16] Kaiser Commission on Medicaid and the Uninsured. Health Care for the Poor: Medicaid at 35. *Health Care Financing Review.* Fall 2000.

[17] Kaiser Commission on Medicaid and the Uninsured. *State Health Facts, 1998.* Kaiser Family Foundation. www.kff.org/docs/state/state.html.

[18] American Academy of Pediatrics, Committee on child health financing. scope of health care benefits for newborns, infants, children, adolescents, and young adults through age 21 years. *Pediatrics* 1997; 100:1040–1041.

[19] Lillie-Blanton, M. A Review of the Nation's Progress and Challenges in Assuring Access to Health Care for Low-Income Americans. *Access to Health Care: Promises and Prospects for Low-Income Americans.* Report of

the Kaiser Commission on Medicaid and the Uninsured. Washington, DC. 1999.

[20] Lyons, B. Welfare Reform and Medicaid Coverage of Low-Income Families. Testimony before the United States House of Representatives Committee on Ways and Means, Subcommittee on Human Resources. May 16, 2000.

[21] Health Care Financing Administration. Impacts of Medicaid managed care on children. *Health Services Research* 2001; 36(1):7–23.

[22] Social Security Administration. Welfare Reform and Childhood Disability Factsheet. February 1997. www.ssa.gov/pubs/wrchild.html.

[23] Hurley, R. E., and M. A. McCue. *Partnership Pays: Making Medicaid Managed Care Work in a Turbulent Environment.* Princeton, N.J.: Center for Health Care Strategies Inc., 2000. Meyer, H. Medicaid: States give up a real turkey. *Hospitals and Health Networks.* November 1997.

[24] Health Care Financing Administration. *A Profile of Medicaid 2000 Chartbook.* U.S. Dept. of Health and Human Services. www.hcfa.gov/stats/2Tchartbk.pdf.

[25] Urban Institute. Unpublished analysis of Medicaid enrollees and expenditures, based on data from Urban Institute as cited in Kaiser Commission on Medicaid and the Uninsured. Health Care for the Poor: Medicaid at 35. *Health Care Financing Review.* Fall 2000.

[26] Hakim, R., et al. Medicaid and the Health of Children. *Health Care Financing Review* 2000; 22(1):133–140.

[27] National Center for Health Statistics. 1999.

[28] Health Care Financing Administration. *The State Children's Health Insurance Program: Preliminary Highlights of Implementation and Expansion.* 2000. www.hcfa.gov/init/wh0700.pdf

[29] Congressional Budget Office. *Budgetary Implications of the Balanced Budget Act of 1997.* CBO Memorandum.

[30] St Peter, R. F., et al. Changes in the scope of care provided by primary care physicians. *New England Journal of Medicine* (December 22) 1999; 341(26):1980–1985.

[31] DeAngelis, C., et al. Final Report of the FOPE II Pediatric Workforce Group. *Pediatrics* 2000; 106(5):1245–1255.

[32] Stoddard, J. J., R. F. St Peter, P. W. Newacheck. Health insurance status and ambulatory care for children. *New England Journal of Medicine* (May 19) 1994; 330(20):1452–1453.

[33] American Medical Association. Nonfederal Physicians in the US and Possessions by Selected Characteristics. www.ama-assn.org/ama/pub/category/2688.html.

[34] National Conference of State Legislatures. The Health Care Workforce in Ten States: Education, Practice and Policy, Interstate Comparisons. Spring 2001

[35] Council on Graduate Medical Education. COGME Physician Workforce Policies: Recent Developments and Remaining Challenges in Meeting National Goals. March 1999. www.cogme.gov/14.pdf.

[36] National Association of Pediatric Nurse Associates. About NAPNAP. www.napnap.org/about.html.

[37] Shogren, J. Children and the environment: Valuing indirect effects on a child's life chances. *Contemporary Economic Policy* 2001; 19(4):382–396. National Academy of Sciences National Research Council. Accounting for Renewable and Environmental Resources. *Survey of Current Business* 80(3):26–51.

[38] Szilagyi, P., and E. Schor. The health of children. *Health Services Research* (October) 1998; 33(4):1001–1039.

[39] U.S. Census Bureau. *Poverty in the United States.* 1999.

[40] Federal Interagency Forum on Child and Family Statistics. America's Children: Key National Indicators of Well-Being, 2001. www.childstats.gov.

[41] U.S. Census Bureau. *Health Insurance Coverage Status by Selected Characteristics: 1990 to 1998.* Current Population Reports. Unpublished data as cited in the Statistical Abstract of the United States: 2000.

[42] Newacheck, P. W., et al. Children's access to primary care: Differences by race, income, and insurance status. *Pediatrics* 1996; 97:26–32.

[43] Montgomery, L. E., et al. The effects of poverty, race, and family structure on us children's health: Data from the NHIS, 1978 through 1980 and 1989 through 1991. *Am J Public Health* 1996; 86:1401–1405.

[44] Schmitt, E. For First Time, Nuclear Families Drop Below 25% of Households. *New York Times.* May 15, 2001.

[45] U.S. Census Bureau. *Poverty in the United States, 1999.*

[46] McLanahan, S. (1995). The consequences of nonmarital childbearing for women, children, and society. In National Center for Health Statistics, *Report to Congress on out-of-wedlock childbearing.* Hyattsville, MD: National Center for Health Statistics. Ventura, S. J., and C. A. Bachrach. Nonmarital childbearing in the United States, 1940–99. National Vital Statistics Reports, 48(16). Hyattsville, MD: National Center for Health Statistics, 2000.

[47] Zahm, S. H., and M. H. Ward. Pesticides and Childhood Cancer. *Environmental Health Perspectives* (June) 1998; 106(Suppl 3): 893–908.

[48] Perry, B. Stress, Trauma and Post-traumatic Stress Disorders in Children. Child Trauma Academy. 5 September, 1999. www.childtrauma.org/ptsd_interdisc.htm.

[49] American Lung Association. Prevalence Based on Revised National Health Interview Survey. www.lungusa.org/data/data_102000.html.

[50] American Lung Association. Trends in Asthma Morbidity and Mortality. January 2001. www.lungusa.org/data/asthma/asthmach_1.html#prevalence.

[51] Center for Disease Control. Facts about Asthma. www.cdc.gov/od/oc/media/fact/asthma.htm.

[52] Evans, R. Asthma among minority children: A growing problem. *Chest* 1992; 101(6):368–371.

[53] Landrigan, P. J., Environmental hazards for children in the U.S.A. *Int'l. Journal of Occupational Medicine and Environmental Health* 1998; 11(2):189–194.

[54] Environmental Protection Agency.

[55] American Cancer Society. Cancer Facts and Figures, 2000. www.cancer.org/downloads/STT/F&F00.pdf.

[56] Chow, W., et al. Cancers in Children. In: Schottenfield, D., et al., eds. *Cancer Epidemiology and Prevention*, 2nd ed. Oxford, MA: Oxford University Press, 1996.

[57] National Institute of Mental Health. The Numbers Count, Mental Disorders in America. www.nimh.nih.gov/publicat/numbers.cfm#23. Shaffer, D., P. Fisher, M.K. Dulcan, et al. The NIMH Diagnostic Interview Schedule for Children Version 2.3 (DISC-2.3): description, acceptability, prevalence rates, and performance in the MECA Study. Methods for the Epidemiology of Child and Adolescent Mental Disorders Study. *Journal of the American Academy of Child and Adolescent Psychiatry* 1996; 35(7):865–877.

[58] Leung, A. K., and W. L. Robson. Children of Divorce. *Journal of Social Health* (October) 1990; 110(5):161–163.

[59] Newacheck, P. W., and N. Halfon. Prevalence and impact of disabling chronic conditions in childhood. *American Journal of Public Health* 1998; 88:610–617.

[60] Centers for Disease Control and Prevention. Measuring Childhood Asthma Prevalence Before and After the 1997 Redesign of the National Health Interview Survey—United States. Morbidity and Mortality Weekly Report, 1998. www.cdc.gov/od/oc/media/mmwrnews/n2k1013.htm#mmwr2.

[61] Halsey, C. L., et al. Extremely low-birth-weight children and their peers. A comparison of school-age outcomes. *Arch Pediatr Adolesc Med.* 1996. 150:790–794.

[62] National Center on Birth Defects and Developmental Disabilities. Developmental Disabilities. www.cdc.gov/ncbddd/dd/default.htm.

[63] Healthy People 2000. Maternal and Infant Health Indicator Review. www.cdc.gov/nchs/about/otheract/hp2000/childhlt/mchb&w.pdf.

[64] Centers for Disease Control and Prevention, 1995. Kiely, John L. Poverty and Infant Mortality—United States, 1988. *Morbidity and Mortality Weekly Report* 44(49):922–927.

[65] National Center for Health Statistics. Faststats A to Z, Birthweight and Gestation. www.cdc.gov/nchs/fastats/birthwt.htm.

[66] Institute of Medicine (IOM). *Preventing Low Birthweight.* Washington, DC: National Academy Press, 1985.

[67] Healthy People 2000. Maternal and Infant Health Indicator Review. www.cdc.gov/nchs/about/otheract/hp2000/childhlt/mchb&w.pdf.

[68] The Alan Guttmacher Institute. Facts in Brief, Teen Sex and Pregnancy. 1999. www.agi-usa.org/pubs/fb_teen_sex.html#tp.

[69] Darroch J. E., D. J. Landry, and S. Oslak. Age differences between sexual partners in the United States. *Family Planning Perspectives* 1999; 31(4):160–167.

[70] The Alan Guttmacher Institute. Sex and America's Teenagers. 1994. Abma, J., A. Driscoll, and K. Moore. Young women's degree of control over first intercourse: An exploratory analysis. *Family Planning Perspectives* 1998; 30(1):12–18. www.agi-usa.org/pubs/journals/3001298.html.

[71] National Institute on Drug Abuse, National Institutes of Health. High School and Youth Trends. www.nida.nih.gov/Infofax/HSYouthtrends.html.

[72] Centers for Disease Control and Prevention, National Center for Chronic Disease Prevention and Health Promotion. *Women and Smoking: A Report of the Surgeon General.* 2001. www.cdc.gov/tobacco/sgr/sgr_forwomen/Executive_Summary.htm.

[73] U.S. Department of Health and Human Services. Child Maltreatment 1999: Reports from the States to the National Child Abuse and Neglect Data System. www.acf.dhhs.gov/programs/cb/publications/cm99/index.htm.

[74] Meek, J. G. Juvenile Violent Crime Lowest in 10 Years. November 24, 1999. www.apbnews.com/newscenter/breakingnews/1999/11/24/juvenile1124_01.html.

[75] Centers for Disease Control and Prevention, National Center for Health Statistics. *Health, United States.* 2000.

[76] Kaiser Family Foundation/Children Now. Talking with Kids About Tough Issues: A National Survey of Parents and Kids. 1998. www.talkingwithkids.org.

[77] Morreale, M., and H. Grason. Health Services for Children and Adolescents: "Non-System" of Care. In: Stein, R.E.K., ed. *Health Care for Children: What's Right, What's Wrong, What's Next.* New York: United Hospital Fund, 1997.

[78] Adler, M. ASPE (Assistant Secretary for Planning and Evaluation) Research Notes: Disability Among Children. January 1995. aspe.hhs.gov/daltcp/reports/rn10.htm.

[79] Szilagyi, P., and E. Schor. The health of children. *Health Services Research* (October) 1998; 33(4):1001–1039.

CHAPTER 14

Health and Health Care of America's Seniors

The Future Awaits Us

There's a big change coming. The largest generation in recent history, the baby boomers, is aging into the most service intensive and therefore expensive health care period of their lives. Although the first of the baby boomers will not be turning 65 until 2011, this chapter focuses on them and the future of health and health care for America's seniors because they are expected to transform the health care delivery system. In this chapter we first describe seniors in terms of changing demographic, economic, health, and social trends. We then describe the health care delivery system they will encounter. The final section addresses some of the implications of this meeting.

THE DEMOGRAPHICS OF AN AGING POPULATION

Americans have witnessed incredible advances in health care during the 20th century. Technological advances in imaging, vaccines, pharmaceuticals, and surgery have combined with social and public health infrastructure changes, such as sanitation, to improve health and health care and enable people to live healthier, longer lives. Life expectancy

has increased dramatically in the 20th century and will continue to increase, though less dramatically, over the next decade.[1]

The largest generation of the 20th century, the baby boomers, is moving into the final third of their lives and the time when their health care utilization increases with senescence, the natural decline of our bodies. This section forecasts the demographic changes in America with special attention to the baby boomers. Though baby boomers are not the only people who will be aging in America through 2010, their sheer numbers will test the capacity of the health care system and much of the next 10 years will be spent preparing for their needs. Additionally, the baby boomer generation has transformed every institution they have interacted with throughout their lives—and health care is next.

THE BABY BOOM GENERATION: DEFINITION AND IMPACTS

Low fertility rates during the 1930s Depression were followed by high fertility rates after World War II and the birth of 76 million baby boomers from 1946 to 1964. Fertility rates began declining after 1964 and were accompanied by increasing longevity.

Described by the Census Bureau as a "human tidal wave," the baby boom generation is technically defined as those born between 1946 and 1964. This cohort is 70 percent larger than the generation born during the prior two decades and it is expected to live longer than any cohort before. Now in their most economically productive years (aged 39 to 57 in 2003), these "boomers" currently comprise more than one-third of the U.S. population.

WHY 2010 IS A BENCHMARK YEAR

As the baby boom generation ages, U.S. society will be transformed. While those over 65 years of age are now a relatively small part of the population—12 percent—by 2030 this age group will constitute fully one-fifth or 20 percent of the population—a sizable segment of all consumers, voters, home owners, and patients. Increasingly, every social institution and sector will be required to accommodate the needs of older people. Resources will have to be mobilized to serve them.

A critical concept in preparing to manage this sweeping transformation of society is the recognition that the transformation itself will happen suddenly, not gradually or incrementally, over the coming decade. It may seem common sense to say that the shape of the "age wave" will match that of the baby boom from which it was spawned. But many health care planners do not fully appreciate that the period from now through 2010 is, relatively speaking, a "quiet before the storm." Because the baby boomers will not begin reaching the retirement age of 65 until 2011, the dramatic changes in population aging will not occur until after 2010—the benchmark year around which many issues in this chapter revolve.

Thus, those considering the future of health care for the elderly must plan for two distinct time frames:

1995 to 2010

■ *Older growth rate is declining.* Between 1990 and 2010, the average growth rate of the older population will actually be lower than at any equivalent period since 1910.

■ *Elderly population is increasing.* Over the 15-year period 1995 to 2010, the population aged 65 and over will, however, increase 17.5 percent, from

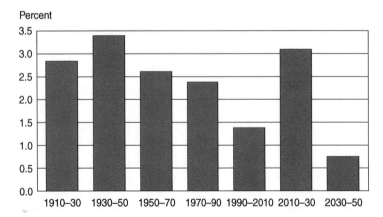

Figure 14-1. Average annual growth rate of the elderly population, 1910–2050

Percent

Source: U.S Bureau of the Census. General Population Characteristics, PC80-1-B1. Washington, DC: USGPO, May 1983; 1990. Census of Population and Housing, CPH-L-74, *Modified and Actual Age, Sex, Race, and Hispanic Origin Data; Population Projections ot the United States by Age, Sex, Race, and Hispanic Origin: 1995 to 2050.* Current Population Reports, Series P-25, No. 1130. Washington, DC: USGPO, 1993.

Chapter 14: Health and Health Care of America's Seniors

*Figure 14-2. U.S. demographic profile, 1995:
Middle-age spread of the baby boomers*

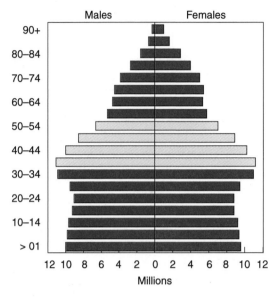

Source: U.S Bureau of the Census. *Population Projections ot the United States by Age, Sex, Race, and Hispanic Origin: 1995 to 2050.* Current Population Reports, Series P-25, No. 1130. Washington, DC: USGPO, 1993.

*Figure 14-3. U.S. demographic profile, 2010:
Baby boomers reach AARP territory.*

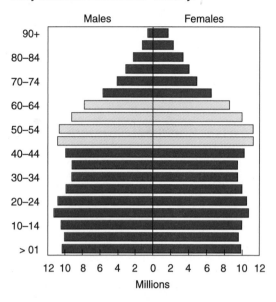

*Figure 14-4. U.S. demographic profile, 2030:
Top-heavy baby boomers*

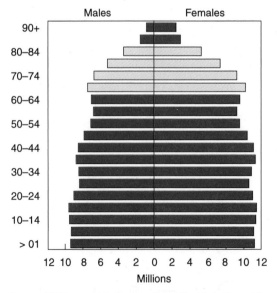

Source: U.S Bureau of the Census. *Population Projections ot the United States by Age, Sex, Race, and Hispanic Origin: 1995 to 2050.* Current Population Reports, Series P-25, No. 1130. Washington, DC: USGPO, 1993.

33.5 million to 39.4 million or from 12.8 percent to 13.3 percent of the total population. In the year 2010, half of the U.S. population will be 37 years or older, and the baby boomers will be aged 46 to 64.

- *Watershed year.*   In 2010 the first *half* of the baby boom population (i.e., those aged 55 to 64) will be poised to initiate the real "tidal wave of aging." By 2020, the population of these near-elderly will have grown to 31.4 million from their 1995 level of 21.1 million

2010 to 2030

- *Period of most rapid growth.*   Over this 20-year period, the elderly population will increase from 39.4 million to 69.4, the most rapid growth period for the elderly of the 21st century.

- *One in five.* By 2030, as the last of the baby boom cohort reaches retirement age, one out of five persons will be at least age 65 and comprise slightly over 20 percent of the total population.[2]

Figure 14-5. Projection of the elderly population by age, 1995–2030

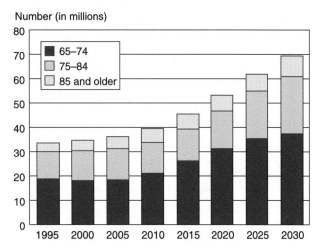

Number (in millions)

Source: U.S Bureau of the Census. *Population Projections of the United States by Age, Sex, Race, and Hispanic Origin: 1995 to 2050.* Current Population Reports, Series P-25, No. 1130. Washington, DC: USGPO, 1993.

Figure 14-6. Centenarians in the United States, 1995–2030

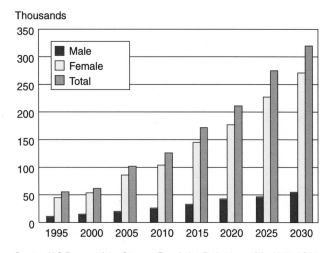

Thousands

Source: U.S Bureau of the Census. *Population Projections of the United States by Age, Sex, Race, and Hispanic Origin: 1995 to 2050.* Current Population Reports, Series P-25, No. 1130. Washington, DC: USGPO, 1993.

THE "OLDEST OLD" AND CENTENARIANS: A NEW FORCE

who are they?

Of particular significance in developing health care strategies for the elderly is the projected growth in the "oldest old," the population aged 85 and above. The health and income status of a large proportion of this age group will be significantly compromised, raising serious questions related to funding for the health, social service, and long-term care (LTC) needs of this population. Thus, estimating the future size of this high-utilization group is critical.

In 2000, 4.2 million people had reached age 85, and approximately 337,000 were 95 and older. By 2010, the number of people aged 85 and older will increase to 5.7 million and the number aged 95 and older will more than double to 666,000. By 2030, the number of people aged 85 and older will have grown to 8.5 million.

The number of centenarians in the United States is already rapidly growing and will rise from approximately 50,000 in 2000 to 131,000 in 2010, by which year women centenarians will outnumber men by more than five to one. According to the middle series projection, by 2030 the number of centenarians will nearly triple to 324,000 (271,000 women and 53,000 men) (see Figure 14-6).

GENDER CONSIDERATIONS

Women constitute the largest segment of this fast-growing aging population. In 2000, there were 20.6 million women aged 65 and older in the United States versus 14.4 million men, making 70 men

who are

for every 100 women. This gender disparity increases with age: at ages 65 to 74 years, there are 82 men for every 100 women; at ages 75 to 84, 65 men per 100 women; and beyond 85 only 41 men per 100 women. Although life expectancy for men is projected to improve slightly over time, the gender disparity is not expected to change throughout the period 2010 to 2030, leaving many very old women without spousal income and/or care (see Figure 14-7).

DIVERSITY IN AGING

Over the long term, the aging population will be increasingly diverse due to higher birth and immigration rates of ethnic and racial minority groups (see Figure 14-8). Many of these diverse populations will be low-income, and/or require specialized health care services as they age.

The older Latino population will grow significantly between 2000 and 2010, rising from 1.7 to 2.8 million. By 2050, this population will nearly triple to 7.8 million. The elderly African American population will rise from 2.8 to 3.4 million between 2000 and 2010, reaching 6.9 million by 2030. The number of elderly Asian Americans will grow as well, from 819,000 to 1.3 million by 2010. In spite of these changes, Caucasian Americans will remain the dominant ethnic and racial proportion of those over 65 years old and will grow by 4 million from 30 to 34 million between 2000 and 2010.[3]

Figure 14-7. Number of men per 100 women by age, 1995 and 2030

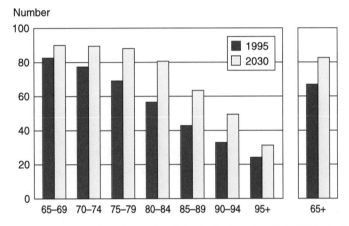

Source: U.S Bureau of the Census. *Population Projections of the United States by Age, Sex, Race, and Hispanic Origin: 1995 to 2050.* Current Population Reports, Series P-25, No. 1130. Washington, DC: USGPO, 1993.

Figure 14-8. Percent of population, 65 and older, by race and ethnicity, 1995 and 2030

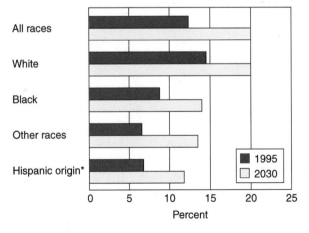

*Hispanic origin may be of any race

Source: U.S Bureau of the Census. *Population Projections ot the United States by Age, Sex, Race, and Hispanic Origin: 1995 to 2050.* Current Population Reports, Series P-25, No. 1130. Washington, DC: USGPO, 1993.

SUMMARY

The overall message to be taken from U.S. Census–based estimates of elderly population growth is that the full impact of aging will hit after 2010. Between 2000 and 2010, the United States will remain in a period of quiet buildup to the crescendo of population aging. During this anticipatory period of relatively modest population growth, the most rapid growth patterns will be seen in the oldest old (those 85 and older) and older Latinos.

After 2010, the first of the baby boom cohort will reach retirement age. Beginning in 2010 and going until 2030, "there will be an unparalleled increase in the absolute number of older persons [as the] baby boom cohorts . . . place tremendous strain on the myriad specialized services and programs required of an elderly population."[4] Health and social service systems will face accelerated pressures due to this unprecedented increase in the elderly population.

It will be the post-2010 demographic tidal wave that challenges the nation to adjust its health and social service systems, but it will be the planning and policy work done pre-2010 that determines U.S. success—private, public, and personal—in meeting this challenge.

THE ECONOMIC STATUS OF SENIORS

Income, assets, and retirement timing are interrelated factors associated with health status—and health care service use—of the elderly. This section provides an overview of these topics.

The overall economic picture of the elderly has improved significantly since 1970 when 4.8 million persons 65 years of age and older (24.6 percent of the total elderly population) lived below the poverty level. By 2000, the percentage had dropped to 3.2 million (9.7 percent of the total), an historic low.[5] Neverthe-

less, economic discrepancies remain. Older women, minorities, and singles are at the lowest end of the income scale, and over the next decade, these disparities will not diminish. If anything, the income gaps will grow larger with older women, minorities, and non-married elders receiving lower incomes than men, whites, and those who are married.[6] The linear relationship between socioeconomic status and health and illness is well established. As more elderly fall into poverty, we can expect more of them to be in poor health.

In 1999, 66 percent of the 55- to 64-year-old men and 52.1 percent of the women in the same age group were in the labor force. For people age 65 and older, the labor rates were 18.6 percent for men and 10 percent for women.[7] Although the trend over the past decade has been toward early retirement, the Bureau of Labor Statistics (BLS) projects that labor force participation rates for those aged 55 years and older will increase by 5.5 percentage points from 1998 to 2008.[8]

The retirement age will start to increase for a number of reasons. By congressional mandate, beginning in 2000, the normal retirement age for collecting a full Social Security pension will increase incrementally from its current level of 65 years to 67 years in 2022. At the same time, the amount of reduced pension benefits one can collect at age 62 also will be lowered. In addition, Congress recently eliminated the earnings limit on the amount that Social Security recipients between the ages of 65 and 69 can earn before having to forfeit part of their Social Security benefits. Together, these rule changes should keep people in the workforce longer.[9]

Another reason the retirement age is likely to rise in the future is the trend toward companies offering defined contribution pension plans instead of defined benefit plans. A Bureau of Labor Statistics survey of medium to large employers showed that, among full-time employees, participation in defined benefit pension plans declined from 59 percent in 1991 to 50 percent in 1997.[10] Defined benefit plans provide the maximum benefits when taken at the earliest possible age of eligibility. In contrast, under defined contribution plans such as 401(k)s, the amount of benefits accrued depends on the amount contributed to the plan by employers and employees, as well as on the rate of growth of the investments in the retirement fund.[11]

A study by the American Association of Retired Persons (AARP) provides further evidence of prolonged labor force participation, finding that 8 in 10 baby-boomers plan to work during their "retirement years," although not necessarily at the same job and not necessarily full time.[12] Declining age discrimination and increasing labor force participation among women also should contribute to raising the retirement age in the future. To the extent that these changes occur and the retirement age rises, the BLS estimates may overstate the number of retirements occurring over the 1998–2008 period.

The increasing age of eligibility for Social Security (and potentially for Medicare) will have particularly deleterious effects for racial and ethnic minorities whose health and life expectancy is lower than that for whites. Most disadvantaged by this policy change are minority males, many of whom may not live long enough to receive their retirement benefits.

The higher age of eligibility will also have negative repercussions for women in particular. With fewer years in the labor force, women often have more "zero" years of income under Social Security and therefore receive depressed benefits under this program.[13] Further, because women live six to seven years longer than men, over time they are more at risk for developing chronic illnesses. Already meager incomes will be stretched to cover the associated costs of these illnesses.

Taking early retirement to caregive (again, predominantly performed by women) will compound the dire financial situation for women dependent on Social Security. Although those who retire early are eligible for Social Security benefits on a reduced basis at age 62, they do not qualify for Medicare until age 65. As a result, for those not working or married there is a gap in health insurance between retirement and age 65. If the retirement itself is triggered by poor health, this insurance gap can be a major concern.

INTERGENERATIONAL ISSUES

Conflict between the generations is drawing increased media attention. Much of the new media focus is based on concerns voiced by policymakers and analysts over how the rapid aging of the population will affect health and retirement programs. Some analysts and advocacy groups claim that older persons benefit from Social Security and Medicare at the expense of workers and children; thus, these programs are called "unfair" and become a flashpoint for intergenerational conflict. The critics also say U.S. policy fails at "generational equity."[14,15]

Others say that "generational interdependence" in financing programs such as Social Security is essential. They point to factors beyond individual control (e.g., demographic and economic booms and busts) that, without intergenerational exchange, would result in unequal retirement incomes for different generations. Retirement health and income should not, they say, depend on the luck of the historical draw and, therefore, multiple generations should share responsibility for the current elderly population's retirement.[16,17]

The central question in this ongoing debate is whether the "ties that bind"[18] will hold together generations in some type of interdependence or whether the hypothesized "age wars"[19,20] and projected "age-race collision" will materialize for the demographic buildup period from the present to 2010.[21]

Apart from the intergenerational hot-button issues centered on the large governmental social and health programs, other forms of intergenerational exchange involve more personal and family-level mediums of exchange such as money, time, and space (e.g., shared living arrangements). Recent trends in these areas indicate that some concerns over intergenerational friction may be

misplaced.[22] For example, contrary to myth, data indicate a very low incidence of financial transfers to older parents. In fact, there seems to be a far greater likelihood that older parents will be giving financial help to children and grandchildren rather than receiving it.[23]

Recent data also confirm that competing intergenerational exchanges may have the highest personal financial stakes for women. This is because caregiving for dependent children and/or parents is most likely to diminish a woman's—rather than a man's—formal work, with "distinct [negative] implications for pension eligibility, saving, asset accumulation and ultimately post-retirement income."[24]

THE SUPPORT RATIO

The complex and multilevel exchanges between generations are more than topics for magazine articles and talk shows. The magnitude and direction of these transfers of time, money, and space will directly influence the environment of aging over the next several decades. How can we quantify, and therefore predict and plan for, the pace-setting factors in this fast-evolving environment?

One measure that is widely used in discussing the present and future support of the elderly is the "support ratio" (sometimes called the "dependency ratio") characterized by the following formula:

Those in need of support : Those capable of providing support

A number of caveats regarding interpretation of this ratio should be made clear.

First, not all youth and elderly require support, nor do all working age persons provide direct support to youth and elderly family members. Also, the number of working age adults does not equal the number of adults actually participating in the labor force. A support ratio, in other words, simply lays out the numbers of one dependent population compared to the numbers of a working age population.

A support ratio is just a starting point that requires further interpretation based on other—often quite changeable—inputs and assumptions. For example, many interpretations of support ratios may overestimate the degree of intergenerational support (often termed "the burden") required. This occurs because they do not take into account the increasing labor force participation of women, the effect of economic growth, or the potential of older persons to work longer.

Nevertheless, the support ratio is a useful crude indicator of potential changes in the future levels of economic support needed. The ratio described here provides a snapshot of the intergenerational burden likely to be created in the coming demographic transformation.

The combination of child dependency and old age dependency is a good measure of the overall dependency burden on the working age population. This total support ratio will actually decline between 2000 and 2010, from 69.8 to 60 older persons and children per 100 persons of working age.[25] The largest changes in the total support ratio will occur in the period post-2010 when the baby boomers reach retirement age. From 2010 to 2030, the total support ratio is projected to increase 32 percent, rising from 60 to 79 children plus elderly per 100 workers.

The overall economic outlook for the elderly is mixed. People will be living and working longer, but disparities in economic status will exacerbate differences in health status over time. In spite of media attention to intergenerational conflict, most people seem to understand that all generations have a common stake in social and economic policies that meet differing needs across the life cycle conflict.[26,27] The challenge now is meeting the needs of all generations without trading off the needs of one age group for those of another. The full effect of public policy changes for the elderly can only be determined with time.

HEALTH STATUS OF SENIORS

Seniors' health status depends on a combination of their economic circumstances, access to health care, their genetic makeup, the environment in which they live, and their risk behaviors. By all of these measures, the health status of Americans has improved greatly this past century and will continue to improve. Nonetheless, as individuals age and the wear and tear of daily life begins to take its toll on most bodies, the average person is more likely to suffer from a chronic condition that increases his or her utilization of health care products and services. This section describes those chronic conditions and the prevalence and shape of age-related morbidity.

LEADING CAUSES OF DEATH

In 2000, the leading cause of death among persons age 65 or older was heart disease (1,712 deaths per 100,000 persons), followed by cancer (1,127 per 100,000), stroke (422 per 100,000), chronic obstructive pulmonary diseases (310 per 100,000), pneumonia and influenza (173 per 100,000), diabetes (150 per 100,000), and Alzheimer's disease (139 per 100,000 persons). In 2000, among persons age 85 and older, heart disease was responsible for 38 percent of all deaths.[28] Recently, reductions in mortality occurred for all of the above-listed diseases except pneumonia and Alzheimer's disease.

CHRONIC CONDITIONS

Chronic conditions can affect individuals at any age, but it is the single most important factor influencing the health, independence, and life expectancy of seniors. Chronic conditions are those that have persistent or recurring health consequences over many years. They are illnesses or impairments that cannot be cured, and in some cases can interfere with a person's ability to accomplish activities of daily living (ADLs.)[29] Although trends indicate that the prevalence of those whose lives will be limited due to chronic conditions may be decreasing, because people will be living longer, the absolute number of people living with chronic conditions is expected to increase.[30]

Eighty-eight percent of those over 65 years of age live with some type of chronic illness or condition[31] and as peo-ple age, the probability of suffering from more than one chronic condition increases.[32] Although many people who suffer from chronic conditions over age 65 live productive, full lives, 34 percent of those age 65–74 and 45 percent of those 75 years and older are limited in their daily activities because of chronic illness.[33]

For Americans 70 years of age and older, the most common chronic conditions reported include arthritis, hypertension, and heart disease (see Figure 14-9).[34] In 2000, one-quarter and one-third of the population 70 years and older suffered from visual and hearing impairments respectively.[35] A full 63 percent of women and 50 percent of men over 70 suffer from arthritis. Women also lead men in the prevalence of hypertension at age 70 and older, although men take the lead in heart disease.

Depressive symptoms are an indicator of general well-being and mental health among older Americans. Higher levels of depressive symptoms are associated with higher rates of physical illness, greater functional disability, and higher health care resource utilization.[36] In 1998, about 15 percent of persons aged 65 to 69, 70 to 74, and 75 to 79 had severe symptoms of depression, compared with 21 percent of persons ages 80 to 84, and 23 percent of persons age 85 or older.[37] This is much higher than the approximately 8 percent (19 million) of the general public that suffer from depressive disorders.[38]

The negative or disabling effects of chronic illness often develop slowly over

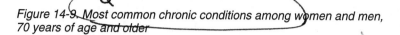

Figure 14-9. Most common chronic conditions among women and men, 70 years of age and older

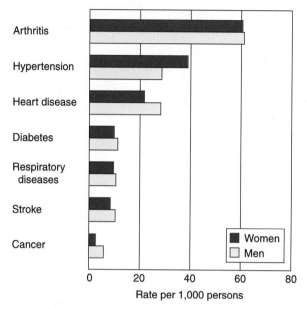

Source: Centers for Disease Control and Prevention, National Center for Health Statistics. 1994 National Health Interview Survey, Second Supplement on Aging. Based on interviews conducted between October 1994 and March 1996 with non-institutionalized persons. Percents are age adjusted.

time. Although assistance is available for those who suffer from chronic conditions, the demand for these services outweighs the supply[39]. Informal caregivers—volunteers who provide valuable and uncompensated care—often provide necessary assistance. The issue of caregiving and social support networks for the elderly will be discussed later in this chapter. For a further discussion on chronic conditions, please see Chapter 15.

THE "COMPRESSION OF MORBIDITY" FACTOR

After 2010, with increased numbers of elderly, the economic burden of chronic diseases will undoubtedly grow even heavier. But beyond the increased size of the at-risk population, will an extended life span within this larger population also contribute to a greater prevalence of chronic disease? This has been a topic of considerable debate. Some argue that the prevalence of chronic disease and disability will indeed increase as life expectancy increases, leading to a "pandemic of mental disorders and chronic diseases."[40] They predict that the extension of life will bring a concomitant extension of disease and disability—and related higher medical costs. Increased longevity is seen as "the price of our success at surviving." The anticipated boom in the 85+ population is cited as a particularly explosive factor in the projected increased rate of frailty and dependency.[41]

However, many others say that the burden of illness can be reduced by postponing the onset of chronic infirmity relative to average life expectancy. Thus, the period of morbidity is compressed between an increased age of onset and a relatively fixed life expectancy.[42] In other words, we may have more elderly people with arthritis in 2020 than we do now, but new therapies and improved lifestyles will allow a higher percentage of these people to live infirmity-free lives for longer periods. This compression of long-term disability into a shorter period or proportion of life expectancy is called "compression of morbidity."

Such predictions regarding changing morbidity—although still extremely controversial—could play an important role in estimating future illness patterns, in developing population projections, and in policy development. The evidence

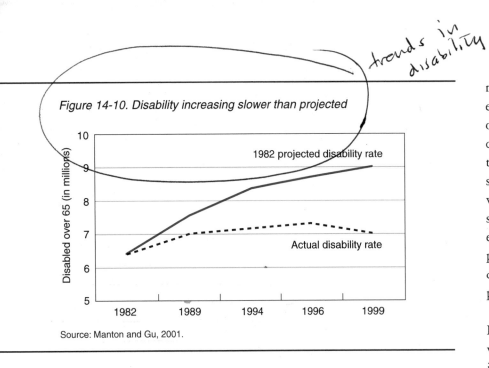

trends in disability

Figure 14-10. Disability increasing slower than projected

Source: Manton and Gu, 2001.

to date for these two ideas seems to support many of the ideas put forward by the "compression of morbidity" advocates. For example, for the period from 1982 to 1999, the prevalence of chronic disability among the elderly declined from 24.9 to 19.7 percent or 7 million disabled over the age of 65.[43] (See Figure 14-10). Even assuming some continuing trend toward more disease-free or disease-delayed aging, however, the sheer growth in the number of very old persons will clearly continue to boost demand for medical and long-term care services.

THE DELIVERY SYSTEM AND PROVIDERS FOR THE ELDERLY

New technologies and the drive to contain costs will reshape the health care delivery system for the elderly. Most of the infrastructure that determines the nature and structure of the health care delivery system is well established and reinforced by reimbursement mecha-

nisms, policies, and patient and provider expectations. However, the availability of new technologies and treatments, in combination with high patient expectations, will drive the health care delivery system toward new methods of delivery within well-established parameters. This section focuses on the health care delivery system and the personnel and provider needs required to meet the demands the elderly population will place on the system.

Health care for the elderly encompasses a wide range of systems and services, including acute, chronic, skilled nursing, ambulatory, short-term, long-term, and socially oriented community-based personal care. This diverse system of publicly and privately financed services is fragmented and highly uncoordinated. The juncture between acute and long-term care is especially wide and variable. Regulations, licensing requirements, and nonuniform reimbursement mechanisms contribute to the lack of coordination across the system. Cost-shifting among programs is a financial symptom of the disjointedness.

Recently, efforts to contain rapidly rising health care expenditures and to integrate health systems have led to a gradual restructuring of this fractured terrain of care for the elderly. Growth in capitated health care and home health care have become two of the largest forces reshaping health care for the elderly today.

The devolving role of the federal government is another significant force altering the systems of health and social services for the elderly. As state and local governments assume more financial and programmatic responsibilities for health and long-term care, authority for priority setting and resource allocation is becoming decentralized. The result—with all the new opportunities for locally controlled trade-offs between programs, population groups, and services—is more variability and less certainty in the scope and duration of delivered services for the elderly.

THE HEALTH CARE WORKFORCE OF THE FUTURE

Although the first baby boomers will not reach retirement age until 2011, changes in Medicare and other restructurings of delivery systems are already occurring. Many questions remain—for example, about the magnitude and extent of chronic disability in the elderly in coming years and about changes in medical technologies. However, even with the considerable uncertainty, several baseline predictions about the composition of the future health care workforce can be safely ventured. These predictions, mainly extrapolations of current trends, include:

- more medical group practices; fewer solo practices

- more inter- or multidisciplinary systems; fewer single specialty practices or nonintegrated provider groups

- more inclusion within health networks of nurse practitioners (NPs), physician assistants (PAs), social workers, and physical therapists (PTs)

- an ongoing shift from hospital-based to ambulatory and office-based care

The current concentration of physicians and nurses in metropolitan areas is another general trend with implications for elderly people. This uneven geographic distribution of medical personnel means that necessary care may be delayed for those who live far from medical facilities and who must depend either on public transit or rides from friends, family, or caregivers. Since mobility is an issue for many in the elderly population, such delays may become more common. Telehealth demonstrations indicate that remote service delivery is a good way to "bridge the gap" and provide health services to the elderly. Reimbursement and technology infrastructure will determine the effectiveness of this approach long-term.

Several of the top issues related to the supply and training of specific health care providers are discussed in the following sections.

PHYSICIANS

The biological, psychological, pathological, and socioeconomic factors that define the aging process are not self-evident. That is, the elderly are not just people with more illness. Yet, many doctors treat them this way. Today, in fact, most primary care physicians and specialists rely on their informal and anecdotal clinical experiences to shape their view of what constitutes adequate care for the elderly. Recent research into the chronic disabilities and special health-related circumstances of the elderly shows that attention to the whole constellation of age-related health parameters is often necessary for a positive clinical and economic outcome.

To provide physicians with the broad view of age-related health matters, formal training in geriatrics is necessary. In coming years, increased attention to such training will be needed in order to furnish adequate numbers of primary care and consultative physicians with the expertise to meet the unique health care demands of an aging population. Trained geriatricians, for example, would be the preferred providers for assessing patient function and treating functional disability.[44] Their special training allows them to help elderly patients maintain the highest degree of function and independence and avoid costly institutionalization. Beginning to boost the supply of geriatricians now will also allow time for development of an adequate core of medical school faculty and researchers with special knowledge of aging issues.

In 1999, Florida State University commissioned a study of geriatric education in the United States. Forty of 140 U.S. medical schools responded to the survey and 39 of those schools reported including geriatric education in their undergraduate medical curriculum, a huge increase over 1995 when only 11 U.S. medical schools required geriatric education. Thirty-eight of the responding schools reported that their school had a department and/or division of geriatrics.[45]

The Alliance for Aging Research and UCLA's Dr. David Reuben believe that by 2010 the United States will need approximately 25,000 geriatricians (see Figure 14-11).

Currently, there are just 9,000 certified geriatricians out of a total U.S. physician population of more than 700,000. Most of these aging specialists today are internists or family practitioners who

were certified under a 1988 grandfather clause that allowed practicing physicians with experience in geriatrics to sit for a qualifying exam rather than obtain formal training. Since this post-1988 influx, many of these physicians have themselves reached retirement age. States such as Florida and California are taking significant legislative steps to increase geriatric training in medical schools, with apparent success as the number of students that chose geriatrics as a specialty exceeded 200 in 2000. The federal government is also paying attention to the need for an increase in geriatric education by considering the Geriatric Care Act of 2001, legislation to increase geriatric incentives and improve Medicare reimbursement for geriatric care, as well as Health Resources and Services Administration's (HRSA) recent establishment of Geriatric Education Center grants to strengthen the multidisciplinary training of health professionals in the diagnosis, treatment, and prevention of disease in older Americans.[46,47]

Once physicians leave medical school, the opportunities for formal geriatrics training diminish. Today, most managed care plans and HMOs do not have additional time or resources to expend on the board certification process. Some managed care plans can barely allocate the time needed to train new physicians with the skills to operate in a managed care environment. The time crunch will likely continue. Within the formal managed care structure, however, various physician groups (e.g., independent physician organizations, multispecialty practices) may eventually take the lead in postgraduate geriatrics education. The possible venues for such education include mentoring within the group practice itself, or training in community settings, LTC facilities, hospitals, or nearby medical schools.

DENTISTS

More dentists trained to serve elderly patients will be needed as well. These dental providers will require a special knowledge of, and clinical training in, the aging oral cavity—including preventive, restorative, and rehabilitative approaches.

Financial disincentives in the current health care delivery system indicate that the underlying demand for skilled geriatric dentists is unlikely to be met. In 1987, 80 percent of dental expenses for elderly Americans were paid out of pocket. According to an HRSA report, "Inadequate reimbursement or lack of sources of payment for dental care is a

substantial barrier for greater dental provider involvement." This lack of insurance coverage may explain why only about 55 percent of all older adults visit the dentist annually.[48] In addition to this cost-reimbursement constraint, many elderly shun dental services for a more painfully obvious reason: they have not retained their teeth. This sizable population of Americans over age 65 without teeth—30 percent—is much less likely to visit the dentist.[49]

If the delivery of dental services to older persons remains economically unfavorable, it will of course remain unattractive to dentists-in-training who carry an interest in the geriatric specialty. This economic reality not only drives potential future specialists away from the field, it also affects decisions about educational program development and funding for clinical training sites. Since additional government subsidies for dental services or training are not on the horizon and the majority of patients will continue to pay for dental services out of their own pockets, it is unlikely that the number of geriatric dentists will increase.

Current statistics support this bleak view. According to HRSA, "Clinicians with added competency in geriatric dentistry and geriatric dental academicians are not being developed in adequate numbers to meet current and projected workforce needs."[50] In a 1987 report, DHHS projected a need for 7,500 dental practitioners with advanced preparation in geriatric dentistry in the year 2000, and 10,000 in the year 2020. About 1,500 geriatric dental academicians would be needed in the year 2000, and 2,000 in 2020. However, in the last two

Figure 14-11. The growing gap: Anticipated number versus projected need for physicians trained in geriatrics

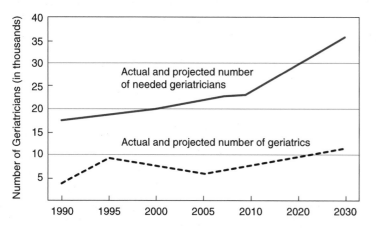

Source: Alliance for Aging Research. *Ten Reasons Why America Is Not Ready for the Coming Age Boom.* Washington, DC: Alliance for Aging Research, 2002.

decades just 100 dentists completed advanced geriatric dentistry fellowships or master's level training programs.

NURSES, NURSE PRACTITIONERS, AND PHYSICIAN ASSISTANTS

As providers for much of the day-to-day care given to elderly patients in acute- and chronic-care settings, nurses and physician assistants (PAs) likely will also be in short supply in the decades ahead. The supply of those with special geriatrics training is almost certain to be inadequate, mainly because the current system is woefully unprepared to deliver such training. Consider these statistics from a 1992 HRSA survey:

- 40 percent of nursing faculty had no gerontology or geriatrics preparation.

- 77 percent of schools lack gerontology-qualified clinical preceptors.

While the number of full-time positions for RNs is expected to increase 18 percent overall by 2010, the demand for full-time RNs in nursing homes is projected to increase by 30 percent, while the demand in community health settings will increase by 44 percent.[51] Some predict that the supply of RNs will keep pace with increased demands if, as in the physician workforce, nurses shift away from hospital skill sets toward expertise more appropriate for the primary care setting, nursing homes, and skilled nursing facilities.[52]

That's a big "if" given that recruiting and retraining qualified personnel to provide direct care in long-term care remains a critical problem. Currently,

federal and state regulations require very few RNs in nursing homes and thus facility owners tend to hire more lower-pay nursing aides, licensed practical nurses (LPNs), and licensed vocational nurses (LVNs). In the early 1990s, RNs working in nursing homes received just 86 percent of the typical acute-care wage and, not unexpectedly, the 5-year retention rate was just 40 percent. Data demonstrated that as pay increased, retention rates increased accordingly.

These lower retention rates in LTC apparently are closely related to lower pay, and this becomes a particular problem for younger nurses. Thus, both opportunity and economic incentive are failing to attract RNs into community and LTC facilities.

As if these barriers were not enough, nurses are also being squeezed out of the elder care environment from the "high end" by the more highly trained nurse practitioners (NPs) and physician assistants. Demand is currently strong for these advanced care "physician extenders," especially among large health plans, hospital systems, and medical groups looking to control costs. Managed care programs are leading the way in supporting the use of non-physicians, including nurse specialists and nurse practitioners, as members of health care teams fostering interdisciplinary care for elderly members.[53] This use of nonphysicians in a team approach will increase. In fee-for-service settings, however, political pressures can more easily influence licensing requirements, and physicians are often reluctant to cede any responsibility or remuneration to those other than doctors; these turf issues mean that use of NPs and PAs will probably not grow as fast in the shrinking fee-for-service sector.

In summary, without new economic incentives or legislative controls to retrain or retain nurses in LTC facilities and nursing homes, the role of the RN in health care for the elderly may diminish. Unless the current trend toward displacement from acute care hospitals accelerates, RNs will not naturally migrate toward LTC facilities, and LVNs, LPNs, and nurse's aides will be left to meet the bulk of the growing elder care demand.

PHYSICAL THERAPISTS

The rapid growth in demand for rehabilitation therapies by the elderly and nonelderly is already outpacing the supply of physical therapists (PTs).[54] In 1993, the Bureau of Labor Statistics projected physical therapy to be one of the fastest growing occupations in the country, with rapid growth expected to continue well past 2000. Even with growth somewhat tempered by cost-driven managed care access restrictions, the sharply increased demand for geriatric physical therapy services at nursing homes and in home care settings should intensify the overall physical therapy shortage as baby boomers move into retirement.

According to the American Physical Therapy Association, 39 percent of current patients treated by PTs are over the age of 65. However, the training of most PTs is void of any significant formal geriatric component. Only 19 percent of PT programs report at least 75 percent of their students complete a geriatric

clinical internship.[55] Barriers to creation of clinical PT internships include low student interest in, and poor attitudes about, the elderly; inadequate numbers of qualified geriatric sites with knowledgeable practitioners; inadequate numbers of PTs on staff; and an insufficient variety of elderly patients in a single geographic area.

Geriatric Physical Therapy was approved as a specialty in 1989, with first exams administered in 1992. In 1998, there were 78 board-certified Geriatric Clinical Specialists in the United States and only 50 new specialists will be added annually. The expectation that these specialists will fill the anticipated demand for geriatric services is unrealistic. However, the new generation of board-certified specialists may serve as the nucleus for a more widespread continuing education effort in PT geriatrics. Only if specific coursework relating to rehabilitative methods for elderly patients is incorporated into the training curricula of all PTs will the supply of adequately trained PTs be sufficient.

LONG-TERM CARE

Currently, the nursing home remains the main option for formal long-term care (LTC). An estimated 53 percent of all elderly now require nursing home care in their lifetime, with the highest use occurring after age 85.

Of the more than $100 million spent on all LTC today, Medicaid pays 37.8 percent, out-of-pocket costs account for 42.6 percent, Medicare pays 19 percent, and LTC insurance covers 1 percent.[56] Nursing home costs still comprise the overwhelming share of the public bill, constituting 85 percent of Medicaid LTC expenditures in 1995.[57] Medicaid expenditures per elderly resident for all services averaged $967 in 1995, with a range from $383 to $2,444. Medicaid nursing home expenditures per recipient averaged $7,821, with a range from $3,593 to $15,785.

The U.S. approach to LTC relies heavily on unpaid care by family members and other informal caregivers.[58] Approximately 70 percent of disabled elders rely exclusively on help from spouses, children, or other informal sources,[59] with the greatest burden and indirect cost of this informal care falling heavily on women.[60]

BEYOND THE NURSING HOME: GROWING DEMAND FOR COMMUNITY-BASED SERVICES

The elderly express a clear preference to remain in the community; thus non-institutional services have grown substantially in recent years. Despite this demand, home and community-based services are far from universally available and serve only a small percentage of the potential LTC population.

The rate of growth of these alternative LTC programs may depend on demonstrated reductions in expenditures that would otherwise have gone into nursing home care. However, such cost savings are far from a certainty.

The next decade will bring a major shift in LTC emphasis toward home and community settings, a shift that will lay the groundwork for even more significant changes beyond 2010. The future infrastructure for home and community services will need to overcome a LTC system that is currently fragmented (i.e., without adequate transitions between acute and chronic care) and difficult to access. Truly integrated systems of care will need to include some combination of the following features:

- Combined acute care and LTC service (both financing and delivery) for the elderly

- An organized continuum of services and providers

- Case management to assure care continuity across the acute care and LTC delivery systems

- Training for providers to promote awareness of patient-focused care

- Capitation and other financing incentives to contain costs[61]

A few promising but isolated efforts at providing such integrated acute care and LTC now exist as small demonstration efforts. The PACE/On Lok program and the Social HMO currently reach several thousand people nationwide. Oregon is the sole state providing services to more people in the community than in nursing homes. Clearly, for the majority of elderly persons today, access to a full array of integrated acute-to-chronic and medical-to-social services remains extremely limited. It is unlikely between now and 2010 that managed care will radically change this situation. Instead, most HMOs and other managed care models for the elderly will remain a separate system providing primary and acute care. The search for the ideal LTC financing and delivery system will continue.

THE KEY MULTIGENERATIONAL CHALLENGE: CAREGIVING

Intergenerational issues will also play out in terms of caregiving for the elderly. As already described, the increased longevity and an increase in the size of the aging population will result in more people living with chronic care needs. In the past, care giving for an elderly parent has been done by family members. We forecast that caregiving for the elderly will stress the health care system and social support networks for a number of fundamental intergenerational shifts that have already been set into motion.[62]

- The average American has more parents than children.

- A growing percentage of elders have children who themselves are over 65.

- Most married couples aged 51 to 61 have living parents, children, and grandchildren.

But what do the various comparisons and descriptions of generational shift tell us about the future of the typical American family? By far, the greatest implication of all current intergenerational trends is that the United States will become a nation preoccupied by caregiving (see Figure 14-12). The multiple forces driving the coming caregiving crunch are clear:

why do we face a cgc?

- Increasing numbers of elders in quadruple-generation families [63]

- Increasing age-related health problems affecting both health care receivers and caregivers

- Modestly increasing growth in the participation of women in the labor force[64]

- Continuing moderately low fertility rates

As the baby boom generation ages and the need for caregiving increases, the supply of family caregivers is projected to decline. This decline can be traced to lower fertility rates in the caregiving generation and to family networks that are getting smaller and are becoming more geographically dispersed. In 1980, there were 11 potential caregivers to every one older person. By 2000, this ratio had already declined slightly to 10 to 1,[65,66] and it will continue to decline as the size of the elderly population grows. By 2030 the ratio of potential caregivers to elders will be reduced to 6 to 1.

Gerontologists report that older persons strongly prefer to live independently of children and relatives, and one-third currently live alone.[67] Because federal health policy for the aged does not cover

Figure 14-12. The shrinking pool caregiving potential caregivers

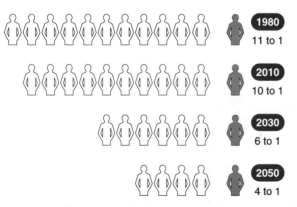

1980	11 to 1
2010	10 to 1
2030	6 to 1
2050	4 to 1

Source: Robert Wood Johnson Foundation. *Chronic Care in America: A 21st Century Challenge*. Princeton, NJ: Robert Wood Johnson Foundation, 1996.

Chapter 14: Health and Health Care of America's Seniors   **269**

long-term care (LTC), the only alternative (other than impoverishment to become eligible for Medicaid) is to seek informal care. The following statistics provide a portrait of who is providing this informal care:

- 75 percent of all elder care is provided by unpaid, informal caregivers.

- 80 percent of caregivers today are female.

- Nearly two-thirds (60 percent) of caregivers of the elderly are themselves either old or approaching old age.[68]

- Fully one-third of caregivers of the elderly are age 65 years and older.

The toll of increased caregiving responsibilities will take many forms. One study shows that "over 40 percent of adult offspring . . . report that the time spent on caregiving tasks was equivalent to the time required by a full-time job."[69] Research demonstrates deleterious financial and health effects for the caregiver.[70,71] Because four of every five caregivers are women, they will be especially exposed to the competing pressure between paid and unpaid work.

In terms of the working age population's responsibility for the elderly, there will be few major changes before 2010. Most significantly, from the present to 2010, the "total societal support ratio" (the combination of child and old age dependency) will actually *decline*. The growing focus of concern is the potential shortage of informal caregivers (primarily women). Already, however, U.S. society is finding the determination, the forums, and the terminology to deal with the growth of multigenerational families and the "sandwich generation" of "women in the middle."[72,73]

Although the overall outlook for the health status of seniors is bright, a shortage of geriatric-trained providers and informal caregivers will stress the delivery system in the future.

ELDER HEALTH CARE FINANCING THROUGH MEDICARE

Public support such as Medicare and Medicaid will continue to be a critical contributor to health care financing for the elderly. This section focuses on our forecast for Medicare.

MEDICARE TODAY

Medicare is financed by a combination of payroll taxes, general revenues, and private premiums. The insurance program focuses almost exclusively on acute care, primarily hospital and physician services. It also covers a limited amount of home health services, particularly skilled care for periods of acute illness. Services such as chronic, long-term nursing home care and outpatient prescription drugs are *not* reimbursed by Medicare.

Medicare patients also incur coinsurance and deductible costs for the care received. In fact, recent data indicate that Medicare covers only 44 percent of the total medical costs of the elderly—a difficult situation given that three of every four Medicare enrollees have annual incomes below $25,000. To help pay for medical coinsurance and uncovered benefits, about 71 percent of elderly

Medicare beneficiaries carry some form of private insurance to supplement Medicare.[74] Other facts about Medicare today include:

- In 2000, 33.2 million elderly persons (95 percent of the total elderly population) were enrolled in the Medicare program.[75]

- About 80 percent of enrollees actually were assisted by Medicare funds; the remaining 20 percent either did not use any covered services during the year or did not reach the deductible amount.

- The largest relative increase in Medicare enrollment since the beginning of the program in 1966 has occurred among those 85 years and older.

- Total Medicare outlays in 2000 amounted to $214.9 billion.[76]

- Medicare payments per enrollee in 2000 were more than 25 times the 1967 amount, rising from $217 in 1967 to $5,490 in 2000, reflecting inflation in the medical care market and market expansion of benefits.

- Medicare costs increase with age: in 1998, payments per enrollee averaged $3,973 for those 65 to 74 years of age and averaged $7,641 for those 85 years and older.[77]

MEDICARE CIRCA 2010

Under current law, annual Medicare spending is expected to approximately double to $431.8 billion by the year 2007. A deficit in the Medicare trust fund is projected to occur before the year 2010. Anticipating such a deficit, Con-

gress adopted Medicare changes in the Balanced Budget Act (BBA) of 1997. According to the Congressional Budget Office,[78] these changes will be phased in over the following decade and will reduce Medicare Trust Fund expenditures between 1998 and 2007 by $385.5 billion. Even with this substantial reduction, however, the projected trust fund deficit in 2007 remains at $30.8 billion. More ominous is the fact that this deficit occurs several years in advance of the increase in Medicare expenditures expected after the 2010 arrival of the Medicare-eligible baby boom generation. This makes it highly likely that further policy changes to increase revenues and reduce costs will be developed and implemented between now and 2010. One of the changes most likely to occur is a shift in expenditures to beneficiaries in the form of increased Medicare Part B contributions, deductibles, and co-payments above those already in the BBA of 1997.

SHIFT OF ENROLLEES TO AND FROM MANAGED CARE

The most striking change affecting the Medicare-eligible population since 1997 has been the rapid growth and subsequent decline in managed care enrollment. Early on it was hoped that offering enrollees HMO plans would result in lower overall costs to the program. The ability of plans to offer older persons low monthly premiums and many benefits, including drug coverage, was possible, to some extent, because those enrollees choosing managed care plans were healthier than the overall Medicare population.[79] Thus, Medicare overpaid the plans relative to the true actuarial risk of their older members.

As market penetration increased, however, and as members grew older, it has become more difficult for Medicare HMOs to "cherry pick" or disproportionately enroll the relatively healthy older population. That is, a higher proportion of HMO members now have multiple chronic problems and disabilities, and consequently are at risk for higher health expenditures. As costs have increased for these members, and premium payments have not, more and more HMOs have pulled out of the program altogether.

If managed care plans are to continue in the Medicare program, they must be able to seek out and retain potentially high-cost Medicare members. To do this, the federal government will need to implement some form of risk adjustment in the per-member reimbursement. This risk adjustment model will require information systems that capture comparative patient data, and will need to be budget-neutral so that there is no increase in overall Medicare expenditures. Only such a budget-neutral system will sustain the financial viability of the Medicare Trust Fund. As payments for high-risk groups increase (e.g., those with heart disease or in nursing homes), the rates for other groups (e.g., those defined as healthy) must decrease.

Even with the introduction of risk-adjusted payments, HMO operating costs may climb faster than reimbursement rates for the elderly. If this occurs, plans are expected either to increase out-of-pocket costs to members (both in the form of higher premiums and co-payments) or to reduce benefits (e.g., reductions in the annual coverage for prescription drugs), or continue to pull out of the program altogether. However, higher rates and reduced benefits also encourage disenrollment of the high-cost users, with movement back into the fee-for-service delivery system—precisely the opposite effect intended by risk-adjusted payments. Policy changes stimulated by the 1997 BBA, such as allowing only annual enrollment or disenrollment from plans (instead of monthly disenrollment), will reduce incentives to leave a plan when the maximum annual coverage (e.g., for prescription drugs) has been reached. There is also the possibility that the federal government will agree to pay higher reimbursement rates to HMOs. In the meantime, co-payments in the fee-for-service Medicare program are likely to rise, forcing even more well-off elderly into HMOs and intensifying the temptation among current plan administrators to compromise the quality of care.

THE MEDICARE DRUG BENEFIT

Over 85 percent (some say as high as 90) of Medicare beneficiaries use at least one prescription drug annually obtained through a supplemental policy, by enrollment in a Medicare+Choice plan, which includes coverage for prescription drugs, through Medicaid or some other public source (e.g., the Veterans Administration and state-sponsored pharmacy assistance programs), or out of pocket. In 1996, 69 percent of Medicare beneficiaries had coverage for prescription drugs for the entire year but in 2000 that had dropped to 50 percent.[80,81] This was due largely to the increase then decrease in Medicare HMO enrollment. However, it is predicted that increases in drug benefits from all sources will decline for the following reasons:

- Fewer beneficiaries will have access to employment-sponsored drug coverage as a result of employers continuing to cut back retiree benefits or requiring enrollees to pay much or all of the cost.

- Medicare HMOs will continue to reduce their drug benefits and/or terminate their contracts.

- Continuing growth in the cost of drugs may cause further reductions in drug benefits and/or increased premiums.

Further, individuals who have no coverage, and must pay for prescriptions out of pocket, do so at a higher price than individuals covered by a plan because plans receive discounts resulting from economies of scale.

Whether to add a prescription drug benefit to Medicare for those in need has been debated for several years. Among the considerations in defining a determination of need are:

- Annual income in relation to the federal poverty level

- Persistent lack of drug coverage over an extended period

- Lack of stable drug coverage

- High out-of-pocket spending

- Total drug expenditures

- Chronic disease burden

Many experts believe that a new "part" to the Medicare program (e.g., Medicare Part C) would be the most financially viable and politically feasible. This plan would work much the same as Part B in which beneficiaries sign up for drug coverage and pay a premium. However, to work, the premium would have to be set so that enrollment would be near-universal and high-cost users could still be covered.

IMPLICATIONS

Today, 20 percent of Florida's population is over 65 years old. By 2030, we will be living in a nation of Floridas. The elderly health and health care challenges that Florida faces today will be challenges for the entire country. Implications from this forecast point to some of the challenges to the future health of American seniors.

- *Be prepared for a larger population of seniors and larger numbers of chronic illnesses.* With an overall increase in life expectancy comes an overall increase in chronic disease. Today's system, which focuses on acute conditions, is just beginning to learn how to manage individuals with multiple comorbid conditions. A shift *away* from acute, curative care of already-existing ailments *toward* prevention of ailments common to the elderly and disease management across the continuum of care would improve the efficiency and efficacy of care interventions.

- *Be prepared to replace free "daughter care."* The caregiving burden is increasing, but working women are too busy to stay home with their family members. The caregiving drought will become increasingly apparent as women find alternatives to leaving the workforce and alternative funding for home health care.

Chapter 14: Health and Health Care of America's Seniors   273

- *Train geriatricians and other clinicians properly.* There are fundamental differences between health care needs of seniors and those of younger adults. Seniors are more likely to suffer from multiple, comorbid conditions. They are more likely to be taking multiple prescriptions. Many illnesses present differently in seniors. The window of opportunity to alter the education of the health care workforce to recognize and integrate these differences before the age wave bears down on the system is quickly closing.

- *Prepare for the elder boomers.* The baby boom is promising to revolutionize consumer demands on health care. They'll demand a more customer-friendly system; organizations that provide better service will win boomer loyalty.

- *Align Medicare incentives.* To encourage a focus on prevention, Medicare funding should support a holistic approach to medicine that encourages early diagnosis, upstream in the disease process. Screening initiatives, such as mammograms for women over 50 years of age, that currently exist should be expanded to include more diagnostics and more diseases.

- *Swallow the pill sooner rather than later.* We all age one year at a time, but 75 million Americans are steadily moving toward a time in their lives when they will need more care. Foundational policy change and a focus on prevention, disease management and the continuum of care take time. The sooner we start planning, the better prepared we will be.

ENDNOTES

[1] National Center for Health Statistics. *Health, United States, 1999, with Health and Aging Chartbook*. Hyattsville, MD: National Center for Health Statistics, 1999

[2] U.S. Census Bureau. *Population Projections of the United States by Age, Sex, Race and Hispanic Origin: 1995 to 2050*. Current Population Reports, Series P-25, No. 1130. Washington, DC: U.S. Government Printing Office. 1992.

[3] U.S. Census Bureau. *Age: 2000*. Census 2000 Brief. September 2001

[4] U.S. Census Bureau. *65+ In the U.S.* Current Population Reports, Series P-23, No. 190. Washington, DC: U.S. Government Printing Office. 1996.

[5] Administration on Aging. Profile of Older Americans. 2000. www.aoa.gov/aoa/stats/profile/#figure7.

[6] Meyer, M. Harrington. making claims as workers or wives: The distribution of social security benefits. *American Sociological Review* 1996; 61:449–465.

[7] U.S. Census Bureau. The Older Population in the United States: March 2000 Detailed Tables (PPL-147). www.census.gov/ population/www/socdemo/age/ppl-147.html.

[8] Dohm, A. Gauging the Labor Force Effects of Retiring Baby-Boomers. *Monthly Labor Review.* July 2000.

[9] U.S. Department of Labor. Employee benefits in medium and large private establishments, 1997. USDL 99-02. January 7, 1999.

[10] U.S. Department of Labor. Employee benefits in medium and large private establishments, 1997. USDL 99-02. January 7, 1999.

[11] U.S. Department of Labor. Employee benefits in medium and large private establishments, 1997. USDL 99-02. January 7, 1999.

[12] American Association of Retired Persons. Baby Boomers Envision Their Retirement: An AARP Segmentation Analysis. February 1999. http://www.aarp.org

[13] Ross, J. *Implications for Women's Retirement Income*. Washington, DC: United States General Accounting Office (GAO-HEHS-98-42), 1997.

[14] Peterson, P. *Will America Grow Up Before It Grows Old?* New York: Random House, 1996.

[15] Longman, P. *The Return of Thrift*. New York: Free Press, 1996.

[16] Quadagno, J. The Myth of the Entitlement Crisis. *The Gerontologist* 1996; 36:391–399.

[17] Binstock, R. The Oldest Old and 'Intergenerational Equity.' In: Suzman, R., D. Willis, and K. Manton, eds. *The Oldest Old*. New York: Oxford University Press. 1992.

[18] Kingson, E., J. Cornman, and B. Hirschorn. *Ties That Bind: The Interdependence of Generations in an Aging Society*. Cabin John, MD: Seven Locks Press, 1986.

[19] Binney, E. A., and C. L. Estes. The Retreat of the state and its transfer of responsibility: The intergenerational war. *International Journal of Health Services* 1988; 18(1):83–96.

[20] Dychtwald, K. The 10 physical, social, spiritual, economic and political crises the boomers will face as they age in the 21st century. *Critical Issues in Aging* 1997; 1:11–13.

[21] Hayes-Bautista, D., W. O. Schinck, and J. Chapa. *The Burden of Support: The Young Latino Population in an Aging Society*. Palo Alto, CA: Stanford University Press, 1988.

[22] Soldo, Beth J., and M. S. Hill. Family structure and transfer measures in the health and retirement study: Background and overview. *Journal of Human Resources* 1995; 30:S138–S157.

[23] Rosenthal, C., A. Martin-Andrews, and S. Mathews. Caught in the middle-occupancy in multiple roles and help to parents in a national probability sample of canadian adults. *Journal of Gerontology: Social Sciences* 1996; 51B:S274–S283.

[24] Soldo, Beth J. Cross pressures on middle-aged adults: A broader view. *Journal of Gerontology: Social Sciences* 1996; 51B(6):271–273.

[25] Table V. A2 Social Security Area Population as of July 1 and Dependency Ratios, by Broad Age Groups, Calendar years 1950–2000. Historical period. www.ssa.gov/cgi-bin/cgcgi/@ssa.env

[26] AARP, Public Policy Institute, and The Urban Institute. *Coming Up Short: Increasing Out-of-Pocket Health Spending by Older Americans.* Washington, DC: AARP, 1994.

[27] Jacobs, L., and R. Shapiro. Myths and Misunderstandings About Public Opinion Toward Social Security. Paper presented at the National Academy of Social Insurance, January 29–30, 1998. Washington, DC.

[28] National Center for Health Statistics. *Health, United States, 1999, with Health and Aging Chartbook.* Hyattsville, MD: National Center for Health Statistics. 1999.

[29] Chronic Conditions: A challenge for the 21st century. *National Academy on an Aging Society.* November 1999.

[30] Manton, K., and X. L. Gu. Analysis from the National Long Term Care Survey. *Proceedings of the National Academy of Sciences.* May 8, 2001.

[31] Hoffman, C., D. Rice, and H. Sung. Persons with chronic conditions: Their prevalence and costs. *Journal of the American Medical Association* 1996; 26(18):1473–1479.

[32] Van Norstrand, J. F., S. E. Funer, and R. Suzman, eds. *Health Data on Older Americans: United States, 1992.* National Center for Health Statistics, Vital and Health Statistics, Series 3, No. 27. DHHS Pub. No. (PHS) 93–1411. Hyattsville, MD: Public Health Service, 1992.

[33] Trupin, L., and D. Rice. *Health Status, Medical Care Use, and Number of Disabling Conditions in the United States.* Disability Statistics Abstract Number 9. National Institute on Disability and Rehabilitation Research, June 1995.

[34] National Center for Health Statistics. *Current Estimates from the National Health Interview Survey: United States, 1994.* Vital and Health Statistics, Series 10, No. 193. DHHS Pub. No. (PHS) 96-1521. Hyattsville, MD: Public Health Service, 1995.

[35] National Center for Health Statistics, 2001 Fact Sheet. Series of Reports to Monitor Health of Older Americans.

[36] Wells, K. B., et al. The functioning and well-being of depressed patients. Results from the Medical Outcomes Study. *Journal of the American Medical Association* 1989; 262:914–919.

[37] Health and Retirement Study, Older Americans, Key Indicators of Well-Being. 2000.

[38] National Institute of Mental Health. Depression Research at NIMH. www.nimh.nih.gov/publicat/depresfact.cfm.

[39] Robert Wood Johnson Foundation. *Chronic Care in America: A 21st Century Challenge.* Princeton, NJ: Robert Wood Johnson Foundation, 1996.

[40] Kramer, M. The rising pandemic of mental disorders and associated chronic diseases and disorders. *ActaPsychiatrica Scandinavica* 1980; 62:382–396.

[41] Cassel, C. K., M. A. Rudberg, and S. J. Olshansky. The price of success: Health care in an aging society. *Health Affairs* 1992; 11(2):87–89.

[42] Fries, J. F. Natural death and the compression of morbidity. *New England Journal of Medicine* 1980; 303(3):130–135.

[43] Manton, K. G. and X.L.Gu. Changes in the prevalence of chronic disability in the United States black and nonblack population above age 65 from 1982 to 1999. *Proceedings of the National Academy of Sciences.* 2001; 98:6354–6359.

[44] Alliance for Aging Research. *Meeting the Medical Needs of the Senior Boom—The National Shortage of Geriatricians.* Washington, DC: Alliance for Aging Research. 1992.

[45] Florida State University. A Study of Programs that Train Physicians to Care for the Elderly. November, 1999.

[46] The American Geriatrics Society. Geriatric Care Act Gains Support. Press Release. www.americangeriatrics.org/policy/from_ cap_4_01.shtml.

[47] American Dental Association. HRSA Grants Target Improvement in Geriatric, Rural Health Care. July 2001. www.ada.org/prof/pubs/daily/0107/0725hrsa.html.

[48] National Center for Health Statistics. 2001 Fact Sheet, New Series of Reports to Monitor the Health of Older Americans. www.cdc.gov/nchs/releases/01facts/olderame.htm.

[49] National Center for Chronic Disease Prevention and Health Promotion. Oral Health for Older Americans. www.cdc.gov/nccdphp/oh/adultfacts2.htm.

[50] National Center for Health Statistics. 2001 Fact Sheet, New Series of Reports to Monitor the Health of Older Americans. www.cdc.gov/nchs/releases/01facts/olderame.htm.

[51] National Center for Health Statistics. 2001 Fact Sheet, New Series of Reports to Monitor the Health of Older Americans. www.cdc.gov/nchs/releases/01facts/olderame.htm.

[52] National Center for Health Statistics. 2001 Fact Sheet, New Series of Reports to Monitor the Health of Older Americans. www.cdc.gov/nchs/releases/01facts/olderame.htm.

[53] National Center for Health Statistics. 2001 Fact Sheet, New Series of Reports to Monitor the Health of Older Americans. www.cdc.gov/nchs/releases/01facts/olderame.htm.

[54] National Center for Health Statistics. 2001 Fact Sheet, New Series of Reports to Monitor the Health of Older Americans. www.cdc.gov/nchs/releases/01facts/olderame.htm.

[55] Nieland, V., N. Farina, and C. Edwards. *Enhancement of the Age-Related Content and Learning Experiences in Physical Therapy Curricula: A Resource Manual*. Fairfax, VA: APTA, Department of Accreditation, 1990.

[56] Levit, K. R., et al. Data view: National health expenditures. *Health Care Financing Review* 1996; 18(1):175–214.

[57] Wiener, J., and D. Stevenson. *Elderly People*. Baltimore, MD: Johns Hopkins University Press, 1997.

[58] Pepper Commission, U.S. Bipartisan Commission on Comprehensive Health Care. *A Call for Action*. Washington, DC: U.S. Government Printing Office. 1990.

[59] Liu, K., K. Manton, and B. Liu. Homecare Expenses for the Disabled Elderly. *Health Care Financing Review*. 1996. 18(1):175–214.

[60] National Center for Health Statistics. 2001 Fact Sheet, New Series of Reports to Monitor the Health of Older Americans. www.cdc.gov/nchs/releases/01facts/olderame.htm.

[61] Stone, R. *Caregivers of the Frail Elderly: A National Profile*. U.S. Department of Health and Human Services, Public Health Service, National Center for Health Services Research and Health Care Technology Assessment. Washington, DC: DHHS, 1987.

[62] National Institute on Aging and the Survey Research Center. *Study of Health, Retirement and Aging*. Bethesda, MD: University of Michigan. 1997.

[63] Soldo, Beth J. Cross Pressures on Middle-Aged Adults: A Broader View. *Journal of Gerontology: Social Sciences* 1996; 51B(6): 271–273.

[64] Fullerton, H. Labor Force 2006: Slowing Down and Changing Composition. *Monthly Labor Review*. November 1997.

[65] Hoffman, C., D. Rice, and H. Sung. Persons with chronic conditions: Their prevalence and costs. *Journal of the American Medical Association* 1996; 26(18):1473–1479.

[66] Robert Wood Johnson Foundation. *Chronic Care in America: A 21st Century Challenge*. Princeton, NJ: RWJ Foundation, 1996.

[67] Falcon, R., M. O'Hara-Devereaux, and J. Stewart. *The Future of Growing Old in California: The Current Context, 1997–2000*. Menlo Park, CA: Institute for the Future, 1997.

[68] Stone, R., G. Cafferata, and J. Sangl. Caregivers of the frail elderly: A national profile. *The Gerontologist* 1987; 27:616–626.

Chapter 14: Health and Health Care of America's Seniors

[69] Feldblum, C. R. Home health care for the elderly: Programs, problems and potentials. *Harvard Journal of Legislation* 1985; 22(1):193–254.

[70] Brody, E. Parent care as a normative family stress. *The Gerontologist* 1985; 25:10–29.

[71] Brody, E. *Women in the Middle: Their Parent-Care Years*. New York: Springer. 1990.

[72] National Center for Health Statistics. 2001 Fact Sheet, New Series of Reports to Monitor the Health of Older Americans. www.cdc.gov/nchs/releases/01facts/olderame.htm.

[73] National Center for Health Statistics. 2001 Fact Sheet, New Series of Reports to Monitor the Health of Older Americans. www.cdc.gov/nchs/releases/01facts/olderame.htm.

[74] Komisar, H. L., et al. *Medicare Chart Book*. Menlo Park, CA: The Henry J. Kaiser Family Foundation, 1997.

[75] National Center for Health Statistics. 2001 Fact Sheet, New Series of Reports to Monitor the Health of Older Americans. www.cdc.gov/nchs/releases/ 01facts/olderame.htm.

[76] National Institute on Aging Fiscal Year 2002 Congressional Justification. www.nia.nih.gov/fy2002_congress/index.html#reducing.

[77] Health Care Financing Administration, Office of Strategic Planning. Health Care Financing Review: Medicare and Medicaid Statistical Supplements for years 1996 to 2000.

[78] U.S. Congressional Budget Office. CBO Memorandum: Budgetary Implications of the Balanced Budget Act of 1997. Washington, DC: CBO, 1997.

[79] Brown, R., et al. Do health maintenance organizations work for Medicare? *Health Care Financing Review* 1993; 15(1):7–24.

[80] National Center for Health Statistics. 2001 Fact Sheet, New Series of Reports to Monitor the Health of Older Americans. www.cdc.gov/nchs/releases/ 01facts/olderame.htm.

[81] The Commonwealth Fund. Prescription Drug Coverage Is Fragile for Beneficiaries. www.cmwf.org/media/releases/stuart_drug_release02022000.asp?link=11.

CHAPTER 15

Chronic Care in America

An Evolving Crisis

The story of chronic care in the United States is the story of mismatched incentives. Health care in the United States has historically been built on Big Science and dramatic technological interventions directed at acute episodes of disease. That's how we see health care, and that's how we fund it. The better the drugs and more expensive the machinery, the better the care. But chronic illnesses require a longer-term approach, an approach that includes early diagnosis, patient education, lifestyle change, home monitoring, and the prevention of severe crisis. Americans are loath to give up our belief in the quick fix of science and technology, even when faced with evidence that it isn't always appropriate or effective.

Nearly a century after the threat of death from acute disease has been wrestled to its knees by treatments, vaccines, and public health measures, our tax dollars and health care policies still support a research and treatment industry dedicated to acute care.

Chronic illnesses now account for nearly 70 percent of all deaths in the United States. Heart disease, cancer, and strokes were responsible for 59 percent of all deaths in 2000.[1] Moreover, the number of people living with chronic conditions will increase in the next decade, reaching 157 million by 2020 (see Figure 15-1).[2] Approximately 50 million of these people will have some activity limitations, including 15 million who will be unable to perform a major activity associated with their age group. Inadequate care of these chronic conditions not only affects the quality of life for millions of people, it also exacts tremendous costs from society at large.

As a result, every sector of the health care industry—from pharmaceuticals to community providers—is preparing to treat the chronically ill, but currently these efforts are diffuse and uncoordinated. How can such an advanced nation have a health care delivery system so ill-prepared for treating the health care needs of its growing chronically ill population? This chapter identifies the key trends shaping the current chronic care system and explores the outlook for the future.

CHRONICALLY MISUNDERSTOOD: THE WHO, WHEN, AND WHAT OF CHRONIC ILLNESS

In its simplest definition, a chronic illness is one with a long and indefinite duration that has little prospect of immediate change, either for better or

Figure 15-1. Prevalence of chronic conditions

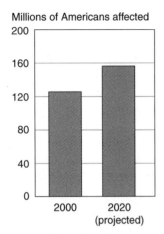

Millions of Americans affected

Source: Anderson, G., and J. R. Knickman. Changing the Chronic Care System to Meet People's Needs. *Health Affairs.* Vol. 20, No. 6, 2001.

for worse, even though symptoms of disease may not always be apparent.

The National Health Interview Survey (NHIS) defines a chronic health condition as one that has persisted for three or more months. For analyses based on the National Medical Expenditure Survey (NMES), the term "chronic condition" encompasses both chronic illness (the presence of long-term disease or symptoms, usually lasting three months or more) and chronic impairment (a physiological, psychological, or anatomical abnormality of bodily structure or function, including all losses or abnormalities, not just those attributable to active pathology).

A large and diverse population of people suffers from a variety of chronic maladies, including pediatric asthma, mental retardation, blindness, diabetes, and terminal cancer. In 2000, an estimated 125 million people were living with chronic conditions in the United States.

Chronic conditions are very individual in terms of symptoms or type of care required, but they do share the following critical elements:

- Chronic conditions cannot be "cured" in the traditional sense of the word. People with such conditions will carry the disease or disability with them for months, years, or a lifetime.

- The goal of treatment for people with these conditions is to improve their ability to live productive and pain-free lives, not to rid them of the condition.

- If people with these conditions receive medical treatment, lifestyle education, and support early in their disease, many acute care episodes can be avoided.

- Some chronic illness leads to disability, or the long- or short-term reduction of a person's activity as a result of an acute or chronic condition.

Many people who have chronic conditions lead active, productive lives, but some experience significant difficulties as a result of their chronic conditions. Approximately 50 million of the almost 125 million people who have chronic conditions have a disability and 15 million are limited in their activities by their condition. The prevalence of disability due to chronic illness increases with age because the conditions common among the elderly tend to be more disabling.

Those who study the people who experience disabling effects of chronic illness categorize them by their dependence on others. In other words, they distinguish the effects of chronic conditions that limit people from being productive themselves, from limitations that require the time and assistance of other individuals. The Activity of Daily Living (ADL) measurement scale allows researchers, care providers, and policymakers to better understand the needs and challenges of the disabled population. The ADL scale categorizes the disabled population based on people's ability to successfully accomplish the activities of daily living within their limitations. This can be a proxy for the severity of illness and the expected needs. A person with a high number of ADL limitations will need the most assistance. Specifically:

- *Major Activities of Daily Living* (ADLs) include eating/nutrition, dressing, personal hygiene, mobility, toileting, and behavior management.

- *Instrumental Activities of Daily Living* (IADLs) include preparing meals, shopping, using the telephone, managing money, taking medications, doing light housework, and other measures of independent living.

As with most measurement scales, there is discrepancy among researchers regarding how to capture and categorize ADLs.

Differences in criteria and measurement can affect the estimated size of the population. Agreement among policymakers, researchers, and advocates concerning how to measure and assess the needs of the chronically ill will be critical to informing policy and programs in the future.

THE CHRONICALLY ILL ARE DIVERSE

Perhaps one reason chronic care doesn't get the attention it deserves is the common misperception that equates chronic illness with the elderly and disability. Data from 1996 showed that although 88 percent of the elderly suffered from one or more chronic conditions[3] and approximately 40 percent of the chronically ill were disabled, the bulk of chronic care patients were under 65 and did not experience disability due to their chronic condition (see Table 15-1). For example, more than half of the 40 million Americans affected by arthritis and other rheumatic conditions were younger than 65.

Each age group is affected by a different set of chronic conditions. Eight percent of children between the ages of 5 and 17 suffer from some ADL limitation due to chronic disease.[4] Asthma is one of the most common chronic ailments for kids; in 1996, 6.2 percent of children under the age of 18 suffered from asthma.[5] Approximately 400 children die of asthma each year during severe asthma attacks that could have been prevented with adequate diagnosis and treatment. On the other hand, arthritis and cardiovascular disease, two of the seven most

Table 15-1. Most noninstitutionalized individuals with chronic conditions are under age 65.

Age	0–17	18–44	45–64	65+	All ages
Percentage	14	31	29	26	100

Source: Hoffman, C., D. Rice, and H. Sung. Persons with Chronic Conditions: Their Prevalence and Costs. *Journal of the American Medical Association* 1996; 26(18):1473–1479.

prevalent chronic conditions, primarily affect older adults.

The type and prevalence of chronic conditions differ not only by age, but also by race and economic status. More members of minority ethnic and racial groups and more poor people die from chronic conditions than those who are Caucasian and wealthy. African Americans have higher mortality rates from heart disease, stroke, cancer, cirrhosis, and diabetes than do Caucasians. There is also a widening gap in health outcomes between African Americans and all other races for some chronic conditions, including asthma, diabetes, and several forms of cancer. For example, the 5-year survival rate for cancer among African Americans diagnosed between 1986 and 1991 was 42 percent, compared to 58 percent for Caucasian Americans. Although the death rate from breast cancer among all women in the United States fell 10 percent between 1990 and 1995 (from 23.1 to 21 per 100,000), the rate for African American women remained

high at 27.5 per 100,000. A considerable proportion of the mortality differences may be attributed to social phenomena, for example, later diagnosis, lack of access to appropriate medical care, and other health determinants such as socioeconomic status and environmental conditions.

THE CHRONICALLY ILL USE MORE SERVICES AND ARE OFTEN AFFLICTED BY MULTIPLE DISABILITIES

People with chronic illnesses not only die earlier than their "healthy" counterparts; they often face higher rates of illness and hospitalization. Chronically ill patients spend more time in doctors' offices, emergency rooms, and hospital beds, but often don't receive the kind of care they need when they need it—that is, before the need for care becomes acute. Specifically, chronically ill people account for 55 percent of all emergency room visits, 70 percent of all hospital admissions, and 80 percent of all hospital stays. In a large study of health maintenance organization (HMO) enrollees, the average annual number of office visits for people with chronic conditions was between 68 and 154 percent higher than for people without chronic conditions, with the greatest number of visits attributed to respiratory conditions (see Table 15-2).

Individuals with chronic illnesses are also at greater risk for comorbidities, defined as medical conditions that exist in addition to the most significant chronic condition from which a person suffers. For example, diabetes is the seventh leading cause of death in the

Table 15-2. Annual per-person office visits

Status/condition	Number of office visits
Healthy	2.57
Asthma	5.12
Depression	4.74
Diabetes	4.83
Emphysema	6.52
Hypertension	4.34

Source: Sachs Group, Inc. Tracking Usage Patterns of the Chronically Ill. *Hospitals and Health Networks* 1994; 68(20):84.

United States, increases the risk of heart attack or stroke twofold to fourfold, and is the leading cause of new blindness, end-stage renal disease, and loss of lower limbs. Approximately 85,000 diabetes-related, lower-extremity amputations were performed in 1996.[6]

CHRONIC ILLNESS AND DISEASE ARE EXPENSIVE

The direct costs of chronic illness alone in 1996 added up to $564 billion (in 1996 dollars), or more than 60 percent of all personal health care expenditures in this country.[7] Add to that the lost productivity resulting from disability and premature death and the total bill increases by $234 billion.

The onset of many chronic illness complications can be delayed by early detection, clinical treatment, and lifestyle changes and environmental improvements. Diabetes is an excellent example of how some of the pain and costs of chronic illness could be avoided by early detection and treatment. Early detection and treatment measures could reduce some of the ill effects of diabetes. For example, detection and treatment could eliminate 90 percent of the new cases of blindness among adults age 20 to 74.[8] In 1995, an estimated 16 million people in the United States had diabetes, although only 8 million were diagnosed with the disease. As much as half of the diabetes population is undiagnosed due to two factors: the disease symptoms vary so widely that without a blood sugar or glucose tolerance test even a physician may not be able to diagnose diabetes in the early stages; and the cost of testing is not covered for a large part of the population (including the millions of under-insured or uninsured Americans).[9]

A second approach to limit the indirect costs of chronic illness is to provide home care to assist the disabled among the chronically ill in their daily activities to enable them to work. However, people with disability often don't have access to home care or community-based services, and when they do, those services are inadequate. For example, between 31 and 55 percent of people who require assistance with an activity of daily living do not obtain such assistance (see Figure 15-2). As a consequence, between 37 and 71 percent of adults aged 18 to 64 years were unable to perform one of the six daily activities evaluated (see Figure 15-3). Inability to get assistance can potentially lead to further disability; 49 percent of adults aged 18

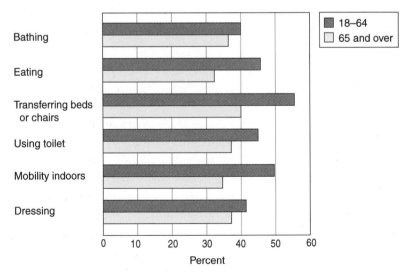

Figure 15-2. Prevalence of unmet need for assistance among persons with need for ADL help, by age group

Bathing
Eating
Transferring beds or chairs
Using toilet
Mobility indoors
Dressing

■ 18–64
□ 65 and over

0 10 20 30 40 50 60
Percent

Source: Robert Wood Johnson Foundation. *Chronic Care in America: A 21st Century Challenge*. Princeton, NJ: Robert Wood Johnson Foundation; 1996.

Chapter 15: Chronic Care in America   283

Figure 15-3. The consequences of unmet need for help, by age group

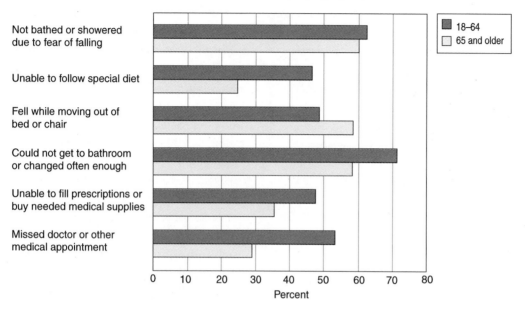

Source: Robert Wood Johnson Foundation. *Chronic Care in America: A 21st Century Challenge*. Princeton, NJ: Robert Wood Johnson Foundation, 1996.

to 64 fell while moving in or out of bed or chair, as did 58 percent of those over 65 years old.

Increased prevalence of chronic disease as the population ages only begins to explain why chronic illness is a major public policy concern. The cost of lost economic productivity is high, considering the large number of people whose work is restricted or terminated by a chronic disease, and adding in the time of those who tend to the chronically ill. People with serious chronic conditions, such as severe mental retardation, need constant attention of a caregiver to avoid injury and illness. Less obvious or severe chronic illness, such as arthritis or chronic obstructive pulmonary disease, can interfere with a person's ability to perform normal activities and may

require more limited assistance. Getting chronic care "right" is not just a matter of increasing the quality of life of those who suffer from chronic conditions—it can also bring about a more efficient use of resources for society at large.

CHRONIC CARE TODAY: HOW WE GOT HERE

The number of people living with chronic disease is increasing due to medical and social advances that allow us to live longer, both with and without chronic disease. As a result, providing treatment for the chronically ill in the future will only grow more important as the afflicted populations continue to increase. Several trends are contributing to the increase in chronically ill people and the growing importance of treatment.

Chapter 15: Chronic Care in America

TRENDS LEADING TO MORE CHRONIC ILLNESS

The population is aging. After 2010, when the first wave of the baby boom reaches traditional retirement age, about one-third of the U.S. population will be over the age of 65. Although there are good reasons—lifestyle changes and better drugs among them—to believe that elder boomers will be healthier than their parents, there will also be a greater number of elder boomers. New medical treatments for the leading causes of chronic disease and disability are expected to extend the life span of patients with conditions such as heart disease and cancer. The number of extended lives with managed—but not eradicated—chronic illnesses will mean that, though the *share* of those with chronic illness may decrease, the absolute *number* will actually increase.

New treatments allow people to live longer with their disease. New treatments will allow people to live longer with their disease, and some diseases previously identified as terminal can now be treated as chronic illnesses. Both of these trends contribute to a growing population of the chronically ill. For example, new pharmaceuticals for treating osteoporosis help people to maintain their bone mass and prevent fractures. Although osteoporosis isn't fatal, illnesses that might result from a fracture, such as pneumonia, can be life threatening. Even for HIV/AIDS and cancer, where finding a "cure" has been evasive despite rigorous research, new treatments are beginning to offer hope. Some HIV/AIDS patients are now able to return to work and pursue other endeavors due to recently developed drugs. Cancer treatments such as chemotherapy allow some patients to live in remission for years. Such new procedures, pharmaceutical treatments, and patient self-management have enabled people to live longer, healthier lives and mitigate some of the negative impacts of chronic disease.

Many patients are not effectively managing chronic disease. Despite the advances that help people live longer, patients diagnosed with chronic conditions don't always have the ability, will, or support to carefully follow the regimen of diet, exercise, and medication their doctors prescribe. Because the effects of chronic illness often are not felt acutely from day to day, it is tempting to overlook them.

The number of patients who do not adhere to strict, recommended treatment regimens is not surprising, given the lack of support for sustained behavior modification, and the reliance on bio-medical and scientific breakthroughs for treatment. As a society, we believe in the promise of science to save, to cure, to fix, to forge a path to the future. In addition, many individuals increase their risk of developing a chronic illness by smoking, drinking heavily, eating and sleeping poorly, not exercising, and working and worrying too much for their own good.

Poor dietary patterns, physical inactivity, and other high-risk behaviors are key risk factors for heart disease and cancer and major contributors to chronic disease-related morbidity and mortality in the United States.[10] More and more people are putting themselves—and often others—at risk by working in high-stress positions, driving dangerously, and failing to practice safe sex.

Chapter 15: Chronic Care in America 285

Suggested solutions to these problems have been many, including:

- Educating people about the dangers of their high-risk behaviors

- Charging high risk-takers more for insurance coverage

- Making the products associated with high-risk behaviors prohibitively expensive

- Providing people with financial incentives to abandon their high-risk behaviors

- Focusing on long-term changes by educating children and young adults intensively.

Why haven't these solutions had a powerful effect? The answer lies in two distinct cultural forces. First is the belief in science as a solution. Medical research has brought us to the brink of a cure for cancer; to safe, effective, and available liver transplants; to medications that reduce the suffering of substance abusers; and to surgical procedures that suck away unwanted fat. Why should we behave ourselves when we can do as we wish, then let the health care system bear the burden of a cure?

Second, for every "take-good-care-of-yourself" message would-be patients receive from health care professionals and loved ones, they are bombarded with at least 20 conflicting product advertisements. Ads hawking the desirability of smoking cigarettes, drinking alcohol, enjoying rich foods, severely dieting, and gaining wealth and power by working in high-pressure positions pervade our society. Add the fact that our society also allocates tax subsidies to tobacco growers and sanctions the trade of American produce for South American cigars. Now *that* is a mixed message.

Our medical system is not geared toward acute care. A focus on treating discrete, acute medical episodes and infectious diseases has created a U.S. health care system badly suited to the needs of a chronically ill population. Scientific breakthroughs in the 19th century, particularly the developments of germ theory, water purification, and pasteurization, dramatically reduced illnesses and premature deaths caused by external forces. Indeed, the virtues of medical science have been many. In this century, medical research has resulted in safer and more effective surgical practices, the virtual annihilation of polio in the developed world, and antibiotics that kill microorganisms at the root of pneumonia and other bacterial infections.

Unfortunately, these scientific breakthroughs have been almost too successful. While the discovery and availability of life-saving drugs, early disease-detection technologies, and surgical techniques have increased, so have our expectations that all maladies can be cured or surgically removed. As a society, we have put our money and our policies behind those beliefs, fueling growth in medical, surgical, and pharmaceutical research. The focus on treating acute disease is further exacerbated by a finance system that favors reimbursable procedures and devices over treatment regimens that are complex and for which long-term outcomes vary, depending on the individual.

Because of scientific breakthroughs, the leading causes of illness and death have changed through the century from infectious to chronic diseases, which, by definition, cannot always be cured. Our beliefs about what medicine can do, however, have not evolved similarly. We still make funding decisions that support medical and technological research based on what scientists believe is possible rather than what ordinary citizens need to lead healthier lives.

Even individual providers are inadequately prepared to treat chronically ill patients. Most physicians' training leaves them in a poor position to provide prevention and health promotion counseling. A recent study, for example, noted that most doctors do not counsel their patients about behavior modifications that could reduce their risk for heart disease. The physicians counseled patients about exercise during only 19 percent of office visits, about diet during only 23 percent of visits, and about weight reduction during only about 10 percent of visits. Further, only 41 percent of cigarette smokers were advised during office visits to quit smoking.[11]

Are these doctors always the best caregivers for the chronically ill? People with chronic conditions do require the services of highly trained medical specialists at certain critical points. However, most of the time these patients' needs could be met adequately by other trained caregivers such as nurse educators, home care providers, social workers, and even informal unpaid caregivers—often family members. This is already the case in a number of situations. In 1990, 83 percent of the disabled population under the age of 65 and 73 percent

of the elderly population relied exclusively on informal caregivers. Not only would an increase in prevention and primary care interventions reduce the frequency and extent of hospitalizations, but greater and better organized utilization of home and community-based services would provide a more appropriate mix of care and reduce the cost of care overall.[12]

Funding does not support integrated, long-term care for the chronically ill. The financing structure of America's health care system clearly encourages the provision of acute care services at the expense of comprehensive services over time for people with chronic conditions. The greatest amount of federal support is devoted to acute, episodic care that aims to cure. Private insurance and government programs cover 92 percent of all hospital expenditures and 81 percent of charges for physician services.[13] To date there has been little insurance coverage for the nonmedical services and nontraditional sites of care that assist people with chronic conditions (see Figure 15-4).

The federal government, the single largest payer of health care services and the major insurer for the elderly, does not finance a program specifically designed to cover long-term care. Home health care, homemaker services, adult day care, nursing home care, help with activities of daily living, housing with supportive services, and other social services are not included in most health benefits plans. Even when these services are included in a benefits package, the coverage is limited by number of days or hours of service. In the case of medical

Chapter 15: Chronic Care in America   287

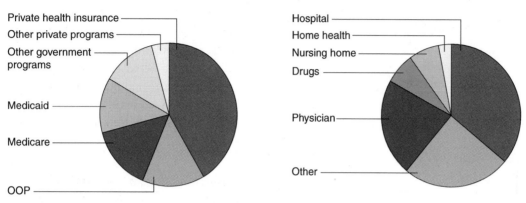

Figure 15-4. Who pays for what? 2000 national health expeditures

Private health insurance
Other private programs
Other government programs
Medicaid
Medicare
OOP

Hospital
Home health
Nursing home
Drugs
Physician
Other

Source: Medicare and Medicaid Statistical Supplement, Health Care Financing Review, 1996.

equipment, dental services, and nursing home care, for example, consumers pay on average 26 to 52 percent of total expenditures out of pocket.

The lack of incentives for organizations and individuals that would provide services to the chronically ill is felt not only in the relatively small total financial commitment, but also in the fragmented nature of the funding. Small pockets of funds to support chronic care can be found in government and private standard coverage, special grants and programs funded by disease-specific charities, national and local foundations, special legislation for programs in certain states, and local churches and nonprofit organizations. Some providers who treat a high number of chronic patients employ part- or full-time grant writers whose sole function is to find and apply for these special funds.

With each funding source come limitations on the types of services covered (hospital care, rehabilitation, home health) and eligibility requirements that must be met by the provider and the patient (providers can be required to be nonprofit organizations, patients can be required to demonstrate financial need or have a specific ethnicity, gender, age, health status, or employment status).[14] With these types of funding comes the knowledge that the financial support is temporary, subject to shrinking during times of economic uncertainty, or evaporating entirely with changes in the latest funding priorities of an organization's board.

The fact that most health insurance is employment-based also contributes to the inaccessibility of health care services for the chronically ill. People with disabilities, the majority of whom are disabled due to a chronic condition, represented roughly 15 percent (5.5 million people) of the uninsured in 1994, including one million disabled children under the age of 18 (see Figure 15-5).[15] People over 65 are not included in this number, with the exception of the small

Figure 15-5. Source of health insurance coverage for persons with any disability, by age

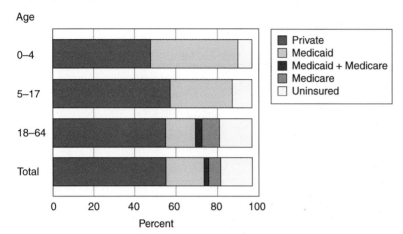

Source: Meyer, J. A., and P. J. Zeller. *Profiles of Disability: Employment and Health Coverage*. Economic and Social Research Institute for the Henry J. Kaiser Family Foundation's Commission on Medicaid and the Uninsured. Washington, DC: Henry J. Kaiser Family Foundation, September 1999.

percentage that does not qualify for Medicare. High premiums, coverage denial for pre-existing conditions, and restricted eligibility for public programs are some of the reasons people with chronic conditions lack health insurance.

Lack of health insurance, inadequate coverage, temporary funding, and higher premiums all translate into higher out-of-pocket costs for chronically ill patients. The per capita costs of care for people with chronic conditions are three times higher than those for people without chronic conditions and the costs for individuals with comorbidities are two-and-a-half times higher than those for people with only one chronic condition. Out-of-pocket expenditures on health care for older disabled persons (45–64 years old) were expected to consume nearly 30 percent of their annual income in 2000.[16]

One of the biggest challenges facing people who have chronic conditions is the integration of care across three continua—time, providers (physicians, nurses, home care providers, social workers), and service settings (hospitals, nursing facilities, home health agencies, community-based programs). The fragmented funding of providers and services usually means that health care professionals who are working with a chronically ill patient have no system and no expectations for communicating with each other. Requiring the patient to transmit information about treatment and services often means that information is lost. Even the most knowledgeable, intelligent, observant patient would have difficulty communicating all of his or her medical information to all providers. These problems are particularly severe for patients with multiple chronic conditions, a good portion of all patients with chronic illness. Of people 55 years and older who have arthritis, for example, as many as 48 percent also have hypertension, 16 percent also have heart disease, 11 percent also have cancer, and 11 percent also have diabetes.[17]

At best, the state of chronic care today is unfocused and uneven. What will it be like in 2010?

FORECAST

How is chronic care likely to evolve in the rest of this decade? As in the general health care forecast in Chapter 1, some forecasts call for "Stormy Weather," and others are "On the Sunny Side of the Street."

STORMY WEATHER

Public health will continue to be financially strapped and undervalued. The public health sector, with its concentration on populations, prevention, and the non-medical determinants of health, potentially has a lot to offer in the detection and prevention of chronic conditions. However, this sector will continue to face financial pressure, even in the absence of a federal deficit, especially now that the economy is slowing down. Efforts to deliver personal health care services to uninsured populations will continue to divert attention and resources from public health providers, as the number of uninsured rises each year. The extent to which particular public health agencies focus on population-based approaches to chronic disease will depend on local community support, both in terms of finances and vision, and the charisma of their individual leaders.

Underinvestment in long-term prevention strategies will persist. The majority of the commercial market, including health plans, insurers, and employers, will limit prevention efforts to specific diseases—those that either help insurers gain National Committee for Quality Assurance (NCQA) accreditation or those that show a quick financial return on investment. In evaluating the effectiveness of chronic care provided by managed care organizations, NCQA is concentrating on four conditions: childhood asthma, diabetes, coronary artery disease, and major depression. In order to meet NCQA's quality standards, many health plans will ensure that their screening rates for all four conditions are high. Because people change employers and health plan membership with greater frequency than ever before, however, employers and health plans will continue to be reluctant to make large investments in prevention measures that provide only long-term payoffs—no matter how important they are to the patient.

Teens will still think they're immortal. While the smoking rate among adults is declining, smoking rates among teenagers are on the rise. Each generation of youths find new threats to ignore. For each generation, we can only try to reduce the number of youths who ignore threats and try to keep them alive until their judgment improves.

Sick baby boomers will find themselves home alone. The availability of informal caregivers is projected to decrease in the future, even as the demand for their services increases. Smaller family networks and the increasing participation of women—the traditional caregivers—at higher levels in the workforce will contribute to the decline. Current studies indicate that many of the remaining caregivers are in poor health themselves, with increased risks of stress-related disorders such as hypertension and heart disease.[18] All such caregivers report requiring support, information, and occasional respite from caregiving in order to continue providing care.[19] The availability of formal and informal caregivers will become critically important as the baby boomers age. As of 2010, this country will face no fewer than 18 years in which approximately one-third of its population will be 65 or over.[20] Given inadequate funding for home health care workers and long-term care, increased prevalence of chronic conditions, and reduced availability of unpaid informal caregivers, the baby boom generation faces the very real possibility of being sick and left home alone.

Disparities in health status by race and ethnicity are expected to persist. Despite significant health and health care advances that will benefit all chronically ill individuals, disparities in health status by race/ethnicity are expected to persist. This trend is attributable to a number of factors, including access to health care, and lifestyle and environmental factors.

ON THE SUNNY SIDE OF THE STREET

Those with chronic disease will live longer. More people will live longer, more fulfilling lives with chronic disease. This is the result of a number of converging trends, from increased life expectancy to increased availability of pharmaceutical products that treat chronic illnesses.

The prevalence of disability among the chronically ill will decrease. The projections given for the growth in chronic disease are calculated by applying the most recent rates of chronic disease and disability to projected changes in the U.S. demographic distribution, implicitly assuming that the rates of disease and activity limitations by gender and age will remain constant. There is some evidence that the prevalence of disability among the elderly is declining.[21] It is not surprising, considering the advances in overall health status achieved during the past century, that as younger cohorts age, they will have fewer health problems than their parents. If the trend continues, the prevalence of disability for the elderly population is expected to

decline from 21.3 percent in 1994 to 17 percent in 2010. Keep in mind, however, that the absolute number of people with chronic conditions is likely to reach well over 125 million by 2010.

There will be more investment in long-term disease management and coordinated care. Some hope for growth in truly integrated services can be pinned on insurers' interests in disease management— the coordination of inpatient, outpatient, education, home, and community services after a patient has been identified as high risk for certain conditions. In the end, there are two critical factors that will influence the success of coordinated disease management.

First is the cost-benefit trade-off for the payer, whether public or private. The closer the relationship between cost outlay and financial benefit for the payer, the more likely that payer will pursue disease management. For example, cardiac programs that coordinate postsurgical monitoring, education, and home care and show short-term results in reduced risk of rehospitalization or second surgery have an outstanding chance to thrive. However, smoking cessation and weight management programs have a much looser and longer-term relationship with financial benefit, therefore a much lower likelihood of being funded. In order for these programs to be effective, they require constant support and, if successful, may reduce an individual's risk of a variety of chronic diseases that would be costly to treat 20 years from now. Although many insurers report that they offer disease prevention programs,[22] a series of interviews with health plan medical directors and employer groups across the nation indicate that most are not investing in prevention measures that provide a long-term payoff. Most organizations are looking for cost savings within the first 18 to 24 months of introducing a program.

The second critical factor is the capacity for disease management techniques to manage patients with a wide variety of comorbidities. If an arthritic asthma patient and an arthritic diabetic must be "coordinated" through one continuum of care for arthritis and another for the other diagnosis, and those providers do not communicate with each other, it's not really a continuum of care from the patient's perspective.

Early intervention and disease management will reduce the personal and financial cost of chronic illness. Prevention and behavior changes can delay the onset of and disability related to chronic diseases. There is some evidence that middle-aged and older adults are more likely than are younger adults to invest in behavioral changes that may improve their health outcomes.[23] Even for those who already suffer from a chronic condition, behavioral changes may delay the progression of their illness and related disability. For example, recent studies indicate that an exercise routine, even one for the frail elderly, increases muscle mass and bone density and reduces the risk of falling. There's a ray of hope: Even if young people feel immortal, they can change their ways later in life, and reduce their risk of becoming chronic patients.

Of course, even the best detection and disease management procedures can't eliminate all the effects and costs of chronic care, but they can be reduced if we diagnose chronic illnesses earlier, intervene more consistently, and unlock the secrets to prevention and successful patient education. To use diabetes disease management as an example once again, the Diabetes Control and Complications Trial, a national 10-year study that involved 1,441 volunteers with insulin-dependent diabetes, confirmed that careful control of blood sugar prevented the onset or delayed the progression of eye, kidney, and nerve damage by at least 50 percent. Another program, the Michigan Diabetes Control Program's Upper Peninsula Diabetes Outreach Network (UPDON), showed that improvements in the quality of diabetes care and education reduced hospitalizations by 45 percent, lower-extremity amputations by 31 percent, and the death rate by 27 percent for program participants, compared to nonparticipants.

Health systems will attempt to organize around the patient's chronic disease. Many hospitals and health systems have attempted to create "integrated" delivery systems over the past 10 years. However, plans for service integration are more often based on the demands for physical plant and personnel and the potential for reimbursement than on patient needs.

There is, however, the National Chronic Care Coalition (NCCC), a 37-member group of nonprofit health systems working together to provide high-quality care for people with chronic conditions. Initiated by hospital systems, members are required to have integrated care networks already in place in their service areas, to have a reputation for innovation, and to have full board and CEO support for active NCCC participation. NCCC offers free online information and care guidelines and is involved in at least two large demonstration projects of national significance. The consortium has partnered with the State of Minnesota's Department of Human Services, and with the help of the Robert Wood Johnson Foundation, has proposed and been awarded a 5-year demonstration project waiver from the Health Care Financing Administration (HCFA). The project allows Medicare and Medicaid funds to be combined to provide a continuum of care for the elderly in the seven metropolitan counties of Minneapolis/St. Paul. NCCC also has teamed with the Alzheimer's Association to create a project testing the effectiveness of managed care for Alzheimer's patients.[24]

Sensors will allow remote monitoring and facilitate disease management. As the size of remote sensors decreases, and their ability to detect small changes in environments increases, sensors will become an increasingly integral part of most disease management treatments. For a diabetic patient, for example, sensors will provide constant and passive communication between the patient and a provider about blood sugar levels as well as blood pressure and pulse. This will enable providers to conduct remote monitoring of their patients' health status and potentially manage a component of disease without any extra effort for a patient.

Belief structures can be changed. In the previous chapter, we discussed the critical importance of Americans' belief that sci-

ence will save us from our bad behavior. The promising news is that belief structures can and do change. They don't change quickly or easily, but the pace of change should not be confused with the direction of change. The following are examples of repeated, sustained actions turning the tide:

- *If Moms are against it, it must be bad.* One of the most effective campaigns in the United States to change societal acceptance of a particular high-risk behavior has been Mothers Against Drunk Driving (MADD). MADD's campaigns at the public information and legislative levels have, in 19 years, significantly contributed to changing attitudes and laws about the acceptability of driving when intoxicated. This movement succeeded in gaining support, in part, because it targeted the effect of drunk driving on the safety of innocent bystanders, particularly children.

- *The Marlboro Man and Joe Camel go on indeterminate leave.* Several states have taken aggressive stances against cigarette smoking. They actively prosecute retailers who sell tobacco to minors, heavily tax the sale of cigarettes, and use the tax dollars almost exclusively on tobacco-related research and high-profile antismoking campaigns. Some states, such as California, have banned cigarette smoking in most public places. Preliminary data reveal that these efforts do indeed reduce tobacco consumption, albeit more slowly than some might hope.[25] The critical factor in these programs is their ability to slowly change the American mind-set about the acceptability of smoking. We forecast that by 2010, smoking in public will have the same stigma currently associated with drunk driving and the reduction in smoking will contribute to a further reduction in tobacco-associated chronic conditions.

■ *It's hip to be aware.* What began as a 1960s hippie revival of consuming natural foods and eschewing animal flesh has become, with some twists and turns, a part of most Americans' consciousness. Today in most social circles it is acceptable, if not commendable, to be aware of the fat content, fiber, cholesterol, and processing of the foods we eat, and to drink mineral water instead of alcohol. The widespread European outrage over bioengineered food products has not reached across the pond with full force, but that is a next step for a growing number of Americans who want to know where and what their food was before they eat it.

IMPLICATIONS

In the next decade, there is both hope and despair for changing the U.S. health care system to better meet the needs of its citizens, especially regarding chronic care. The evolution of chronic care in the next 10 years will have the following implications:

■ *Here come the elder boomers.* The impact of the baby boom generation will continue to be strong as boomers age, influencing attitudes, services, products, and the success of new technologies—the toys and tools of this generation. At the same time, however, aging boomers will increase demands and financial stress on a health care system already weak in payment and personnel devoted to long-term and chronic care. Political priorities are unlikely to change dramatically until boomers feel the full effects of a system unable to support good chronic care. By then, it may be too late to develop a coordinated system able to deliver the high-quality care they demand.

■ *Profit will drive many initiatives.* The power of profit, or the lack thereof, will continue to be a strong influence on the decisions of health plans, insurers, and employers' support of disease management programs. Those that show a short-term profit (heart disease programs) will get funded, and those that don't (smoking cessation) won't. The long-term cost savings due to disease management programs are difficult to capture and do not factor well into a short-term budgeting cycle. The mind-set that a return on investment must be immediate if funding is to continue must change before the system will change.

■ *Support for home care and less formal caregivers will be needed.* With the unpaid, informal caregivers of America (primarily women) leaving for the workforce, those left at home to care for the chronically ill will be older people susceptible to chronic illness themselves. Without some type of organized home care system, the chronically ill will continue to use the more expensive care and technology required for acute episodes.

■ *Health insurance is not enough.* Even the chronically ill who are fully insured pay as much as half their health care costs out of pocket. Medicare and Medicaid do a poor job of funding long-term, chronic care. Already, many people can't afford to be chronically ill and those numbers can only be expected to grow.

■ *Kids these days . . .* The pressure to "behave badly" will still be the initiation dance of youth. We can't afford to give up on programs targeted toward youth, however. The earlier they get the message, the better prospects they have of avoiding chronic illness. Society-wide programs for restricting tobacco use and treating alcohol abuse can also go a long way toward limiting the self-destructive behaviors of youth.

■ *Get over the blame game.* Why have efforts to increase early detection, educate patients and the public, and provide continuous monitoring not become the cornerstone of the U.S. health care delivery system? Some activists blame members of Congress for funding high tech over high need. Others blame health care providers for not taking greater interest in the needs of chronically ill patients. And of course there are those who blame the patients themselves for not taking a more aggressive role in preventing illness and promoting their own health. Each of these fingers of blame points at the result, not the source, of our current dilemma. The true source is the system itself, and these attitudes won't change until the system changes.

■ *The chronically ill and disabled can be productive.* Only a small percentage of chronic illnesses need to claim the productivity of patients and those caring

for them. Depending on the type of work they do, many people who require help dressing or living independently may be gainfully employed if they receive assistance. For example, developments in voice-activated computers allow paraplegics to write anything from interoffice memos to novels. Minor adjustments in signs and office procedures can allow a sight-impaired person to be an active participant in many different types of knowledge work. A study published by the Economic and Social Research Institute reveals that 57 percent of Americans with any disability and more than one-third of those with a chronic disability that limits major life activities are employed or seeking work. Even though some of these workers may need help dressing themselves or transporting themselves to work, the great majority of disabled workers (87 percent) need no accommodation or special equipment once at work. If limitations were more easily accommodated or social/personal support easier to come by, many more Americans could be "productive" once again.

■ *The poor need more help with chronic care.* Poor people suffer disproportionately from chronic illness. Prescription drug benefits available through Medicaid provide a strong foundation to manage one aspect of chronic disease, but more social support must be available to enable sustained behavior change and to assist people who otherwise would not be able to work. In addition, affordable long-term care strategies must be in place to mitigate and postpone the negative impacts of chronic disease.

■ *Funding must be harmonized.* Any funding that does support chronic care in the current system often comes from so many disparate sources that no one person can keep track of them all. Something must be done to centralize, if not the funding itself, then at least the way it's managed, to give chronically ill patients as close to one-stop shopping as possible. Disease management programs will be central to achieving this coordination, as well as to providing social support for people suffering from chronic disease. As previously stated, funding cycles must be extended. This will help capture the benefits of disease management and ultimately rationalize their effectiveness in terms of cost-savings.

Perhaps the greatest hope for improvements in chronic care and reducing the negative impacts of chronic disease in America lies in a sea change of beliefs and attitudes toward science, health, and wellness. Policies and programs that expand the definition of health, and health care to include lifestyle and environmental factors have the potential to transform individual and community health and, ultimately, reduce the burden of chronic disease in America.

ENDNOTES

[1] Minino A. M., and B. L. Smith. Deaths: Preliminary data for 2000. National Vital Statistics Reports 49(12). Hyattsville, MD: National Center for Health Statistics, 2001.

[2] Anderson, G., and J. R. Knickman. Changing the chronic care system to meet people's needs. *Health Affairs* 2001; 20(6).

[3] Hoffman, C., D. Rice, and H. Sung. Persons with chronic conditions: Their prevalence and costs. *Journal of the American Medical Association* 1996; 26(18):1473–1479.

[4] Forum on Child and Family Statistics. *America's Children: Key National Indicators of Well-Being, 2000.* Vienna, VA: National Maternal and Child Health Clearinghouse, 2000. childstats.gov/ac2000/ac00.asp.

[5] National Center for Health Statistics. *Current Estimates, From the National Health Interview Survey, 1996.* (PHS) 99-1528. GPO stock number 017-01471-8.

[6] Centers for Disease Control and Prevention. *Diabetes Surveillance, 1999.* U.S. Department of Health and Human Services. www.cdc.gov/diabetes/.

[7] Trupin, L., D. Rice, and W. Max. *Medical Expenditures for People with Disabilities in the United States, 1987.* Washington, DC: U.S. Department of Education, National Institute on Disability and Rehabilitation Research. 1995.

[8] Centers for Disease Control and Prevention. *Diabetes: A Serious Public Health Problem.* Atlanta, GA: CDC, 1999.

[9] Diabetes Public Health Resource. *Diabetes: A Serious Public Health Problem At-A-Glance 2000.* National Center for Chronic Disease Prevention and Health Promotion. 2000.

[10] Health Insurance Association of America. *Source Book of Health Insurance Data.* Washington, DC: Health Insurance Association of America, 1996.

[11] Physician and other health-care professional counseling of smokers to quit—United States, 1991. *Morbidity and Mortality Weekly Reports* (November 12) 1993; 42(44): 854–857.

[12] Alecxih, L., et al. *Estimated Cost Savings from the Use of Home and Community-Based Alternatives to Nursing Facility Care in Three States.* Pub. No. 9618. Public Policy Institute/AARP. 1996.

[13] National Health Expenditures Projections: 2001-2011. Health Care Financing Administration. Office of the Actuary. National Health Statistics Group. www.hcfa.gov.

[14] Interviews with San Francisco Bay Area providers, 1997.

[15] Meyer, J. A., and P. J. Zeller. *Profiles of Disability: Employment and Health Coverage.* Economic and Social Research Institute for the Henry J. Kaiser Family Foundation's Commission on Medicaid and the Uninsured. Washington, DC: Henry J. Kaiser Family Foundation, September 1999.

[16] Maxwell, S., M. Moon, and M. Segal. *Growth in Medicare andOut-of-Pocket Spending: Impact on Vulnerable Populations.* Urban Institute, December 2000.

[17] Van Norstrand, J. F., S. E. Funer, and R. Suzman, eds. *Health Data on Older Americans: United States, 1992.* National Center for Health Statistics. Vital and Health Statistics, Series 3, No. 27. DHHS Pub. No. (PHS) 93–1411. Hyattsville, MD: Public Health Service, 1992.

[18] Gaynor, S. E., The long haul: The effects of home care on caregivers. *Image Journal of Nursing Schools* 1990; 22(4):208–212. Given, B., and C. W. Given. Family caregiving for the elderly. *Annual Review of Nursing Research* 1991.

[19] Cloonan, P. A. Managing Home Care. *Key Aspects of Caring for the Chronically Ill: Hospital and Home.* New York: Springer Publishing Company, 1993.

[20] Baby Boomer Headquarters. 1999. www.bbhq.com.

[21] Manton, K., and X. L. Gu. From the Cover: Changes in the prevalence of chronic disability in the United States black and non-

Chapter 15: Chronic Care in America

black population above age 65 from 1982 to 1999. *Proceedings of the National Academy of Sciences of the United States* (May 22) 2001; 28(11).

[22] Health Insurance Association of America. *Source Book of Health Insurance Data.* Washington, DC: Health Insurance Association of America. 1996.

[23] Tai Chi for Older People Reduces Falls, May Help Maintain Strength. News release text from National Institute on Aging. Washington, DC. May 2, 1996.

[24] National Chronic Care Consortium. www.nccconline.org.

[25] Centers for Disease Control Tobacco Information and Prevention Source. www.cdc.gov/tobacco.

CHAPTER 16

Disease Management

Weaving Disease Management into the Fabric of Patient Care

What exactly is disease management? It's as much a philosophy and a concept as it is a set of tools for delivering health care in a certain way. For the purpose of this forecast, we have defined disease management as an integrated, systematic approach to delivering care to populations of patients with specific chronic diseases.

Disease management integrates many clinical, business, and technology tools to improve health care quality and patient satisfaction. The core concept is to eliminate unnecessary complications from disease through patient and provider education and clinical protocols, among other approaches.

The number one driver of disease management is cost reduction. Therefore, disease management programs today are provided by, purchased by, or created by whoever is at financial risk for the cost of health care.

DISEASES BEING MANAGED

The most common initial targets for disease management are asthma, diabetes, and congestive heart failure (CHF).

- *Asthma.* More than 14.9 million people suffer from asthma in the United States, and it is the number one cause of pediatric admissions to hospitals. With clinically proven medication and patient-education treatment plans, a patient's asthma can be controlled significantly and the number of emergency room visits and asthma attacks reduced drastically. Disease managers have focused on self-care for asthma patients; patient-education programs are commonly used to help patients manage their own disease with peak flow meters and other self-monitoring techniques.

- *Diabetes.* About 15.7 million people in the United States have diabetes, with 5.4 million undiagnosed. Untreated diabetes can lead to cardiovascular disease, kidney failure, blindness, amputation, and death, but treatment is incredibly expensive. The American Diabetes Association and other health organizations have created guidelines that recommend frequent monitoring of blood glucose, regular foot and eye exams, and other interventions to reduce dramatically the incidence of damaging and costly complications. The challenge for disease managers is to incorporate these proven interventions into the standard practice of the primary care physicians who treat diabetes or to develop and contract for separate programs to ensure that this level of management occurs.

- *Congestive heart failure.* Disease management programs have repeatedly proven to be effective at keeping CHF patients out of emergency rooms and hospitals. CHF affects more than 4.6 million people in the United States. The incidence of CHF is highest in patients over age 65, and CHF is consistently one of the top five causes for hospital admissions of the elderly. Effective CHF disease management programs use appropriate medications, intense dietary therapy, frequent monitoring of early warning signs, and patient-education programs to change lifestyle behaviors and to prevent hospital readmissions.

These definitions and examples give some sense of what disease management is about. The next section explains how disease management is accomplished.

A DISEASE MANAGEMENT PRIMER

It may sound all well and good in theory to manage chronic diseases in order to reduce or avoid acute episodes, but how is it actually done? Disease management is accomplished by using an assortment of tools and techniques. There are four basic steps:

- *Step 1.* Find out who: Patient identification and assessment

- *Step 2.* Figure out what they need, then do it: Care delivery

- *Step 3.* Find out if it's working: Outcomes measurement

- *Step 4.* Bring the learning back to Step 1: Feedback.

PATIENT IDENTIFICATION AND ASSESSMENT

Identifying a population that will benefit from disease management is an important first step. Currently, disease managers search for specific clinical data in insurance data, pharmacy databases, or patient-reported surveys to create a "patient utilization profile."

Once patients have been identified, the next step is to assess each patient's overall health status. It is important to measure the general health of the individual at the time of enrollment in a disease management program to provide baseline data for measuring improvement and, once the data are aggregated, the success of the program

CARE DELIVERY

Most care within disease management programs is delivered according to clinical practice guidelines that outline treatment strategies, including those for patient monitoring and education. Clinical practice guidelines outline standardized processes for managing patient care. Most disease management programs cover all aspects of managing care, including:

- Prevention—education and early identification of the disease

- Clinical evaluation—screening, workup, and diagnosis

- Management—treatment and other interventions

- Maintenance—follow-up assessment and care

An asthma guideline, for example, could cover the use of inhalants as well as educational programs for the family, administration of medication in emergency rooms, and recommendations for ongoing maintenance.

OUTCOMES MEASUREMENT

As the field of outcomes measurement advances, the ability to identify, measure, and track relevant indicators will improve and will play an even more critical role in disease management. Pharmacy Benefit Managers (PBMs) are emerging as leaders in this field. As previously mentioned, it is difficult to integrate data elements from across the spectrum of care for any individual patient or disease. PBMs, however, have created enormous banks of data through their sophisticated networks of pharmacies and mail order systems.

FEEDBACK

Risk-adjusted outcomes data, reported to physicians, have been demonstrated to be effective tools in moving physicians' treatments toward best practices and improving outcomes of care. Provider education and feedback also target physicians' understanding of and compliance with practice guidelines and their overall understanding of the disease and the goals of the disease management pro-

gram. In this way, feedback about financial, performance, or clinical outcomes plays a significant educational role in the improvement and refinement of the tools and techniques of disease management.

INFORMATION TECHNOLOGY IN DISEASE MANAGEMENT

The foundation on which these components of disease management are built is information technology. As health care has become more complex, the data required to coordinate and track the care of patients have grown exponentially. It is beyond the capacity of the human brain to maintain and integrate all of the details of patient care, the latest in medical research, and the applications of new medical technologies. The use of computers and software designed to support clinicians and patients in managing chronic diseases is important. Without information technology, the ability to track and monitor patients and their disease states would be slow, burdensome, and nearly impossible

DRIVERS AND BARRIERS ON THE PATH AHEAD

With the right set of tools, processes, and interventions, disease management can help prevent acute episodes of chronic disease and avoid care in high-cost settings. Given the market imperative to cut costs, together with the push from new entrants to stretch disease management into new areas, the disease management industry is poised to grow.

Even people with a few skeptical bones left in their bodies might be impressed by the disease management cost savings reported in a recent survey by the National Managed Health Care Congress (NMHCC). Coronary artery disease and hypertension savings top the list, with 60 percent savings in the 1996–1997 fiscal year. All together, disease management has saved health costs by 10 to 20 percent, depending on the program. In addition to disease management programs, NMHCC also surveyed managed care organizations and employers, both of which reported savings to date as well as high expectations for their future use of disease management programs.

So is disease management the be-all, end-all solution to what ails health care? Not clear. Our health care system is a melting pot of professionally, administratively, financially, personally, and socially competing demands. In order to understand how any new object thrown into the pot will fare, we must look at the forces that support the survival of the new object—drivers of change—and at the forces that would eject or consume the new object—barriers to change.

DRIVING FORCES

Drivers of change are independent trends that can accelerate the adoption of a product, a service, or a concept. Trends in the availability and use of technology, the physician–patient balance of power, and the aging of the population, for example, will in concert accelerate the adoption of the tools and principles of disease management within the next 5 to 7 years. Significant drivers of change include the following:

- *Surfing the age wave.* The U.S. population is growing older as the baby boom generation ages—a demographic trend that will have far-reaching effects. People 65 years of age and older constitute the fastest-growing segment of the population. Their numbers will grow from 34 million in 1995 to 39 million by 2010, a 15 percent increase. This "age wave" has had and will continue to have a transformational effect on many institutions, levels of government, and segments of society. As baby boomers access and interact with the health care system over the next decade, their expectations and preferences—their demands and sheer numbers—will transform this institution as well.

- *Chronic disease: Number one on the chart.* Chronic disease and illness is the leading cause of death and morbidity in the United States. Already, more than 100 million people are living with chronic disease, and this number will increase to 120 million by 2010—40 percent of the population. With more than half a trillion dollars spent per year on care for these people, the impact of chronic illness on the health care industry will only continue to accelerate.

- *Cost containment: How to succeed in business.* The cost-containment imperative and competition in the business of health care remain strong. National health expenditures are just under 14 percent of gross domestic product (GDP) and are expected to grow at 6.5 percent per year. By 2005, national health expenditures will account for 15 percent of GDP, heading toward 16 percent by 2010. Two important factors affect cost growth: chronic disease and illness and medical technology. Nationwide, direct medical costs for the treatment of chronic disease exceed $500 billion annually and account for 45 percent of national health expenditures

- *Payer demands: Results.* The primary interest of payers is reducing costs for health benefits. With increases in health premiums, these payers will increase pressure for better health and cost outcomes, particularly when many of the costs associated with chronic illness can be avoided. As disease management demonstrates substantial cost benefits, employers and other payers will begin to demand that their insurers and providers use these programs.

- *Regulation: The road to good credit.* Accreditation by the National Committee for Quality Assurance (NCQA) and procedures of the Health Plan Employer Data and Information Set (HEDIS) put in place outcomes and process indicators to demonstrate and track provider accountability for specific disease states (e.g., routine retinopathy exams for diabetics). As managed care organizations respond to accreditation and possibly to regulatory requirements and market pressures to be more accountable, they will most likely accelerate disease management efforts.

- *Information and medical technologies: Success is the sweetest revenge for info-tech.* Information technology, the Internet, and new medical technologies are already having a dramatic impact on society and the health care system. The revolution in communication and information technologies is critical for

moving the site of care out of the hospital and into the patient's home, car, or trailer park. Recent advances in medical technologies are allowing new options in care and chronic disease management to emerge.

- *New health care consumers: A little knowledge, a lot of attitude.* Traditionally, health care consumers have been passive recipients of advances in medicine rather than drivers of change. IFTF has identified an emerging demographic group called "new consumers," who demand choice, control, information, and customer service—and are beginning to make these demands in the health care sector. Although new consumers have not been asking for disease management per se, they are demonstrating increasing interest in managing their own health.

- *Complexity and fragmentation.* Our weakness could be a strength. The melting pot of conflicting demands that is the U.S. health care system is nowhere near the precipice of major structural reform. We will continue to have many payers, many vested interests, and many injustices until and unless economic and political forces present an opportunity for significant change. Until that day, disease management is an approach that individual and competing payers and providers can use to reduce costs, increase quality, and increase patient satisfaction.

BARRIERS TO CHANGE

Despite these driving forces, a number of factors have interfered with adoption of the tools of disease management and will continue to do so. Many of these barriers exist across different settings of care and methods of payment. Some barriers, such as difficulty obtaining reimbursement for services, are financially driven—but not all. Significant barriers to change include the following:

- *Fragmented reimbursement: Too many contracts, not enough time.* Providers and health care organizations follow the incentives they are offered when a large portion of their patient flow springs from the source of the incentive—for example, Medicare. In a world of PPOs and open-panel health maintenance organizations (HMOs), physicians and hospitals frequently manage hundreds of payer contracts. If one payer gets into disease management in a big way but others do not, or if others focus on other diseases or use different protocols, providers have little incentive to change their practice patterns to adapt.

- *Short-term orientation: In the health care business, next Tuesday IS a long-term forecast.* Few health care players (payers *or* providers) have incentives to invest in interventions that will pay off in the long term. Instead, because of employee turnover, health plan churn, and FFS reimbursement, most interventions are oriented toward short-term payoffs.

- *Fragmented delivery system: Is anybody in charge here?* The traditional health care system simply is not a system; it is not user friendly and coordinated. Instead, it is a set of independent businesses, individuals, and entrepreneurs with areas of expertise, business interests, and market segments over which competition rather than coordi-

nation rules. Individual patients are often left to their own devices to navigate and negotiate the waters of covered benefits, preexisting conditions, and incomplete medical records. Until incentives are aligned and a strong business case is presented, health care is likely to remain fragmented rather than integrated into any cohesive system resembling disease management.

- *Physician resistance: Hey, you! Out of my sandbox!.* Most physicians are trained to deliver individual care to individual patients, with no feedback from external sources. The population-oriented, feedback-rich approach of disease management is foreign to many providers. Moreover, these physicians identify *themselves* as the managers of diseases. Physicians often perceive disease management programs, whether from health plans or entrepreneurial companies, as controlling their practices and moving onto their turf.

- *Patient indifference: Self-care is boring.* Patient noncompliance is a strong barrier to implementing effective disease management programs. Fewer than half of all Americans with chronic conditions follow their physician's medication and lifestyle guidance—adding up to more than $100 billion annually in unnecessary medical costs and lost productivity. Although patients may be interested in self-care, concrete lifestyle and behavioral changes are difficult to influence.

- *Inadequate information technology: Does anyone know where the patient went?.* Information technology investment in the health care industry is relatively limited when compared to that in other industries; the banking industry, for example, invests 7 to 10 percent of revenues in information technology, whereas health care invests only 2 to 4 percent. Most of the investment in information technology that does exist in health care goes toward administrative or financial information systems, not clinical. Even when clinical information is recorded electronically, computer systems in different offices are often incompatible and compile disparate data elements, making integration of information across offices difficult.

What does the future hold? To create a forecast, these drivers and barriers must be taken in balance to determine the pace of change. The final section of this chapter offers a forecast of the industry for the next 5 to 10 years.

FORECAST

Disease management is at the crossroads of advances in medical and information technologies and increases in consumer demand and cost consciousness. Each of these forces on its own could power and influence the future. Together, they have the potential to create major breakthroughs in the future of health and health care. When new medical interventions, technologies, and needs meet, watershed events can occur.

A shift in power is occurring in health care. Historically, physicians were the unquestioned owners of medical knowledge, and they had tremendous power and authority in the care process. Many long for those simpler days, when one person, the family doctor, knew all that

there was to know about us, our family, and our ailments. But the knowledge and extent of information now required to know all there is to know about medicine is beyond the capability of the human brain. Computers will be used to integrate much of this information. The Internet makes publicly available massive amounts of information. Consumers want access to this information, and they will want to take advantage of this shift from dependence on the knowledge and experience of physicians to that of multiple information brokers on the World Wide Web. With this shift of power in the form of information control, health care will move from a physician-driven industry to a consumer-driven industry. This shift in power could completely transform the financing and delivery of health care.

By 2005, disease management will:

- *Go where disease management has never gone before:* Move beyond chronic care.

- *Grab 'em when they're young:* Focus more upstream.

- *Wake the patient:* Involve the consumer.

- *Join the Jetsons:* Include more medical and information technologies and the Internet.

- *Not forget who pays the bills:* Continue to be aligned with financial risk.

- *Graduate from trend to tradition:* Be woven into the fabric of much of patient care.

The degree to which each of these characteristics appears in a given regional health care market depends on the balance of power between the drivers for and barriers to change. We forecast that the pace of change will be significant in the first four areas identified and that the other two areas will remain stable. Specifically, here is how we map our forecast.

THE MOVE BEYOND CHRONIC CARE

Disease management programs have focused on high-volume chronic conditions such as asthma, CHF, and diabetes. We forecast that this trend will continue and that the focus will increasingly move beyond single chronic conditions. Programs that have been effective in the management of one chronic condition will apply the tools and techniques they've mastered to other chronic conditions, expanding the scope of the program.

FOCUSING MORE UPSTREAM

To focus more upstream means to intervene earlier in a known disease process with a known outcome. This implies the identification of factors that have led up to or caused that outcome. In the case of CHF, the goal has been to reduce severe disease complications that result in hospitalizations. Years of research have identified the factors that contribute to CHF complications. Now, by focusing on upstream factors, the number of complications can be greatly reduced and many of them eliminated.

As we learn more about disease processes and the causes of poor outcomes, including genetic predisposition of disease (the ultimate in upstream intervention is in vitro or even in the zygote), the management of poor outcomes of disease will move even further upstream.

Cost will remain a driver of this push to move upstream in the disease management process, because moving upstream is often cheaper than an expensive hospitalization. In addition, the need to satisfy the consumer will drive care closer and closer to the home, the workplace, and the school.

INCREASED CONSUMER INVOLVEMENT

Consumers increasingly will become involved in decisions about the management and treatment of their health and medical care. For consumers of health services, the Internet provides a portal to information that has never before been easily accessed. Our forecast is that direct-to-consumer marketing of all health care services will increase. This includes pharmaceuticals, traditional and nontraditional treatment options, medical literature, and providers.

MEDICAL AND INFORMATION TECHNOLOGIES

The explosions in medical and information technologies during the past 10 years are revolutionizing the identification and management of diseases. Computing power and speed of communication among researchers has a ripple effect of more rapid dissemination of research results to the lay community, thereby increasing public understanding and knowledge about many diseases. Advances in medical technology will radically change how we manage diseases in the future, by moving us toward less-invasive therapies and devoting more attention to the behavioral causes of disease.

- *The World Wide Web: Faster than Spider-man.* The ability to communicate information with lightning speed through the Internet provides researchers, providers, and consumers with the latest developments before they hit the printing press. The computing power available to medical researchers today gives them the ability to manage and manipulate larger and more complex databases than ever before.

- *The road map of your genes: The Human Genome Project.* The Human Genome Project will take us further in the management of diseases than any other discovery of the 20th century. The mapping of the human genome opens the doors to early detection, *in utero,* of genetic predisposition to disease. By 2005, medical technologies and new information on inherited diseases gleaned from this project will permit the identification of children who are predisposed to a disease many years in advance of the first symptoms. By 2010, vaccines, research on gene therapy, and the use of more efficient vectors to deliver genetic material to specific targets will radically change current methods of preventing and treating chronic conditions such as diabetes, asthma, cancer, and possibly even neurodegenerative diseases such as Alzheimer's.

- *Sensors: Chips that sense and tell.* Sensors will change not only the way we identify diseases but also the way we communicate information about the status of our health and disease to our selves and our providers. The use of sensors will move the monitoring and treatment of many chronic diseases from the physician's office, emergency room, and hospital to the patient's body and home. Sensors are already being used to monitor insulin levels, blood pressure, and infections

FINANCIAL RISK

Disease management will continue to be provided by those individuals and institutions at financial risk for the care of the patient. Financial risk can reside with the patient, the provider, or the insurance company. We forecast that disease management will be recognized as an important strategy to reduce costs associated with avoidable disease complications. Providing disease management services will be easier in the future as advances in information and medical technologies improve our ability to communicate and increase our level of accessible information about patients and their diseases.

THE PATIENT CARE PROCESS

Disease management—the systematic, integrated delivery of health care to a defined population—will be most cost-effective when applied where current care processes are inconsistent and focused on physician office–and hospital-based care. Our forecast is that disease management will continue to expand across comorbid and chronic conditions and move to high-volume, routine primary care problems such as urinary tract, respiratory, ear, and other localized infections. As the concepts and techniques of disease management gain wider acceptance, disease management will become part of the fabric of the care delivery process and cease to exist as a separate care strategy.

Chapter 16: Disease Management   307

THE PACE OF CHANGE

T|F

Most care delivered today (approximately 90 percent) does not incorporate disease management strategies. Most patients are seen by independent physicians in solo or small-group practices, in settings that rarely lend themselves to the type of organization, management, and information systems required for effective disease management. Many are in the process of doing so, but few have been able to adopt disease management across the board for all patients with chronic diseases: the investment is too large, and the near-term benefits have not been sufficiently proven to warrant a complete shift. Moreover, only so much "organizational capital" exists, and managers have to choose their priorities.

As a result, the pattern we see now—initially targeting narrowly defined populations for disease management and then expanding into other diseases—will continue for the next 5 years. This will take place primarily as a collaboration between established organized delivery systems and entrepreneurial companies, whose strengths and weaknesses are complementary—they need each other in the near term.

Here's a breakdown of the evolution of disease management in different settings.

HEALTH INSURERS

Most health insurers have not been in the position of managing diseases actively; they have either managed costs through utilization management or (in certain regions) delegated the responsibility for management to IPAs or medical groups. Health insurers' interest in disease management is increasing, driven by benefits consultants who are putting disease management into requests for

Table 16-1. The pace of adoption of disease management

Fast Movers	Slow Movers
Large medical groups	Small-group or solo practices
Integrated delivery systems	Independent practice associations or preferred provider organizations
Health plans with delivery system	
Capitated reimbursement/other risk-bearing organizations	Fee-for-service reimbursement providers
Organizations in competitive markets	Fragmented care providers
Groups specialized in single-disease focus	
Organizations with capable information technology systems	

Source: IFTF.

Chapter 16: Disease Management

proposals and by the insurer's need to demonstrate both better outcomes and lower costs to their customers.

Forecast: During the next 5 years, disease management activity among health insurers will increase substantially, though from a very small base. Insurers' initiatives will take three main forms:

- *Lease, don't buy.* Most plans will contract with disease management companies for some of their high-cost diseases.

- *Do-it-yourselfers.* A smaller number (20 percent) will purchase tools and components of disease management and apply them to their membership on their own. This will occur primarily in the areas of risk identification and population management—areas that can use data already in an insurer's claims database.

- *Straight to the source.* Some insurers will develop a strong consumer-oriented approach to health and disease management. They will both build and buy components to achieve this. Blue Shield of California's website, mylifepath.com, is an example of this approach.

INTEGRATED DELIVERY SYSTEMS WITH HEALTH PLANS

Large IDSs that include a health plan, such as Kaiser Permanente, Lovelace (Health Systems), and Harvard Pilgrim Health Care, were originally created to reflect the underlying philosophy of what is now known as disease management—involving plan members in keeping themselves healthy with the support of

motivated providers. Yet few IDSs with health plans have fully integrated disease management among their products and services. These organizations have moved slowly because of the difficulty of changing entrenched organizational structures, bureaucracies, and power relationships. Moreover, many IDSs do not have information systems that allow them to integrate and analyze information to intervene in clinical practice.

Forecast: The move toward disease management will happen the fastest in IDSs associated with a health plan. They will be driven by competitive pressures of cost, quality, and accountability. How to undertake disease management will be a make-or-buy decision for these IDSs. Information systems capable of supporting disease management will be a major enabling factor after 2005.

INTEGRATED DELIVERY SYSTEMS WITHOUT HEALTH PLANS

Integrated delivery systems that don't have an affiliation with a health plan—such as not-for-profit hospital chains that have integrated medical groups (e.g., Sutter Health)—are moving considerably more slowly toward disease management.

Forecast: Hospital-based IDSs and other IDSs not associated with health plans will move more slowly toward disease management programs. They will be more open to outsourcing their disease management programs than fully integrated systems. They will base their make-or-buy decisions for disease management mainly on financial considerations, often short-term.

LARGE MEDICAL GROUPS

Large medical groups (of more than 25 physicians) will be slower to adopt disease management than the larger IDSs, because as smaller enterprises, they have less management sophistication and less access to capital to invest in the infrastructure needed for disease management. Their interest in creating disease management programs will hinge to a large degree on how they are reimbursed for services.

Forecast: As medical groups take on more risk (in selected geographic areas and specialties), they will become more focused on the cost equation. Medical groups with strong medical leadership—medical directors and physician leaders who are able to inspire, cajole, or browbeat their colleagues into adopting the techniques of disease management—will move the fastest.

SMALL-GROUP PRACTICES AND INDEPENDENT PHYSICIANS

Finally, small medical groups (of fewer than 10 physicians) and independent physicians are and will be least capable of developing and participating in disease management. They don't have the capital, management sophistication, or critical mass to be significant disease management players. The majority of physicians are in small-group practices of two to six physicians

Forecast: Small-group practices and independent physicians will see more and more of their patients enrolled in disease management programs in which the health plan enrolls the patient and leaves the MD out of the loop. In the long run, information technology could level the playing field by allowing smaller providers to demonstrate outcomes and to manage their practices more effectively.

SUMMARY

Disease management poses opportunities and threats to all players in the health care industry. The opportunities are most obvious for those involved with information and medical technologies. However, the apparent threat to providers, health plans, and others can be seen as an opportunity—albeit one that must be developed and nurtured.

Change in the delivery model of health care is inevitable, just as it has been in every other industry affected by an increase in the use of technology and consumer demand for accountability. How this change is perceived, implemented, and assessed in the future will depend to a great extent on how the current players respond.

CHAPTER 17

Health Behaviors

Small Steps in the Right Direction

Public health researchers in 1993 stated what public health professionals had known for a long time—that the ultimate cause of death for people in the United States is often the consequence of a combination of underlying behavioral and environmental causes.[1] Examining the top ten causes of death in the United States, those researchers illustrated the links between biomedical diseases and their underlying causes (see Table 17-1).

These classifications reveal an underlying complexity in which behavioral, social, economic, environmental, and cultural forces are inextricably related to determinants of mortality. This list of underlying causes of death can therefore be a guide to prioritizing and developing successful prevention strategies for improvement of the public's health.

To that end, it is useful to assess the trends of several of the underlying causes of death. Issues related to toxins and pollutants are discussed elsewhere in this volume as they concern environmental health (see Chapter 11). Poor diet, lack of exercise, and resultant obesity are increasingly acknowledged to be serious health risks to the individual. With widespread recognition of the health risks associated with not only primary

but also secondhand tobacco smoke have come paradigm-shifting public health responses including restrictions on smoking in public and some private enterprises, landmark litigation holding industry accountable for health consequences, and restrictions on advertising.

Without refuting either the substantial effect of those behaviors on public health and society overall or the far-reaching significance of the strategic responses to them, this chapter centers attention on other behaviors associated with major public health problems. These behaviors include the *abuse of alcohol*, the use of *illicit drugs* alone and in relation to the transmission of *infectious diseases*, the use of *firearms*, and the use of *tobacco* as it relates to the adoption of other risk behaviors. These practices are associated with significant injury and loss to both individuals and the general public in terms of mortality and morbidity, economic consequences, and loss of personal and workforce productivity. We focus on these behaviors because we believe they represent the issues that, in the coming decade, will be the most hotly contested, mark the greatest departure from traditional understanding, and spark the greatest innovation in the coming decade.

Table 17-1. Biomedical and underlying causes of death in the United States in 1990

Top Ten Biomedical Determinants

Cardiovascular disease

Cancer

Cerebrovascular disease

Chronic obstructive pulmonary disease

Unintentional injury

Pneumonia and influenza

Diabetes

HIV/AIDS

Suicide

Homicide

Top Ten Underlying Causes*

Tobacco

Poor diet

Lack of exercise

Alcohol

Infectious agents

Pollutants/Toxins

Firearms

Sexual behavior

Motor vehicles

Illicit drug use

*The original list combined poor diet and lack of exercise, for a total of nine causes.

Source: McGinnis, J. M., and Foege, W. H. Review. Actual causes of death in the United States. *Journal of the American Medical Association* (November 10) 1993; 270(18):2207–2212.

ALCOHOL AND DRUG ABUSE IN AMERICA

Alcohol and drug abuse are among the most pervasive health and social problems in the United States today. More than one-half of American adults have a close family member who has or has had alcoholism.[2] In a 1997 survey conducted by the Gallup Organization, 45 percent of Americans reported that they, a family member, or a close friend had used illegal drugs.

Although drugs and alcohol differ in the forms of social dysfunction they wreak, they also have much in common. For example, the abuse of either increases:

- instances of unintentional injury, especially in motor vehicle crashes

- the incidence of morbidity, disability, and untimely mortality

- the danger of harm to the fetus during pregnancy

- the likelihood of engaging in unsafe sexual practices

- the spread of infectious disease—especially HIV/AIDS and hepatitis

- disruptions of family life and household roles and responsibilities

- the incidence of domestic violence, sexual assault, and suicide

- the commission of crimes, including homicide

In addition, alcohol and illicit drugs present special risks for young people, and the number of potential years of life lost to alcohol- and drug-related injuries are as significant as those lost to heart disease and cancer—the two leading causes of death in the United States.

Abuse, addiction, and their consequences appear in every socioeconomic stratum, educational level, geographic region, and ethnic and racial group. The following data are drawn from several major national studies, including the 1999 National Household Survey on Drug Abuse, and the 1998 Health Services Research Outcomes Study, and are consistent with those in several other major studies.[3]

The Scope of the Alcohol and Illicit Drug Abuse Problem in the United States

- Overall levels have remained stable over the past 8 years, but are higher than the lowest levels ever measured.

- Levels among youths fluctuate at high levels, but may have started to decline.

- Use of illicit drugs by people age 18 to 25 is increasing.

- Youths' initiation of marijuana and cocaine are at historically high levels.

- Males, youths, urban populations, and less educated people have the highest levels of drug use.

- Males, urban populations, and more educated people have the highest levels of alcohol consumption.

- Youths and young adults engage in higher levels of binge and heavy drinking.

- The public is well aware of the problem.

Of the 227 million people in the United States age 12 and older in 2001, 48 percent had used alcohol at least once in the past month. Of those 12 and older, about 20 percent engaged in binge drinking, defined as having five or more drinks on the same occasion at least once in the past month; and 5.7 percent were heavy drinkers, who had had five or more drinks on the same occasion at least 5 different days in the past month.

The proportion of people using alcohol in the United States has remained relatively stable overall for the past few years. In 2001, 7.1 percent of those 12 and older were using illicit drugs. That percentage constitutes 15.9 million Americans—although 78 million Americans report having tried illicit drugs at some time in their life. The total number of people using illicit drugs has remained stable since 1992, at levels roughly half the

1979 peak of 25 million users, although patterns by age category vary dramatically (see Figure 17-1).

Marijuana is the most frequently used illicit drug (see Figure 17-2). Among current drug users, 75 percent reported marijuana use, and 18 percent of marijuana users also used other drugs. An estimated 1.5 million people—0.7 percent of the U.S. population—were current users of cocaine in 1999. That percentage has remained fairly stable over the past few years, and it represents a 74 percent decrease from the 1985 peak of 5.7 million users. The estimate of current crack users was 413,000 in 1999.

WHO IS USING AND WHO IS ABUSING?

- *Age.* According to 2001 figures, the highest rates of illicit drug use were among young people age 18 to 25 (18.8 percent). The levels then decline in successively older and younger age groups. In contrast, a majority of people 18 and older use alcohol, but rates of binge drinking and heavy drinking are significantly higher in the 18-to-25 age group than among older adults.

- *Race.* Illicit drug use for African Americans (6.9 percent) is slightly higher than that for whites (6.8 percent) and Hispanics (6.8 percent)—although among the young there are no differences across those racial groups. Among youths aged 12 to 17, the rate of illicit drug use was highest among American Indians/Alaskan Natives (23 percent). Whites have the highest rates of alcohol use (31 percent), followed by Hispanics (24 percent) and African Americans (19 percent).

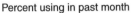

Figure 17-1. Prevalence of illicit drug use by age cohorts (percentage of age cohort, 1979–1997)

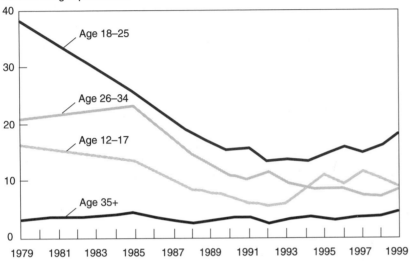

Source: Substance Abuse and Mental Health Services Association, National Household Survey on Drug Abuse, 1998.

Figure 17-2. Marijuana is the drug of choice.

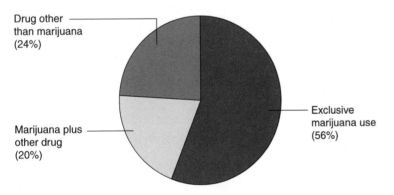

Source: Substance Abuse and Mental Health Services Association, National Household Survey on Drug Abuse, 2001.

■ *Gender*. Males consume higher levels of both illicit drugs and alcohol than do females (8 versus 4.5 percent for drugs, and 59 versus 45 percent for alcohol).

■ *Education*. Illicit drug use is highly correlated with educational status. Young adults who have not completed high school have the highest rate of illicit drug use (10 percent) and college graduates have the lowest (5 percent). Conversely, the higher the level of education, the higher the proportion of people in the group who use alcohol. In 2001, 65 percent of college graduates used alcohol as compared to 33 percent of people who had not graduated from high school.

■ *Interactions*. The level of alcohol use was strongly associated with illicit drug use in 1999, as in prior years (see Figure 17-3). Within each educational level, the more a person drinks alcohol, the more likely it is that the person will also take drugs.

Concern for the Young

Alcohol use among young people has insidious consequences because youths who drink alcohol are at greater risk for the development of a serious alcohol disorder. For example, youths who initiate alcohol use when they are 15 years old are 4 times more likely to become alcohol dependent as people who start drinking at or after the age of 21 (see Figure 17-4).

Especially as it affects the young, the interaction of alcohol, drug, and tobacco use should be considered. Young smokers are 12 times more likely to also take illicit drugs and are 16 times more likely to drink alcohol heavily than are young nonsmokers. Among young people who were heavy drinkers in 1999, 66.7 percent were illicit drug users; among nondrinkers, only 5.5 percent used illicit drugs (see Figure 17-5).

Figure 17-3. Association of alcohol and illicit drug use (Percentage of drinkers also using illicit drugs, by level of alcohol consumption)

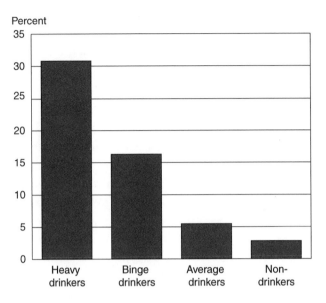

Source: IFTF; Substance Abuse and Mental Health Services Association, National Household Survey on Drug Abuse, 2001.

Figure 17-4. Prevalence of lifetime alcohol dependency or abuse, and age of drinking onset

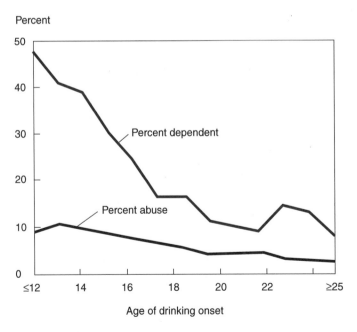

Source: National Institute on Alcohol Abuse and Alcoholism, Office of Policy Analysis, 1998.

In 2001, 28.5 percent of all those 12 to 20 years old reported that they used alcohol. These young people are more likely to engage in binge drinking and heavy drinking. In the young adult population of 18- to 25-year-olds, levels of binge and heavy drinking have fluctuated over the past few years, but remain high.

Illicit drug use among 12- to 17-year-olds, after increasing for several years, declined slightly from 11 percent to 9 percent between 1997 and 1999. However, use of illicit drugs by young adults 18 to 25 years of age rose to its highest level, increasing to approximately 19 percent in 1999 from 14.5 percent in 1997.

Adolescents' perception of risk associated with drug use is another factor to monitor in evaluating trends in drug use. The trend in perceived risk mirrors the trend in the use of marijuana among youths. Over the years, as the perceived risk decreased, drug use increased—and vice versa (see Figure 17-6).

THE CONSEQUENCES OF SUBSTANCE ABUSE

The Toll in Injuries Caused by Substance Abuse

Injuries, both intentional and unintentional, are a major contributor to untimely death, disability, and lost productivity. The two leading causes of death from injury are motor vehicle accidents and firearms, together accounting for more than half of all injury-related deaths, and much of the time, alcohol and illicit drugs are on the scene.

Alcohol- and drug-related injuries accounted for 638,484 emergency room

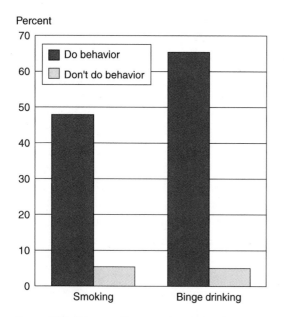

Figure 17-5. Interaction of drugs, tobacco, and alcohol
(Percentage of illicit drug use among youths who do and do not smoke and drink heavily)

Source: IFTF; Substance Abuse and Mental Health Services Association, National Household Survey on Drug Abuse, 1998.

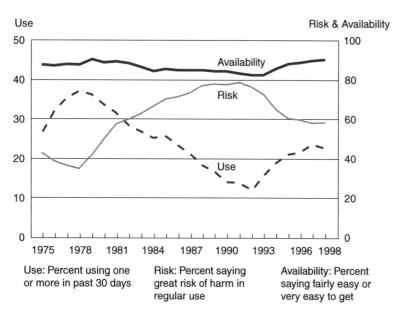

Figure 17-6. Trends in perceptions of availability and risk of regular use, compared with 30-day prevalence for twelfth graders

Use: Percent using one or more in past 30 days

Risk: Percent saying great risk of harm in regular use

Availability: Percent saying fairly easy or very easy to get

Source: Monitoring the Future Study, University of Michigan, 1998.

visits in 2001. Alcohol is a factor in almost 60 percent of all fatal falls and, together with other drugs, figures in 40 percent of all fatal automobile crashes and up to 65 percent of adult drownings.[4,5] In fact, alcohol is implicated in 100,000 deaths each year, mostly from unintentional injuries, homicides, and suicides. The estimated relative risk of accidental death is 2.5 to 8 times greater among males who are heavy drinkers or alcohol dependent than among the general population.[5] Trauma victims are often found to be intoxicated, and a history of trauma is a marker for the early identification of alcohol abuse. Risk-function analysis for social consequences, which assesses the probability of occurrence of specific consequences at specified levels of alcohol consumption, associates alcohol with diminished social functioning and increased harm.

Alcohol and Drugs Causing Morbidity and Untimely Death

After smoking and obesity, substance abuse is the third leading preventable cause of mortality in the United States today. As many as 11 percent of preventable deaths in the United States are related directly to alcohol and illicit drug use. Alcohol accounts for 5 percent of premature deaths, and cirrhosis, alcoholic psychoses, and nondependent abuse of alcohol make alcohol a major contributing cause of hospitalizations.

The National Highway Traffic Safety Administration reports that 40 percent of fatal motor vehicle accidents in 1999 involved alcohol. Illicit drug use is a major contributor to deaths due to overdose, suicide, homicide, motor vehicle injuries, and HIV/AIDS. Furthermore, drug-related deaths increased 42 percent from 1990 to 1995, reaching 14,218. As Figure 17-7 shows, both drug-related visits to the emergency room and levels of heroin- and cocaine-related visits have increased.

Domestic Violence

Violent behaviors between family members causing physical and emotional harm are prevalent throughout the world. More than 1 million children in the United States are known victims of abuse and neglect, one-quarter suffering physical abuse and another quarter being sexually abused or emotionally mistreated.

Spousal and child abuse are as clearly related to alcohol abuse as are motor vehicle injuries. Alcohol and/or illicit drug use is a factor in more than 50 percent of all incidents of domestic violence.

A 1993 study of more than 2,000 American couples showed that rates of domestic violence were almost 15 times higher in households where husbands were often drunk than in homes where husbands were never drunk. Alcoholism and child abuse, including incest, are tightly intertwined as well. Between 25 and 50 percent of men who commit acts of domestic violence have substance abuse problems. Not only do abusers tend to be heavy drinkers, but also the people they abuse are more likely to abuse alcohol and other drugs over the course of their lifetime. Battered women are more likely to abuse alcohol and other drugs, suffer depression, attempt suicide, and abuse their own children.[6,7,8]

Drugs, Alcohol, and Crime

Violent crimes now affect some 11 million victims annually, and drugs, alcohol, and crime go together.[9] Of the 1.7 million men and women in the nation's jails and prisons in 1997, 4 out of 10 reported using alcohol, and 6 out of 10 reported being under the influence of illicit drugs at the time of their offense. The U.S. Department of Justice reports that 35 percent of violent assaults involve the use of alcohol. Each year, 37 percent of all rapes and sexual assaults involve alcohol use by the offender, as do 15 percent of robberies, 27 percent of aggravated assaults, and nearly 25 percent of simple assaults.

Not only is substance abuse a cause of crime, it *is* a crime. More than a million arrests—over one-third of all arrests in the United States—are made each year for intoxicated driving, liquor-law violations, drunkenness, and other statutory crimes concerning alcohol and drugs. America

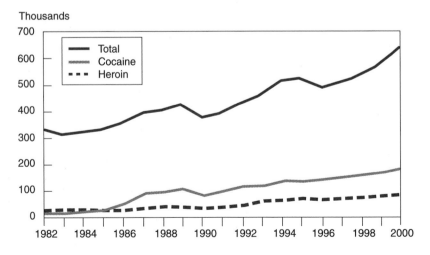

Figure 17-7. Trends in drug-related emergency room visits, 1982–2000

Thousands

Source: Substance Abuse and Mental Health Services Administration, Health and Human Services Drug Abuse Warning Network, 1997 and 2001.

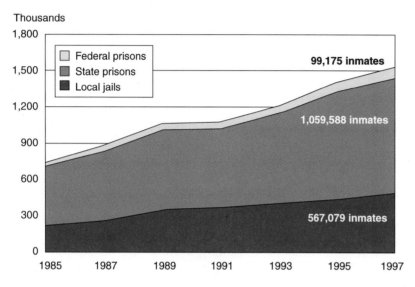

Figure 17-8. Incarcerations in federal and state prisons and local jails, 1985–1997

Thousands

Federal prisons
State prisons
Local jails

99,175 inmates

1,059,588 inmates

567,079 inmates

Source: IFTF; Substance Abuse and Mental Health Services Association, National Household Survey on Drug Abuse, 1998.

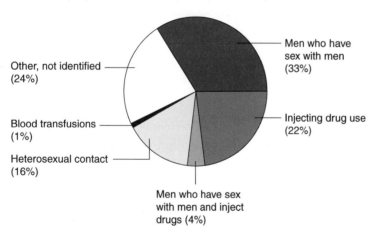

Figure 17-9. Drug use and AIDS (Percentage of new AIDS cases by exposure category, June 2000; 43,293 total cases)

Other, not identified (24%)

Blood transfusions (1%)

Heterosexual contact (16%)

Men who have sex with men and inject drugs (4%)

Men who have sex with men (33%)

Injecting drug use (22%)

Source: Centers for Disease Control and Prevention. *HIV/AIDS Surveillance Report,* Mid-Year Edition, 2000.

has one of the highest incarceration rates in the industrialized world (868 per 100,000 population), and drug violations alone accounted for three-quarters of the growth in the U.S. inmate population between 1985 and 1995 (see Figure 17-8). According to FBI records of arrests from 1970 through 1997, arrests for drug abuse violations reached their highest levels ever in the United States. The number of arrests for drug abuse violations almost doubled for adults (from 629,196 in 1985 to 1,019,621 in 1997) and more than doubled for juveniles (from 68,122 in 1986 to 154,761 in 1997).[10]

HIV/AIDS and Sexually Transmitted Diseases

Alcohol and drug use contribute to the spread of HIV/AIDS and other sexually transmitted diseases. Impaired judgment about having sex and about condom use increases the risk of spreading an infectious disease. Behaviors associated with drug use, such as the exchange of sex for drugs and needle sharing, increase exposure to infectious diseases. More than 40 percent of AIDS cases among women are drug related. There is also evidence that alcohol and other drugs weaken the immune system, thereby increasing susceptibility to infection and disease. In fact, drug use is now the second-largest risk factor for HIV infection in the United States. As of mid-2000, approximately one-fifth of all new AIDS cases were among people using drugs by injection (see Figure 17-9).

THE COSTS

It is difficult to put a monetary value on the human suffering and loss of life associated with alcohol and other drug prob-

Figure 17-10. Economic costs of alcohol and drug abuse

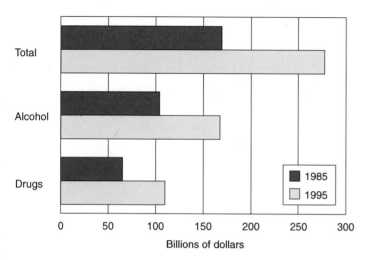

Note: Comparison reflects results of cost of illness studies.

Source: IFTF; Substance Abuse and Mental Health Services Association, National Household Survey on Drug Abuse, 1998.

feel the burden. The economic problems, which are increasing annually in absolute and proportionate terms, include:

- rising share of total health care expenditures related to alcohol and drug use

- diminished workforce productivity

- lower household incomes, in turn affecting family members

- diversion of government funds from other programs into alcohol and drug treatment

THE HEALTH CARE SYSTEM

A large part of the national health care bill is for medical expenses related to the use or abuse of alcohol, tobacco, and other drugs. Many general hospital beds are occupied by patients with alcohol-related medical conditions. When hospital admissions are related to alcohol or illicit drug use, the disorders tend to be more severe and more expensive than in other admissions. Health care costs related to substance abuse do not stop at the abuser. Children of alcoholics average 62 percent more hospital days, 24 percent more inpatient admissions, and 29 percent longer stays than do other children.

National health care expenditures related to alcohol and drug abuse totaled $11.9 billion in 1997, with $6.4 billion for alcohol abuse and $5.5 billion for drug abuse. That cost was small compared to the social costs of $294 billion in 1997 that can be attributed to substance abuse. It is primarily the public that pays for these expenses: 64 percent ($7.6 billion) of total spending on alcohol and drug abuse came from public sources,

lems, but other, more direct costs add up to big dollars. Alcohol and other drug use is a factor in many of this country's most serious and expensive problems, including—in addition to the injuries, health risks, and crimes just described—teen pregnancy, failure at school, escalating health care costs, low worker productivity, and homelessness.

Alcohol and illicit drug abuse in the United States cost society $276.3 billion in 1995, reflecting a 90 percent increase from 1985. Alcohol abuse accounted for 60 percent of the total and drug abuse accounted for the remaining 40 percent (see Figure 17-10).

Most of the costs are borne by the government and the individual substance abusers, although families, businesses, the health care system, and society also

Chapter 17: Health Behaviors

including Medicare, Medicaid, and other federal, state, and local agencies.

THE WORKPLACE

Drug and alcohol abuse costs U.S. businesses more than $110 billion a year in lost workdays, accidents, and increased insurance rates. Although illicit drug users are less likely to be employed than people who do not use drugs, about 76 percent of all current adult illicit drug users and heavy drinkers are employed full or part time. The overall rate of current illicit drug use among full-time employees dropped from a high of 17.5 percent in 1985 to a low of 7.4 percent in 1992, and since then has remained stable; it was 6.9 percent in 2001.

High employment levels among drug and alcohol abusers is good news for the substance abusers, but it is bad news for the workplace. Compared to other workers, employees reporting current alcohol or drug abuse were 2 to 2.5 times more likely to have worked for three or more employers during the past year and to have skipped one or more days of work during the past month. Compared to their drug-free or alcohol-free coworkers, alcohol and drug users generally are less dependable, are less productive, have more unexcused absences, are more frequently fired, and switch jobs more often (see Figure 17-11). The abuse problem is most serious among workers in the restaurant, construction, and transportation industries.

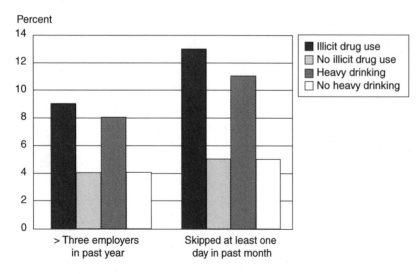

Figure 17-11. The workplace consequences of drug and alcohol abuse: Employment history and absenteeism

Source: IFTF; Substance Abuse and Mental Health Services Association, National Household Survey on Drug Abuse, 1998.

THE POLITICS OF PROBLEMS RELATED TO ALCOHOL AND DRUG ABUSE

It is clear that alcohol- and drug-related problems are profound and seem intractable. An overview of U.S. policy efforts to reduce alcohol and drug abuse in the 20th century highlights the foundations of future directions for substance abuse politics and policies.

U.S. policies on alcohol and drugs are best understood in their historical and social context. Before Prohibition ended in 1933, the alcohol policy was dominated by judgments concerning an individual's behavior rather than by an understanding of alcohol abuse as both a disease and a social phenomenon. Prohibition's policy legacy is a supply-side

Chapter 17: Health Behaviors

approach that incorporates criminal law, drug interdiction, and incarceration more frequently than rehabilitation. Despite ever growing awareness that these Prohibition-based strategies are largely ineffective and economically unsustainable, they have been the cornerstones of national policy for more than 80 years—culminating in the national War on Drugs of the 1980s.

Accompanying this approach were arrests, fines, property forfeiture, and imprisonment for producers, sellers, and buyers. The cost to arrest, try, sentence, and incarcerate people found guilty for the more than 4 million alcohol- and other drug-related offenses committed each year is over $60 billion annually. This expenditure is a tremendous drain on U.S. resources. Incarcerating prisoners is now the most rapidly growing expense faced by governors and state legislatures.

Policy on the control of drugs and alcohol continues to be inadequate. Two particular pressures help to explain the policy impasse.

The Bifurcation of Alcohol and Drug Policy

Although both alcohol and drugs are addictive agents, U.S. policy and prevention strategies approach them quite differently, starting with the distinction in their legal status. Each has its own set of stakeholders, advocates, and opponents. Efforts to develop a comprehensive, coordinated policy are debilitated primarily by a lack of coordination between the criminal justice system and the public health field.

The Dominance of the Criminal Justice System

From 1991 to 2001, federal spending for drug control programs increased from $11 billion to more than $18 billion. The criminal justice system has consistently received about half of these funds, whereas treatment and prevention receive a third of total funding, and other supply-side strategies and interdiction consume the remaining amount. No change to these strategic and spending priorities is in sight.

DETERMINING THE SOLUTIONS: THE PROMISE OF PUBLIC HEALTH

Although the legacy of the War on Drugs still dominates alcohol and drug policy in the United States, there are signs of preliminary shifts in national policy. The National Drug Control Strategy of 2001 attempts to approach drug control as a continuous process rather than a battle with a definitive end. It also addresses the interaction of drug, alcohol, and tobacco use. It emphasizes prevention and treatment efforts and makes a priority of tobacco and alcohol use by underage youths. The National Drug Control Strategy may finally be viewing alcohol and drug problems through a public health lens. But once the politicians and the public focus on public health, what will they see?

Ecological Approaches

The public health community has begun to shift emphasis away from individual-based strategies toward broader ecological approaches. The main goal of individual-based strategies is to increase the individual's knowledge and change his or her behavior. Although they are important, individual-based interventions are ultimately limited by the greater environment, where social drinking and experimentation are encouraged. In contrast, ecological public health strategies address alcohol and drug abuse as an interplay of individual, biological, community, family, environmental, and policy influences. For example, by working in concert, education and rehabilitation programs, peer support groups, regulation of alcohol outlets, restriction of advertising, media advocacy, and taxation can reduce alcohol and drug abuse risks for an entire community. The success or failure of an ecological approach to alcohol and drug abuse is held in the balance by several key issues that are highly controversial and unresolved. They include youth-targeted interventions, funding for treatment and rehabilitation, and the economic dynamics that shape the use and abuse of alcohol.

Youth Focus: Prevention Strategy or Politics?

With high levels of illicit drug use among 12- to 17-year-olds prevailing, and with mounting evidence that early use increases the risk of addiction, helping young people to stay away from alcohol and drug abuse is one of the most urgent issues on the substance-abuse agenda. Public sentiment supports the science. Recent survey data on American attitudes toward children's health issues show respondents citing "drugs/drug abuse" and "alcohol" among the top five serious problems

facing children in America today. However, *how* to address youths' alcohol and drug use is highly controversial. Effective, environmentally based, youth-focused strategies must break through current controversy if they are to shape the future.

Demand for Treatment Is Increasing, but Who Will Pay?

Research shows that treatment not only reduces substance abuse but reduces crime as well. Criminal activity, including income-producing crimes and violent and disorderly offenses, declines by 23 to 38 percent following substance-abuse treatment. Each dollar spent on drug treatment saves Americans $7 by reducing or avoiding costs related to criminal justice, health care, and welfare activities.

Despite these findings, there is a serious gap between the need for and the provision of rehabilitation services. In 1997, 1.9 million people were enrolled in treatment programs and another 7.4 million were on waiting lists. To fulfill the potential of alcohol and drug rehabilitation, the chasm between this need and the resources available to meet it must be bridged (see Figure 17-12).

Economic Forces in Alcohol Use and Abuse

Two main factors are evolving in the understanding of economic forces in alcohol use and abuse. The first is the mounting evidence that the public's consumption of beer, wine, and spirits is sensitive to tax, and ultimately price, increases. The second is the evidence suggesting that alcohol abuse and dependence correspond with lower earnings

Figure 17-12. Reported past year illicit drug or alcohol problem relative to treatment (millions of people, 1998)

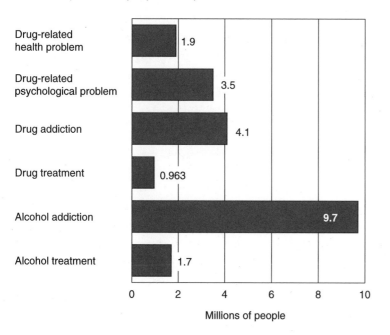

Source: IFTF; Substance Abuse and Mental Health Services Association, National Household Survey on Drug Abuse, 1998.

and income levels. The effects of economic forces differ between moderate and heavy drinkers, and strategies and conclusions must consider variations in alcohol consumption. As more sophisticated methodologies and enhanced data sets develop, approaches can increasingly shape substance-abuse prevention efforts and policy.

THE FORECAST FOR ALCOHOL AND DRUGS

Few of the problems of alcohol and drug abuse in the United States are likely to be resolved within the next 10 years. Improving the overall quality of the social and physical environment holds the greatest promise for reducing the costs of alcohol and drug abuse in society. However, addressing these issues is inher-

ently political, and any future advancements must shoulder the legacies of the past and the problems of today. In this context, we make the following forecasts.

- *Alcohol and drug use and health effects.* Drug use in the teenage and young adult populations will continue to be high, although recent changes in national drug policy may result in some decline. High levels will continue to be driven by marijuana use, conflicting media messages, peer pressure, risk-taking behavior, and the popular sentiment that "all use is not abuse." Alcohol and drugs will continue to be among the leading causes of morbidity, disability, and premature mortality in the United States.

- *Prevention and treatment.* The high levels of new users initiating drug and alcohol use have important implications for substance-abuse prevention efforts and treatment services. Demand for treatment will increasingly place pressure on these already strapped services. As drug-using baby boomers age, they will bring their drug-related problems with them, increasing demands on medical and Medicare services because of their large numbers and because their aging will lead to increased medical complications. Prevention efforts will increasingly target adolescents, both to protect the well-being of individuals and society and to buffer the already overburdened treatment services.

- *Economic and social costs.* Without radical change in policy, overall costs of alcohol and drug abuse—and their consequences in terms of such events as

Chapter 17: Health Behaviors   323

motor vehicle accidents and incidents involving firearms—will remain in the billions. Even with increases in prevention- and treatment-oriented efforts, the time frame for resolution of current problems is likely to exceed this 10-year forecast, especially considering that long-term consequences of alcohol and drug abuse will have a delayed impact on health care systems and government.

- *Community-based organizations.* Expect to see more states and local communities experimenting with ecological approaches and strategies. Citizen-led initiatives will scrutinize local ordinances regarding alcohol sales and advertising, galvanizing local officials, advocates, and parents to seek out ways to reduce the influences of alcohol and drugs in their neighborhoods and to stage community events.

- *The alcohol industry and taxation.* Despite some evidence that increased taxation of alcohol may reduce its purchase by younger and poorer people, future use of this strategy is unlikely, considering the tangled relationship between politics and industry contributions. Industry lobbying will remain strong, as evidenced by the alcohol industry's recent end to its self-imposed ban on advertising of liquor.

- *Strategies.* Although the government will continue to place the bulk of its funding in supply-side and criminal justice measures, prevention strategies will continue. The focus increasingly will be on ecological approaches to

address the problem. Researchers will seek greater understanding of the distinctions in approaches needed for different groups such as youth, women, and heavy drinkers. Concurrently, efforts increasingly will focus on harm reduction, with mounting pressure on the government to work on suppression of consumption.

INJURY PREVENTION: A FOCUS ON GUNS

Accidents don't just happen. Injury prevention experts say that there is no physical event of a health-threatening nature that cannot be avoided or its negative consequences reduced. And yet, in the United States, unintentional injuries and violence are a major cause of death, disability, and lost productivity for people under 55. In 1995, injuries were responsible for nearly 150,000 deaths, 2.6 million hospitalizations, over 36 million visits to the emergency room, and $260 billion in societal costs.[11,12] Motor vehicle injuries, while generally declining, remain the number one injury-related cause of death. Disturbingly, what follows this largely unintentional injury-related cause of death is intentional firearm-related homicide and suicide.

Fortunately, major advances in injury prevention over the past 30 years reduced motor vehicle injury to historically low levels. Epidemiology, the core science of public health, has been a key tool in these efforts by providing the research to prevent and control injuries through legislation, environmental changes, and education. Over the 23 years from 1968 to 1991, the motor vehicle traffic fatality rate declined nearly 30 percent[13] because of developments in legislation, roadway and vehicle design, driver and pedestrian education, protective equipment, and the establishment of emergency medical services systems. Future improvements will result from the use of devices to detect and prevent driver drowsiness, vehicle-mounted sensors to warn of and avert collisions, and stricter laws governing drinking and driving

FIREARMS IN AMERICA

There are over 200 million guns in the United States.[14] Nearly 40 percent of U.S. households have at least one gun and nearly one-quarter have a handgun.[15]

These firearms are not just mounted above the hearth. Rather, many are involved in killing and injuring people: in 1997, there were 32,436 gun-related deaths in the United States—more than 88 deaths every day.[16] Indeed, rates of firearm death and injury are higher in the United States than in any other industrialized country.[17] Particularly chilling, the United States has the highest male teen homicide rate and childhood firearm death rates in the industrialized world.[18]

Solutions to firearm injury, while lying within the public health framework, also present prevention specialists with unique challenges. No other consumer product (except tobacco) remains outside the jurisdiction of a federal agency that can regulate its safety, is embroiled in constitutional and cultural controversies, and is consistently and lethally involved in intentional injury and criminal activ-

ity. In addition, to adequately address firearm injury, public health professionals must coordinate with a complex array of fields and institutions that address criminal justice, violence, mental health, substance abuse, and poverty. These factors have required injury prevention professionals to break new ground and are catalyzing a flurry of policy, litigation, manufacturing, and advocacy actions and reactions. All told, the future of firearm injury prevention is incredibly dynamic, and its unique challenges may generate innovations useful to the broader field of injury prevention.

By 1993, firearm injuries and expenses seemed to be spiraling out of control, and the CDC estimated that by the year 2001, firearms would surpass motor vehicles as the leading cause of injury death in the United States.[13] However, levels of firearm death seem to be cyclical, and gun deaths have declined over 18 percent since 1993, with the decline occurring more in homicides and unintentional injuries than in suicides.[16] If that trend continues, within a few years firearm-related deaths could be at their lowest point since the 1950s.[19]

WHO GETS HURT

Youths, males, and minorities are the main victims of gun injuries. Men, young men in particular, are on average 6 times more likely to die by firearms than are women. African Americans are 2.5 times more likely to be killed by firearms than are whites. African American men 15 to 24 years old are nearly 5 times more likely to die by firearms than white men in that age group.[20]

Figure 17-13. Trends in homicide rates by method, 1985–1999

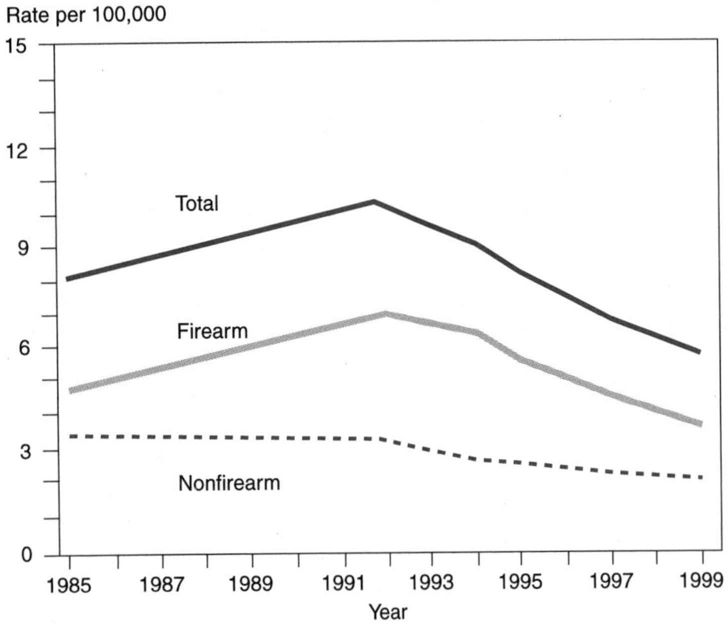

Rate per 100,000

Total

Firearm

Nonfirearm

1985   1987   1989   1991   1993   1995   1997   1999
Year

Note: Variance from the regression line not shown.

Source: U.S. Department of Justice, Homicide Trends in the U.S., Bureau of Justice Statistics, 2001.

related mortality. In 1997, 54 percent of all gun deaths were suicides, and 42 percent were homicides. Guns are the method of choice for nearly 60 percent of people who commit suicide.[16] In homes with guns, the risk of suicide is nearly 5 times higher than in homes without guns.[23] As with homicides, suicide rates have declined since the mid-1990s, but to a lesser degree. Suicide rates among senior adults are consistently the highest, although youth suicide is also at a historical high. Rates for African American youths have increased disproportionately, with firearms accounting for 96 percent of the increase (Figure 17-14).

Unintentional Shootings

Unintentional firearm deaths, representing only about 3 percent of all firearm-related fatalities, have been in steady decline but still firearms killed nearly a thousand people in 1998.[18] It is estimated that over 17,000 people each year are treated for unintentional, nonfatal gunshot wounds in hospital emergency departments. Unintentional shootings are also significant because they may be highly preventable, and because children are often the victims.[24]

At What Price?

The sticker shock of firearm injury—as measured in hospitalization, rehabilitation, and lost wages—is impressive. The cost per firearm-related fatality is higher than for any other class of fatal injury. Firearm injury also tends to generate more costly morbidity.[25] A 1999 study estimated that gunshot injuries in 1994 produced $2.3 billion in lifetime medical costs.[26] Gunshot injuries due to

Homicides

Firearms are the weapon of choice in approximately 70 percent of U.S. homicides, and of these firearm-related deaths, 86 percent involve handguns.[21] In homes with guns, the homicide of a household member is nearly 3 times more likely than in homes without guns.[22] Youth homicide rates climbed sharply until 1994, and while consistently declining since then, remain high, especially among 15- to 19-year-olds (see Figure 17-13).

Suicides

Less recognized than homicide, suicide is a significant contributor to firearm-

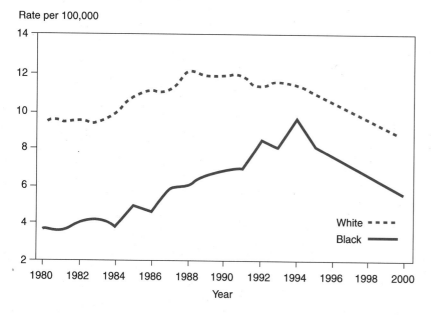

Figure 17-14. Adolescent suicide: A black and white comparison, 1980–2000 (Suicide rates for blacks and whites age 15 to 19, by year—United States)

Rate per 100,000

Source: Centers for Disease Control and Prevention. Suicide Among Black Youths—United States, 1980–1995. *Morbidity and Mortality Weekly Report* (March 20) 1998; 47(10):193–206.

assaults accounted for 74 percent of total costs. Another study estimated that in 1990, total lifetime (medical and indirect) costs of firearm injuries would reach $20 billion.[27] These costs represent a huge potential liability for health care providers and payers, especially since the more serious the injury, the greater the government contribution.

FORCES DRIVING FIREARM INJURY PREVENTION

The future of firearm injury prevention will be shaped by the following factors:

- The past several years have delivered an array of prevention strategies that depart from traditional approaches

and may in fact be the building blocks of real change in the state of firearm injury in the United States.

- Overall firearm mortality is going down, with declines in homicide and unintentional shootings occurring faster than suicide. Young people, males, and minorities experience the greatest firearm injury and mortality burden. Unintentional and nonfatal firearm injuries also cause significant morbidity and mortality. If overall trends continue, gun violence will soon reach its lowest level in decades. With a wide array of interventions recently implemented, there is uncertainty as to the exact causes of the decline, making a forecast of future injury levels unstable. Each firearm injury continues to be expensive, and the associated costs are high for the public sector and for society at large.

- Surveillance and research on firearm use is increasing and will likely be a potent tool for reducing gun use in crime and for understanding the nature of firearm injuries and prevention strategies. However, much more needs to be done before surveillance can be considered truly comprehensive throughout the country.

- A significant number of firearm experts suggest that that debate has reached an impasse on issues such as the Second Amendment right to bear arms or the risks and benefits of gun ownership.[28] Instead, they call for a focus on policy that regulates guns as consumer products, restricts gun ownership based on criminal history, and curtails illegal gun commerce. With broad public support (see Table 17-2), these strategies may shape the prevention framework for the coming decade.

- Firearm regulation tends to lack adequate comprehensiveness and coordination at the federal level, with some important exceptions. Most change in gun policy is originating from state-level activity, but is characterized by great variability: some state regulations strengthen firearm control, while others may weaken firearm injury prevention. Most local regulatory action continues to be limited by state pre-emption laws and public-private business arrangements.

Table 17-2. Support among national poll respondents for policies to regulate firearms

Policy	Percent who favored or strongly favored prohibition	
	All Respondents	Respondents who owned guns
Regulation of guns as consumer products		
Childproofing	88	80
Personalization	71	59
Magazine safeties	82	75
Loaded chamber indicators	73	60
Prohibition of gun purchases for people convicted of crimes		
Violence or illegal use of firearm	83–95	70–91
Alcohol or drug abuse	71–92	59–89
Reduction of the illegal sale of guns		
Tamper-resistant serial numbers	90	85
One-gun-per-month	81	53
Mandatory handgun registration	82	72

Source: IFTF; Teret, S. P., et. al. Support for new policies to regulate firearms. *New England Journal of Medicine* 1998; 339(12):813–818.

- Efforts to reduce firearm injuries are increasingly focused on the distribution and manufacture of firearms, in particular on regulation of handguns as consumer products and reduction of the illegal sale of guns. While some controversy exists concerning specific strategies, evidence is mounting that regulations such as licensing and registration laws, background checks, and purchasing limits can be effective in limiting the distribution of firearms and in decreasing their involvement in crime. At the same time, there is still no federal regulatory agency to provide consumer product oversight and the lethality of guns and ammunition is increasing.

- Lawsuits are increasingly common. Similar to the reframing of guns as consumer products, litigation attempting to hold manufacturers and sellers responsible for the damage their products cause is on the rise. Hoping to imitate the success of tobacco litigation, these suits argue that firearm manufacturers can design and market their products in ways that are less likely to cause death and injury. While the success and implications are uncertain, the reward could be great and the plaintiffs are lining up to sue.

THE FORECAST FOR FIREARMS

Current firearm injury prevention policy will require time to reach its full effect, making precise levels of associated changes in firearm injury uncertain within the 10-year time frame of our forecast. However, a growing body of evidence on the effectiveness of and support for innovative firearm injury prevention strategies makes it likely that improvements in the field will be pronounced in a longer-term, 20- to 30-year, scenario.

The network of surveillance systems across the country is developing, facilitating rigorous evaluation of new prevention programs and policies. Investment in the power of information will shape debate and reduce controversy, ultimately having a major impact on future policy and program development.

Guns will be scrutinized more often by policymakers as "consumer products" and increasing legislative pressure will attempt to control their manufacture and design. While the National Rifle Association will resist these efforts, it is likely that the more fiscally vulnerable manufacturing industry will be receptive to adopting certain standards. However, unless firearms are brought under the purview of a federal consumer product regulatory agency, progress toward safer guns will be slow.

In parallel, the public will gradually unwrap the gun from the American flag, change focus from the final user of firearms to the manufacturer and distributor, and increasingly identify with firearms as consumer products. Increased grassroots organization of victims, such as the Bell Campaign (using the Mothers Against Drunk Driving model), physicians, and police organizations will lead the way, along with increased participation by foundations. This rise in focused community activism, grounded in grow-ing knowledge of which interventions work, may build the bridge between broad public support for reductions in firearm injury and social action.

Lawsuits against the gun industry will continue to increase. The impact of these suits will not be felt immediately and the long-term consequences are uncertain, even if the plaintiffs are successful. For example, it is possible that many gun manufacturers will go bankrupt in the course of these proceedings, which could ironically consolidate gun manufacturer power.

TOBACCO USE AND HEALTH

From decades of research on tobacco use and its negative effects on health, tobacco has been identified as the single greatest preventable contributor to disease and premature death in the nation—greater than illicit use of drugs, motor vehicle accidents, firearms, toxic agents, microbial agents, and alcohol combined.[29] It kills more than 400,000 Americans each year and causes heart disease; cancers of the lung, larynx, mouth, esophagus, and bladder; and chronic lung disease. Approximately $50 billion of total medical costs each year are directly attributable to tobacco use.[30]

Over the past 25 years, significant progress has been made in the health and medical fields documenting the adverse health effects of tobacco use and their related costs. The body of scientific knowledge about tobacco use and its effects on human health is massive and incontrovertible. A causal relationship exists between cigarette smoking and disease; further, nonsmokers also incur serious health problems from environmental tobacco smoke (ETS) or secondhand smoke. Use of smokeless tobacco causes a number of serious oral health problems, including cancer of the mouth, periodontitis, and tooth loss. Cigar use causes cancers of the larynx, mouth, esophagus, and lung. Today, tobacco use is the leading preventable cause of morbidity and premature mortality in the United States.

HISTORICAL OVERVIEW

In the past, helping people quit smoking was the primary focus of efforts to reduce tobacco use. This strategy has been a critical one, since smoking cessation at all ages reduces the risk of premature death. In recent years, however, the focus of tobacco control has expanded to include strategies to prevent kids from starting to smoke, limit exposure to ETS, and stop minors' access to tobacco products.

Efforts to prevent individuals from starting to smoke center on controlling youth access to tobacco products because approximately 90 percent of all initiation of tobacco use occurs among persons 18 years of age or younger.[31] Initiation of smoking at younger ages is associated with a longer duration of smoking and an increased likelihood of nicotine dependence.[31] The decision to use tobacco is nearly always made in the teenage years and about one-half of young people who take up smoking continue to use tobacco products as adults. Therefore, communities have begun taking steps to restrict youth access. Some policies include stepping up enforcement of existing laws, restricting tobacco advertising and licensing, and increasing penalties for selling to minors.

The past two decades have also seen greater recognition of the health hazards resulting from exposure to ETS. ETS is a combination of smoke exhaled by the smoker and the smoke that comes from the burning end of a cigarette, cigar, or pipe. The U.S. Environmental Protection Agency concluded in January 1993 that ETS kills an estimated 3,000 adult nonsmokers from lung cancer each year.[32] What's more, nonsmokers exposed to ETS have higher death rates from cardiovascular disease than unexposed nonsmokers.[33] To help control the effects of ETS, workplaces have begun shifting to smoke-free environments, as have restaurants and bars.

The Tobacco Settlement

On November 16, 1998, the attorneys general of eight states and the nation's four major tobacco companies agreed to settle more than 40 pending lawsuits brought by states against the tobacco industry.

Many supporters of the settlement nationwide worked to ensure that settlement funds were earmarked for health and health care purposes. Unfortunately, in many states this effort was unsuccessful. Instead of creating health-focused tobacco settlement trust funds, many of the first payments are being placed into general funds or going to other social programs. Many believe this outcome to be a huge loss that reflects, in part, the lack of political clout of members of the tobacco control community at large.

TODAY'S CHALLENGES

Racial/Ethnic Disparities

Although lung cancer incidence and death rates vary widely among racial/ethnic groups, lung cancer is the leading cause of cancer death for African Americans, Hispanics, Asian Americans/Pacific Islanders, and Native Americans as well as whites, with rates of tobacco-related cancers high among African American men.[34] Furthermore, it has been observed that immigrant populations, especially Southeast Asian male immigrants, have high rates of smoking that may buoy the smoking rates among racial/ethnic groups.

Nationally, cigarette-smoking prevalence increased in the 1990s among African American and Hispanic adolescents after several years of substantial decline among these adolescents. Educational attainment accounts for only some of the difference in smoking behaviors. Declines in smoking prevalence were greater among African American, Hispanic, and white men who were high school graduates than among those with less formal education. Further, members of racial/ethnic groups are less likely than the general population to participate in smoking cessation groups and to receive cessation advice from health care providers. Research suggests that barriers may include limited cultural competence of health care providers and a lack of transportation, money, and access to health care. Other social and cultural factors are likely to further account for these differences.

Smoking Prevalence Rates Among Children Age 12 to 13 Are Increasing

The continued financial strength of the tobacco industry relies on youth initiation and uptake of smoking as adult smokers either quit or die. The average young smoker begins at age 14.5 and is a daily smoker by age 18. Unfortunately, data indicate that the industry has been successful in reaching its goal. An interesting finding in these data concerns smoking among 12- to 17-year-olds in ethnic communities. Despite the data cited above indicating high rates of smoking prevalence among adult African Americans and Native Americans, in 1997 youths of color experienced lower smoking prevalence rates than whites, with a striking difference of 9 percentage points between white youths (12.5 percent) and African American youths (3.6 percent).

Smokers Are Not Uniformly Counseled to Quit by Health Care Providers

Although smokers cite a physician's advice to quit as an important motivator for cessation, physicians and other health care clinicians, such as dentists, often fail to assess smoking status and even to advise smokers to quit. It is estimated that more than 70 million people are currently enrolled in some type of managed health care plan. Despite the managed care industry's stated interest in prevention, an alarming 68 percent of smokers report getting no help from their doctor or health insurance plan to stop smoking (see Figure 17-15).

Since 1997, national guidelines have been available from the Agency for Health Care Policy and Research regarding smoking cessation. All major health care agencies and associations recommend routine tobacco use cessation counseling for adults and adolescents who smoke.

Chapter 17: Health Behaviors

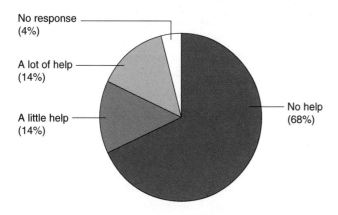

Figure 17-15. Few smokers report getting help to quit smoking.
(Responses to the question: How much help did you get from your doctor
or health insurance plan in the past 12 months to try to quit smoking?)

No response
(4%)

A lot of help
(14%)

A little help
(14%)

No help
(68%)

Source: *California Managed Health Care Improvement Task Force Survey of Public Perceptions and Experiences with Health Insurance Coverage*, UC Berkeley and Field Research Corporation, 1997.

THE IMPACT OF NOT COUNSELING SMOKERS TO QUIT ON PREGNANT WOMEN, THEIR FAMILIES, CHILDREN, AND UNBORN CHILDREN

Women who smoke during pregnancy are more likely to have the following: pregnancy complications, premature birth, stillbirth, and babies with low birth weight, a leading cause of infant mortality.[35] Further, it has been shown that prenatal smoking and ETS compromise the fetal and neonate immune system, thereby leaving a newborn more susceptible to infectious disease.[36] There is also significant evidence that a dose-response relationship exists between prenatal smoking and the incidence of Sudden Infant Death Syndrome (SIDS). ETS exposure in young children has been found to be a significant risk factor for several acute upper and lower respiratory tract illnesses such as bronchitis and

pneumonia, chronic middle ear infections, and greater rates of asthma.

LACK OF STRONG, UNITED LEADERSHIP AMONG TOBACCO CONTROL STAKEHOLDERS TO DESIGN AN EFFECTIVE STRATEGY TO OUTFOX THE TOBACCO INDUSTRY

Throughout communities in America, tobacco control forces are mobilized to counter the tobacco industry. Historically the tobacco control forces in many states have been guilty of infighting that has weakened their effectiveness. And the size of the "force" is small. On the heels of losing the battle to use the tobacco settlement dollars for health, there is a clear need for statewide leadership and replenished resources.

The new leadership could assist in reframing the tobacco control issue to one of population health improvement—highlighting the role of tobacco use in statewide rates of morbidity and mortality. Greater efforts could be made to educate the public and policymakers about effective strategies to decrease tobacco use. For example, coverage of nicotine replacement therapies by health plans is limited, despite the evidence of their role in assuring smoking cessation. Further, many believe that the war against the tobacco industry is over—noting the absence of smoking in public places and the decline of smoking rates from 1955 to 1990.

THE FUTURE OF TOBACCO

The challenges that exist in tobacco control today are legion. Investments in any or all of the areas above could lead to improved health and productivity for many Americans. In addition to these issues, consideration should be given to the following areas:

- *Continue to strengthen local and statewide policy development to prevent tobacco use.* In communities across America, the tobacco industry is making considerable progress in introducing the public, especially young adults, to its products. Tobacco control experts point to problems with continued use of signage in storefronts, sponsorships, and promotions. Of particular concern is bar promotions in which ads are placed in entertainment newspapers to bring young adults to bars where cigarette samples are distributed. Also, on college campuses, students are being recruited to set up parties at which cigarettes are distributed. These are examples of local practices that could be addressed through enforcement of existing laws as well as the adoption of new policies.

- *Support community and statewide efforts to prioritize use of tobacco settlement funds for health and health care programs.* Although efforts to use the tobacco settlement to fund health and health care programs have failed in many states, initial plans are under way in some states to urge the legislatures to reconsider the issue next year. The outcome of this policy change would improve the health of large numbers of people. To achieve this goal, tobacco control stakeholders will need assistance with strategic planning and public education activities, as well as an infusion of new leadership.

WILD CARDS

ALCOHOL AND DRUGS

- Medical technologies, particularly rational drug design, ignite a tidal wave of drug abuse as a new generation of "designer" drugs that bind to specific mood receptors in the brain enter the illegal drug market.

- The alcohol industry follows the tobacco industry—up in smoke. Public opinion turns against the alcohol industries with growing organization of nondrinkers' rights groups.

- A deep economic recession leads to a further loss of access to emergency care that will follow the accompanying erosion of the large municipal hospitals that care for major injuries.

INJURY PREVENTION

- Kids organize a Stop the Pain Campaign, striking a moral chord with the public that even politicians can't resist—comprehensive federal gun control legislation is passed.

- A long economic recession sets in across America: unemployment, crime, and gun violence rise to unprecedented levels.

- A wave of new high-tech weapons, such as laser weapons and polymer guns, hits the streets. Government and emergency systems are not prepared, so initially high injury rates result.

- The United Nations and the WHO create a treaty restricting small arms trade. All but the United States ratify the treaty, resulting in international sanctions against the United States until the gun industry is stopped.

TOBACCO

- The public supports increased taxes on cigarettes. Congress passes a hefty per pack tax that cuts youths' consumption of cigarettes in half.

- The FDA regulates tobacco as a drug. Smoking rates, especially among youths, decline to unprecedented levels.

- The public becomes apathetic about the health consequences of smoking, the media become bored with the smoking issue, the tobacco control movement fragments, and nothing more is done to change smoking behaviors.

ENDNOTES

[1] McGinnis, J. M., and Foege, W. H. Review. Actual causes of death in the United States. *Journal of the American Medical Association* (November 10) 1993; 270(18):2207–2212.

[2] Grant, B., and Dawson D. Age at Onset of Alcohol Use and Its Association with DSM-IV Alcohol Abuse and Dependence. Results from the National Longitudinal Alcohol Epidemiologic Survey. *Journal of Substance Abuse.* 9(January):103.

[3] The National Household Survey on Drug Abuse defines current alcohol or illicit drug use as consumption at least once in the past month; binge drinking as five or more drinks on the same occasion at least once in the past month; and heavy drinking as five or more drinks on the same occasion at least 5 different days in the past month. Results from the study include people living in households and in some group quarters, such as dormitories and homeless shelters.

[4] National Center for Statistics and Analysis, National Highway Traffic Safety Administration, U.S. Department of Transportation. Alcohol Involvement in Fatal Crashes 2000, March 2002.

[5] Eighth Special Report to the U.S. Congress on Alcohol and Health, National Institute on Alcohol Abuse and Alcoholism, 1993.

[6] Collins, J. J., and Messerschmidt, M. A. Epidemiology of alcohol-related violence. *Alcohol Health and Research World.* 17(2):93–100.

[7] U.S. Department of Health and Human Services, National Institute on Alcohol Abuse and Alcoholism, 1993.

[8] Widom, C. S. *Child Abuse and Alcohol Use.* Research Monograph 24: Alcohol and Interpersonal Violence: Fostering Multidisciplinary Perspectives. Rockville, MD: National Institute on Alcohol Abuse and Alcoholism, 1993.

[9] U.S. Department of Justice, Bureau of Justice Statistics, Crime in the United States, Washington, DC.

[10] *Sourcebook of Criminal Justice Statistics.* 25th ed. K. Maguire and A. Pastore, eds. Baton Rouge, LA: Justice Department, Office of Justice Programs, Bureau of Justice Statistics, Claitors Publishing Division, December 1998.

[11] National Vital Statistics System, National Center for Health Statistics, CDC; Johns Hopkins Center for Injury Research and Policy.

[12] Bonnie, R. J., Fulco C. E., and Liverman C. T., eds. *Reducing the Burden of Injury, Advancing Prevention and Treatment.* Committee on Injury Prevention and Control, Division of Health Promotion and Disease Prevention. Institute of Medicine. Washington DC: National Academy Press, 1999.

[13] Centers for Disease Control and Prevention. Deaths resulting from firearm- and motor-vehicle-related injuries—United States, 1968–1991. *Morbidity and Mortality Weekly Report* (January 28) 1994; 43(3).

[14] Guns in America: National Survey on Private Ownership and Use of Firearms, by Philip J. Cook and Jens Ludwig. National Institute of Justice, Research in Brief. May 1997. U.S. Department of Justice. NCJ 165476.

[15] Johns Hopkins Center for Gun Policy and Research, National Opinion Research Center. *Fall 1998 National Gun Policy Survey: Questionnaire with Unweighted Frequencies and Weighted Percentages.* Baltimore, MD: The Johns Hopkins Center for Gun Policy and Research, 1999.

[16] Hoyert, D. L., Kochanek, K. D., and Murphy, S. L. Deaths: final data for 1997. *National Vital Statistics Reports* 1999; 47(19).

[17] Krug, E. G., et al. Firearm-related deaths in the United States and 35 other high- and upper-middle-income countries. *International Journal of Epidemiology* (April) 1998; 27(2):214–221.

[18] Centers for Disease Control and Prevention. Rates of homicide, suicide and firearm-related death among children—26 industrialized countries. *Morbidity and Mortality Weekly Report* (February 7) 1997; 46(5).

[19] Wintemute, G. J. The future of firearm violence prevention: building on success. *Journal of the American Medical Association* (August 4) 1999; 282(5):475–478.

[20] *National Vital Statistics Reports*. June 30, 1999; 47(19).

[21] Federal Bureau of Investigation. *Uniform Crime Reports for the United States: 1997*. Washington, DC: U.S. Department of Justice, 1998.

[22] Kellermann, A. L., et al. Gun ownership as a risk factor for homicide in the home. *New England Journal of Medicine* 1993; 329:1084–1091.

[23] Kellermann, A. L., et al. Suicide in the home in relation to gun ownership. *New England Journal of Medicine* 1992; 327:467–472.

[24] Sinauer, N., Annest, J. L., and Mercy, J. A. Unintentional, nonfatal firearm-related injuries. *Journal of the American Medical Association* 1996; 275:1740–43.

[25] Miller, T. R., and Cohen, M. A. Costs. In *The Textbook of Penetrating Trauma*. R. R. Ivatury and C. G. Cayten, eds. New York: Williams & Wilkins, 1996.

[26] Cook, P. J., et al. The medical costs of gunshot injuries in the United States. *Journal of the American Medical Association* (August 4) 1999; 282(5):447–454.

[27] Max, W., et al. Shooting in the dark: Estimating the cost of firearm injuries. *Health Affairs* (Winter) 1993; 12(4):171–185.

[28] Teret, S. P., et al. Support for new policies to regulate firearms. Results of two national surveys. *New England Journal of Medicine* (September 17) 1998; 339(12):813–818.

[29] Centers for Disease Control and Prevention, Office on Smoking and Health/ National Center for Chronic Disease Prevention and Health Promotion. Adult Tobacco Use in California: Health Impact and Cost 1997.

[30] Smoking Cessation: Clinical Practice Guideline No. 18. Agency for Health Care Policy and Research, U.S. Department of Health and Human Services, Rockville, MD, 1996, p. 5.

[31] Gemson, D. H., et al. Laying down the law: reducing illegal tobacco sales to minors in central Harlem. *American Journal of Public Health* 1998; 88:936–939.

[32] Making Your Workplace Smoke-Free: A Decision Maker's Guide. U.S. Department of Health and Human Services, and Center for Disease Control and Prevention, Office of Smoking and Health, 1996, p. 2.

[33] Steenland, K., et al. Environmental tobacco smoke and coronary heart disease in the American Cancer Society CPS-II cohort. *Circulation* 1996; 94:622–628.

[34] U.S. Department of Health and Human Services. *Tobacco Use Among U.S. Racial/ Ethnic Minority Groups—African Americans, American Indians and Alaska Natives, Asian Americans and Pacific Islanders, and Hispanics: A Report of the Surgeon General*. Atlanta, GA: U.S. Department of Health and Human Services, Centers for Disease Control and Prevention, National Center for Chronic Disease Prevention and Health Promotion, Office on Smoking and Health, 1998.

[35] DiFranza, J. R., and Lew, R. A. Morbidity and mortality in children associated with the use of tobacco products by other people. *Pediatrics* 1996; 4:560–568.

[36] Castellazzi, A. M., et al. Effect of active and passive smoking during pregnancy on natural killer-cell activity in infants. *Journal of Allergy and Clinical Immunology* 1999; 103(1):172–173.

CHAPTER 18

Expanded Perspective on Health
Beyond the Curative Model

Until recently, biomedical understanding of disease and the definition of health as "the absence of disease" provided the fundamental framework in which modern medicine evolved and the curative model of medical care predominated. The curative model narrowly focuses on the goal of cure; that is, the eradication of the cause of an illness or disease. Although cure is unquestionably an appropriate goal, other goals are important as well: restoring functional capacity; relieving suffering; preventing illness, injury, and untimely death; promoting health; and caring for those who cannot be cured.

Cure-oriented medicine reveres the "hard" medical sciences, and it ignores behavioral phenomena that are not entirely explained by biological science. Effective cure is presumed to be contingent on diagnosis gained from knowledge of disordered function. Treatment is supposed to be derived from empirical research on clinical outcomes. In fact, on careful analysis, a significant component of medical practice is neither knowledge-based nor supported by evidence.

The cure-oriented approach to medicine and health is highly invested in a biomedical perspective that values scientifically-

based data over other information and accepts evidence-based approaches to treatment over those less rigorously derived. The curative model has created a hierarchical structure of relationships among health professionals: physicians who command the most biomedical knowledge also command the most authority. Our society has granted this authority to physicians and has entrusted them with the role of granting or denying the legitimacy of matters related to health and disease. Thus, indirectly, the medical profession has defined health in the narrow meaning of disease according to a curative biomedical model.

In the past quarter century, the record of biomedical discovery and progress has been spectacular, and yet on critical analysis our ability to diagnose and treat disease has had no more than a modest impact on the public's health. Despite improved diagnostic and therapeutic capabilities and an unprecedented expenditure of resources, we are not the most healthy of populations among the developed nations. Perhaps an obsession with disease has unintentionally relegated health to a position of secondary importance. The health care delivery system is still organized, staffed, and financed on the assumption that its central task is to use biomedical interventions to provide care for people facing acute episodes of illness.

From many quarters comes evidence that our view of health should be expanded to encompass mental, social, and spiritual well-being. An expanded view of health integrates the concepts of curative medicine (absence of disease) with public health (absence of excessive mortality, morbidity, and risk factors for disease), and adds productive functioning and well-being. This expanded view of health recognizes the importance of mental factors, social support, income, and behavior in avoiding disease and disability. The expanded view of health moves beyond attention only on disease to incorporate the concept of *salutogenesis,* the generation and maintenance of health.[1]

The American public expects accurate and timely diagnosis and treatment of illness and disease, but this same public has new expectations for avoiding illness and disease and wants more attention directed to chronic diseases, aging, and terminal care at the end of life. The public's understanding of health and its interest in healthy lifestyles have advanced remarkably in the past decade. As individuals, each of us wants to be healthy and fully functional. To achieve this, we must adopt an expanded view of health that adds, to physical health, essential mental, social, and spiritual components. This expanded definition of health has three implications:

- For individuals to function at their best, health as defined here is a necessary precondition.

- Impairment of any component of health can predispose to or cause disease and create an unhealthy state.

- Mental, social, and spiritual factors, singly and collectively, influence behavior and therefore health.

An expanded view of health assumes a particular meaning for the elderly, age 65 years or older, who currently constitute 13 percent of the population. Less concerned about life's span than about life's quality during the remaining life span, this cohort embraces all elements of health with the same tenacity of younger generations. Evidence shows that maximum human life span is fixed and that improvements in health can affect only mean life span and not maximum attainable life span. Nonetheless, all adult generations want to postpone the effects of aging and to avoid or mitigate age-related disabilities. Concern about aging thus becomes a largely unarticulated part of the equation for health, and it requires special consideration as we develop a much broader concept of what health and being healthy means to all segments of the population.

Socioeconomic status is a powerful determinant of health and disease. Therefore, recognizing and understanding the relevance of an expanded definition of health to the lower socioeconomic segments of the population will be critical to improving the collective health of the nation. Improving the health of the middle- and upper-income segments of the population is important, but it is clearly insufficient if achieving substantial improvement in our national health status is the goal.

Finally, who can and will integrate an expanded view of health into the planning and delivery of health care, and what should be the roles of government, providers, employers, and consumers in advocating changes that recognize and respect this new definition of health? This multifaceted question will be addressed in a later section of this chapter, but posing the question at this point may heighten sensitivity to the issue.

DEFINITION OF HEALTH

A definition of health must have equal applicability to everyone: to the fully well; to those who are unwell because of disease or illness that is treatable or even curable and for whom the goal is a return to health; and to that growing segment of the population with genetic or acquired impairment, such as those with chronic disease or disability. Furthermore, the definition of health must at the same time represent an objective to be attained and a yardstick by which to judge the state of health. Health can be applied to an individual, a community, or a nation, and in each instance the goal is to be as healthy as possible within constraints that cannot be changed.

Perfect or ideal health is a state of complete physical, mental, social, and spiritual well-being. For the vast majority of our population, being healthy means functioning as fully as possible under present circumstances. Health is a composite of interdependent components that, even if less than perfect, are optimal for the individual. As it is used in an expanded definition of health, each of the four components of health is a necessary contributor. Neglect of any component

of health predisposes one to, or creates, an unhealthy state. Although this may seem to be stating the obvious, the concept is critical to understanding the significance of an expanded view of health and the factors that determine it.

CONTRIBUTORS AND DETERMINANTS OF HEALTH

- *Physical.* In the traditional meaning of health and disease, disease represented disordered form and function whereas health was the absence of disease. Physical health and well-being is essential to good health but taken alone is insufficient. Physical health incorporates functional as well as structural integrity. Impairment of function in the biomedical view of disease is assumed to have an organic basis. "Functional" is used in another way that may be confusing because in clinical practice "functional" describes a set of symptoms that have no organic basis. Thus, in medical practice, a "functional" illness is one that has no known physical (organic) causes and is assumed to reflect mental (including emotional) factors.

- *Mental.* Mental factors include more than the absence of mental illness. They extend to emotional states (e.g., depressed feelings short of clinical depression), dispositions (e.g., hostility, optimism), and beliefs and expectations (e.g., self-esteem, self-control, self-efficacy). Mental factors, such as stress, depression, and inability to change lifelong habits, contribute to the onset of some disorders, the progression of many, and the management of all. Understanding the role of

Chapter 18: Expanded Perspective on Health   **339**

mental factors in health and disease may be the most important contribution of an expanded view of health.

- *Social.* This term has two different meanings in relation to health. Social position or status refers to the tiered structure of society and the activity of its members. This meaning of "social" cannot be dissected neatly from the more descriptive use of socioeconomic status. The position of an individual, a family, or a community in the social order is an ordering of employment, income, wealth, education, voice, and health status. In this context, the multiple social and economic factors that influence health are central not only to the development of disease but also to its treatment and outcome.

  The other meaning of "social," and the one implied in using "social well-being" in the expanded view of health, relates to relationships rather than to social order. This is the term "social" as reflected in "sociable," and refers to companionship, enjoying the company and support of family and friends, and often having intimate and supportive relationships with one or more individuals or groups. The social interaction often takes place in a community of people in the same or a similar socioeconomic stratum.

  A recent body of research has focused on the role of social networks in maintaining individual health. Social networks build communities and contribute to social capital. Social engagement and social support, regardless of an individual's socioeconomic status, are basic human needs

without which a person cannot be fully healthy. Evidence clearly shows the powerful influence of social support on recovery from myocardial infarction and breast cancer.

- *Spiritual.* Spirit is the thinking, motivating, and feeling part of humankind and involves a code of ethics and philosophy. Spirituality usually, but not necessarily, involves belief in a higher power. A spiritual person has a set of beliefs that give meaning to life, and for many this belief provides a basis for faith and trust in an otherwise disorderly and unfeeling world. A growing body of evidence supports religious involvement as an epidemiologically significant protective factor that promotes healthy behavior and lifestyles. When shared in a community, it also provides social support, which buffers stress and enhances coping mechanisms. The consistency and robustness of studies involving the role of spirituality in health have led to the emergence of a growing area of research called the "epidemiology of religion." That spiritual factors promote good health, aid in recovery from illness, and contribute to the state of well-being that characterizes health has generated growing support: the questions are how and why? The mental, social, and spiritual components of health may have distinctive but similar salutary effects mediated through psychoneuroendocrine pathways.[2]

STRESS

Stress is unavoidable, and although the socioeconomically disadvantaged may have fewer means and mechanisms for coping with stress and are thus more vulnerable to it, all of us are exposed to stress on an almost daily basis. Some amount of stress is part of life and is both natural and normal, but when stress is sustained and unrelieved it has deleterious effects on the function of endocrine and immune systems, lowering resistance and increasing vulnerability to illness, disease, and accelerated aging. This mechanistic explanation has garnered scientific support, although any claim for thoroughly understanding this complex series of interactions is premature.

Research is under way to examine how the biological consequences of adaptations to stress interact with other factors and what impact this has on health. Nancy Adler and Bruce McEwen, among others, have promoted the concept of an allostatic (adaptive) system that includes stress-induced activation of the hypothalamic-pituitary-adrenal axis, the autonomic nervous system, the cardiovascular system, the metabolic systems, and the immune system.[3] Allostatic response systems are coupled closely with an individual's psychological makeup, prior experience, and available resources for coping with stress. Stress turns on an allostatic response, and as long as the response is time limited, protection dominates over adverse consequences. However, weeks or years of repeated exposure to elevated levels of stress can result in allostatic load, with resultant damaging physiological consequences. Allostatic load can result from frequent stress, from inability to shut off responses when stress is terminated (a feature of aging), or from inadequate allostatic responses. Inability to control their lives and the daily stresses

on people in lower socioeconomic groups lead to allostatic load, sustained allostatic responses, and a downward spiral toward poor health, illness, and untimely death.

SOCIOECONOMIC STATUS AS A DETERMINANT OF HEALTH

Whether social class is measured by income, education, employment grade, or prestige, it determines the resources that are available to meet life's challenges and thereby influences the control that one has in shaping life. In 1980, the publication of the *Black Report* showed the statistical association between illness and social class in England and Wales. Physical and mental health, the statistics showed, ran parallel to social rank. With the introduction of universal health care through the National Health Service in the United Kingdom, these differences in health status among different socioeconomic groups were not reduced but actually became greater! This observation provided early evidence that the availability of universal health care does not eliminate the root cause of lower health status among the socioeconomically disadvantaged. In England, commoners die sooner than aristocrats, sergeants have more heart attacks than generals, office clerks are more depressed and anxious than office managers. In America, the lower middle class is more mortal, morbid, symptomatic, and disabled than the upper middle class. With each step down the educational, occupational, and income ladders comes an increased risk of health-related symptoms, illness, chronic disease, and early death.

Talking to the Doctor

The relationship between the patient's income, health risk behaviors, the prevalence of physicians' discussion of these behaviors, and patients' receptiveness to advice was examined in a random sample of 6,549 Massachusetts state employees.[4]

- Depression was reported by 31 percent of patients with incomes less than $20,000 and 8 percent of those with incomes greater than $80,000.

- Low-income patients were much more likely to attempt to change behavior on their physician's advice than were those with higher incomes.

- Physicians were more likely to discuss diet and exercise with high-income patients and more likely to discuss smoking with low-income patients.

Socioeconomic status (SES) exhibits a linear relationship to the incidence of illness and avoidable death. Universal health insurance would have an imperceptible effect on reducing the socially driven inequalities in health: SES differences in health are evident in countries with universal coverage; differences can be shown between levels at the upper range of the SES hierarchy; and SES differences appear in a wide range of diseases, some of which are treatable and others that are not.

Cross-national studies have shown the importance of the size of the gap between the wealthy and the less well off. In any given society, the greater the gap in income between the rich and the poor, the lower is the average life expectancy. This consistent observation explains why a country as wealthy as the United States, which spends more money per capita on health care than any nation in the world but has an ever-widening gap between rich and poor, endures an average life expectancy that is conspicuously low among the developed nations.[5]

Research into health and illness has now recognized the contribution of social, economic, and environmental factors to health, and a critical body of evidence is beginning to document the influence of these factors on morbidity and mortality.[6] However, the fact that a group of determinants—social isolation, social class, and depression—predict health outcomes across *all* diseases has been largely ignored in mainstream medical research on disease. Recognizing shared determinants of health rather than only those unique to specific diseases will enrich and modify our understanding of how internal and external factors interact to produce health or lead to illness and disease. Recognition and acceptance of the seminal role of upstream determinants of disease by the medical establishment, policymakers, and funding sources can create a virtual transformation in our approach to creating healthier individuals, communities, and nations.

WHAT'S NEW? WHY NOW?

The answer to "What's new?" is straightforward: dependence on a biomedical model to define disease and health has been rendered insufficient by a growing body of evidence that health involves much more than freedom from active disease or illness and that upstream environmental and psychosocial determinants of disease deserve parity with conventional biological theories. The answer to "Why now?" is more complex, but the reasons revolve around three factors. First, an increasingly empowered public expects more than our existing system of health care provides. When individuals become ill or impaired by

"Alternative," "Holistic," "Expanded": What's in a Name?

The search for a label that adequately captures the essential concepts embedded in an expanded view of health has been a colossal failure. No single word or phrase seems to capture what it means to view health and disease through a wider lens, to define health as a state that moves outside of a biomedical model, and to realize that upstream determinants of disease go beyond genetic endowment and access to care to even more critical socioeconomic, behavioral, social, and environmental factors. Labels in the contemporary lexicon, such as "mind-body" and "holistic," have connotations of their own and further fail the test of descriptive accuracy.

"Alternative medicine," "integrative medicine," and "complementary medicine" merit similar objections as labels, although these descriptors contain elements that pass the test of compatibility with an expanded view of health. The public's acceptance and use of alternative or complementary medical practices must be interpreted as an indication that these alternative providers fulfill some unmet need. Interestingly, much of "alternative" medicine is practiced in a way similar to biomedicine but using different forms of intervention and treatment—for instance, using herbs instead of prescription drugs.

Concluding that no single term or phrase could satisfy the goal, we decided to follow the lead of the Center for the Advancement of Health and use the descriptive label of "an expanded view of health," leaving an open field for creative lexicographers. An expanded view of health maintains and extends beyond the biomedical model. An expanded view of health applies not only to individuals but also to communities and even nations; and each component in an expanded view of health has been validated by evidence submitted to scientific scrutiny. It is the evidence-based foundation of an expanded view of health that makes it such a powerful summons to rethink and then redirect our approach to health, illness, and healing.

full health, greater attention to the management of chronic diseases, and elimination of upstream determinants of diseases that are predicted by socioeconomic status.

A coincidental factor is the new dominance of managed care organizations. Managed care is organized to function according to the fundamental precepts of public health, health promotion, epidemiology, and population-based medicine. Assuming responsibility for the health of a defined population, as capitated managed care organizations do, creates a compelling incentive to improve and maintain the population's health. An expanded view of health is the formulation of the desired goal—good health—for a population as well as for each of its members. An expanded view of health also requires an understanding of upstream determinants of health and illness, which in turn provides insight into the roles of socioeconomic factors, behavior, and social capital. An expanded view of health was no less relevant to the practice of medicine in the era preceding managed care than it is today, but the public's changed expectations of physicians and managed care's new focus on health maintenance and disease prevention have made it appear so.

CONSUMER EXPECTATIONS

Led by health-conscious seniors and a generation of baby boomers who seem to view aging as an option subject to free choice, the medical establishment is confronting a mandate to move beyond the curative model to become engaged in

chronic disease or aging and seek medical care, they want a healing relationship with clinicians. Second, unless corrective measures are implemented very soon, a growing segment of our population, spanning all socioeconomic classes but most severely affecting those at the bottom, will be exposed to avoidable illness and disease and excessive mortality. Third, the nation's bill for health care and health-related disability will continue to rise until an expanded view of health promotes maintenance of

Evidence-Based Studies:
What the Research Shows

Psychological and social factors—how we think, feel, and behave—profoundly influence the onset of some diseases, the progression of many, and the management of nearly all.

- In a large study covering 13 years, depressed and socially isolated persons were four times more likely to have a heart attack than those who were not depressed or isolated.[7]

- A 7-year follow-up of women diagnosed with breast cancer showed that those who confided in at least one person in the 3 months after surgery had a 7-year survival rate of 72.4 percent, as compared to 56.3 percent for those who didn't have a confidant.[8]

- In another study, women with advanced breast cancer who attended weekly therapy groups survived an average of 18 months longer than women who did not get such support. Four years later, one-third of the support group attendees were still alive whereas all of the non-attendees had died.[9]

- In a study examining the correlation of social ties to susceptibility to common cold viruses, increased diversity in types of ties to friends, family, work, and community was significantly associated with increased host resistance to infection.[10]

- In a study examining 232 elderly patients who had elective open heart surgery, those who did not participate in any group and did not receive strength and comfort from religion had three times the risk of dying as those who lacked one or the other.[11]

preserving health and preventing illness and disease. The public believes that medicine has overpromised cure as the be-all and end-all. Preventive maintenance, after all, is standard procedure for other industries. Although the enlightened consumer wants to be healthier and understands the importance of maintaining good health, a quick-fix mentality still encounters difficulty in understanding the hard work of health. Today's physicians were taught nothing about changing their patients' behavior, and with only on-the-job experience as a source of knowledge, most physicians falter when confronted with the conse-

quences of their patients' unhealthy behavior, such as obesity, tobacco use, and sexually transmitted disease. A medical curriculum reconfigured by an expanded view of health would require a course in behavioral psychology.

Their needs unmet in biomedicine, millions of Americans flock to practitioners of alternative medicine in growing numbers. Medical practitioners should not become providers of alternative medicine, and vice versa. Unlike any time in the past, the medical establishment will be more open to adopting an expanded view of health and enlarging the scope of medical practice—not with the intention of introducing alternative methodologies but rather with the goal of providing more comprehensive medical care to patients. Does this mean that for the first time your own physician may ask you about your own social support, spiritual practices, and allostatic load? Quite possibly.

DETERIORATING HEALTH CONDITIONS

The issue most urgently in need of resolution is the deteriorating health status of a growing segment of our population. To argue that this is a socioeconomic problem caused by macroeconomic forces and erosion of social capital, and not a matter of health, indicates a failure to recognize their connectedness and interdependence. In fact, separation of socioeconomic status and health is artificial, and this basic tenet is embedded in an expanded view of health. The emerging reality is that a growing segment of the population in the world's richest nation is unhealthy despite a per capita expenditure on health care that is the largest among developed countries. Health status declines with socioeconomic status, amidst a dizzying array of alarming observations: use of illicit drugs, alcohol, and tobacco by a generation of young people growing up in an environment without social order and support and one in which risky behavior is *de rigueur;* a growing population of underinsured and uninsured, many of whom lack financial resources for access to basic health care as the health care safety net unravels; a rapidly expanding population of the elderly with significant health needs, such as preventive services, social support, and the treatment of depression; and at all levels of society, avoidable illness and disease attributable to ignorance, unhealthy behavior, lack of education, and disintegration of family structure and social support.

Certain mental, social, and spiritual matters fall directly into an expanded scope of health care and can be dealt with by a physician or other health professional without outside intervention. Other socioeconomically driven health concerns cannot be resolved by the health professions, and by their nature these issues will require major shifts in political and social policy and cooperation from other professions for significant change to occur. When the medical profession adopts an expanded view of health, as it almost certainly will, it acknowledges the direct relevance of upstream determinants of health and disease that have received little or no attention because of the profession's historical focus on a bio-medical model of disease.

Quite apart from concern about distributive equity, why should the higher-income classes become concerned about poor health conditions among the less advantaged? The reasons are as follows:

- The cost of preventable illness and disease is enormous and is increasing due to premature births, teenage pregnancies, AIDS, avoidable hospitalizations, communicable diseases, and the consequences of substance abuse and other risky behaviors. To the direct cost of providing health care must be added the indirect costs of lost productivity and chronic disability as a consequence of poor health.

- Communicable diseases are a major public health concern that is amplified by the worldwide emergence of drug-resistant infectious agents, involving not only common infections like *E. coli* and *Staphylococci* but less common infections, such as tuberculosis, HIV, and even plague. Any reservoir of disease constitutes a direct threat to all Americans because we share the same air, water, food, space, and transportation—and even needles and medical devices. We ignore the problem at our own peril.

GLOBAL HEALTH PERSPECTIVE

As we enter the next century, cardiovascular disease, depression, and injury-related death and disability will be major health-related concerns.[12] An individual's behavior and allostatic response to life's stresses create a profile of risk factors for developing and dying from cardiovascular disease. Risk-promoting behaviors—smoking, alcohol abuse, sedentary lifestyle, and unhealthy eating habits—have a dominant role in the evolution of cardiovascular disease, and stress-related factors promote disease progression and affect recovery from acute events such as myocardial infarction. Social and mental factors often contribute to the course of cardiovascular disease, either in promoting its progression or in favoring full recovery from an acute episode of clinical illness.

Depressive illness and risk-taking behaviors are subjects that have been largely excluded from consideration in a traditional biomedical model of disease. Depressive illness—clinically significant but falling short of disabling major depression—affects a surprisingly large proportion of the elderly population, and among the nonelderly, including adolescents, depression directly or indirectly causes poor health. An expanded view of health recognizes depressive illness as a cause of disability to be as legitimate as diabetes, asthma, and peptic ulcer. Because depressive illness looms so large as a major health concern, the rapid adoption of an expanded view of health that addresses its cause and treatment becomes a matter of high priority.

Injury-related death and disability involves the innocent as well as the guilty, the cautious as well as the careless, the abuser as well as the abused. The emergency room log in any major hospital records the consequences of traffic accidents, industrial injuries, personal assaults, alcohol- and drug-related accidents and criminal behavior, in-home injuries, and spousal abuse. The myriad factors in this melange of misery have social, cultural, mental, behavioral, racial, environmental, occupational, economic, and circumstantial elements that with few exceptions have been considered outside the scope of medical education and practice. A study of intentional and accidental injuries inevitably exposes the major role that socioeconomic status plays in causing injury, either directly or indirectly. Social, mental, and spiritual health is incompatible with the risky, antisocial, and violent behavior that often leads to serious injuries and their consequences. The prevention of injuries and injury-related morbidity and mortality, formerly considered the responsibility of public health officials, must become a legitimate concern of medicine and other health professions.

THE FUTURE: SHIFTING PARADIGMS

Thomas Kuhn pointed out that scientific advances come in the form of paradigm shifts only when existing conceptual models break down and are no longer able to explain observable facts.[13] New paradigms will emerge later in this century by expanding the definition of health. An expanded view of health is the engine that will drive the paradigmatic shifts shown in Table 18-1.

The first shift is from rigid adherence to the biomedical model to an expanded, multifactorial view of health. While the scientific model looks only at biological indicators of health, the expanded model goes beyond this to include social, mental, and spiritual, as well as physical, health. This shift in focus will lead to the regular provision of psychosocial and other services that currently are not in the health care mainstream. How the medical community acts to encourage the shift will greatly affect the speed and degree to which it happens.

A second shift will be from attention solely on acute episodic illness to the management of chronic illness. This shift is already beginning in the treatment of certain populations, such as patients with end-stage renal disease, diabetes, and asthma. Chronic disease management programs have evolved rapidly because they provide better care at lower cost across the health care continuum. Protocols, case managers, prevention strategies, and the coordination

of ancillary services have proven the value of chronic disease management by reducing the frequency and severity of acute episodes of illness. In increasing numbers, health plans and large medical groups are forming their own teams to manage populations of chronically ill patients or "carving out" their care to multispecialty networks that assume full responsibility for all patient care needs on a per capita basis.

The shift in focus from individuals to groups reflects several factors. In the traditional model, a physician–patient relationship implied a contract in which physicians vowed to do everything for their patients that might be of possible benefit even if the benefit had marginal value. The terms of this contract recognized no financial restraints, and in a FFS system of care the cost was not a major consideration. As managed care has evolved over the past decade, the principles of population-based health care, already being practiced in the public health system, are beginning to be exploited and adopted by the private sector.

Community-centered health care is population-based medicine as it applies to defined groups of people. As in public health, the central theme is using finite resources to achieve the best health outcome for the entire population. The importance that an expanded view of health assigns to the maintenance of health and prevention of disease fits perfectly into a public health–population-based model of health and health care.

Table 18-1. Paradigm shifts

Biomedical	Expanded View
Rigid adherence to the biomedical model	Expansion to incorporate a multifactorial view of health
Attention solely to acute episodic illness	Chronic illness management
Focus on individuals	Focus on communities and other defined populations
Cure as uncompromised goal	Adjustment and adaptation to disease for which there is no cure
Focus on disease	Focus on diseased person *and* the disease

Source: IFTF.

Cure-oriented medicine recognized a cure as the objective and measure of success, and it used diagnosis and treatment as the means of obtaining it. Palliation—lessening the severity of disease without curing it—was viewed as a compromise and deserving of less interest and attention. Many chronic diseases, such as asthma, diabetes, cardiovascular disease, and multiple sclerosis, and the conditions that accompany the aging process are by their nature incurable. An expanded view of health care promotes individual adjustment and adaptation to live with these conditions comfortably. The functionality and quality of life for those afflicted can be immeasurably improved by using available palliative measures: The aging of our population and the longer survival of patients with chronic diseases will shift greater attention to the health benefits of palliative interventions.

The final shifting paradigm moves from an exclusive focus on the disease to a broader focus on the importance of the person bearing the disease. The diseased person not only has an illness with organic manifestations but is also an individual with unique and relevant social, mental, and spiritual characteristics. Also, many chronically ill patients suffer from multiple comorbid conditions, and the focus on one disease could subordinate the impact of something equally debilitating. Restoration of the patient's health requires elimination of the disease if that is possible, but in addition it requires that attention be directed to the patient's mental, social, and spiritual well-being in keeping with an expanded view of health.

THE PARADIGM SHIFT: EVOLUTION OR REVOLUTION?

Amid signs that the shift is under way, it is sobering to be reminded that institutionalized values and processes change slowly, and that change may not follow a direct linear progression from "what was" to "what will be." To be sure, consumers who want a more personalized relationship with health professionals have spoken, and this message will result in a less formal and more symmetrical physician–patient interchange. However, this manifestation of change may be more cosmetic than fundamental.

With little doubt, by the year 2007, the impact of an expanded view of health will be recognizable although neither dramatic nor widespread. Physicians will be reluctant change makers because the generations of physicians in the current workforce learned, believe in, and practice according to the biomedical, bipolar view of disease and health. Interviews with practicing physicians provide ample evidence that medicine's disdain for soft science—and in their view the psychosocial sciences are soft—is alive and well. In time, many will be converted to proponents of an expanded view of health, but inroads by 2005 will be modest. Economic rewards for attention directed toward social, mental, and spiritual well-being do not exist in current reimbursement guidelines. However, by 2005 the principles underlying an expanded view of health will become general knowledge. This knowledge, reinforced by evidence that health and recovery from disease are profoundly affected by social, mental, and spiritual factors, may create a momentum that could accelerate the paradigm shift in the years following. Unless political forecasts are mistaken, by 2005, no significant legislation will be enacted that will remedy socioeconomic inequities. Health plans may expand mental health benefits in response to consumer pressure, but the impact of this change will be limited.

By 2010, the new physicians entering practice will have been educated in a different school of thought, and this new generation will understand an expanded view of health. Today, almost two-thirds of the nation's 125 medical schools include courses on spirituality, up from only three in 1993. They will need no convincing to practice accordingly, if the practice environment permits. They will augment a growing number of older colleagues in advocating major restructuring of programs to correct socioeconomic ills. The year 2010 will see the beginning of major government initiatives by legislators who understand the interconnectedness of socioeconomic status, the public's health, and the nation's productivity. At the most fundamental level, legislators will have the political will to invest in community-level programs because, for the first time in our history, they can justify the expenditure of public funds for programs that fully benefit the nation's health, productivity, and economic welfare.

This forecast may seem overly optimistic. For certain, change will be incremental and geographically uneven. Although 2010 will look different from

2005, we do not expect major change to occur until the middle of the following decade. It will be an evolution rather than a revolution, the progress of which will be painfully slow unless and until the medical establishment openly adopts an expanded view of health. It will need to bring the full force of its professional position to bear in declaring that mental, social, and spiritual factors are legitimate components of health. Physician-led advocacy is a necessary prerequisite for meaningful change in the way that consumers, providers, employers, health plans, governments, and legislators think about health and its immediate determinants. We bet on physicians to get the ball rolling, but predicting when is a matter of pure speculation.

WILD CARDS

- A major economic recession could postpone crucial legislation and governmental programs and at the same time expand the socioeconomically disadvantaged segment of the population.

- An educated public, a groundswell of community involvement, and a critical number of federal and state legislators with the political will to provide financial support for programs that provide educational opportunities, training for skilled jobs, health care including mental health care, and public health services that focus on behavioral modification could drive the pace of change at a more rapid rate than we forecast.

ENDNOTES

[1] McKinley, J. B. *Preparation for Aging.* Keikkinen, E., et al. (eds.) New York: Plenum Press, 1995.

[2] Kiecolt-Glaser, J. K. Psychoneuroimmunology and health consequences. *Psychosomatic Medicine* 1995; 57:269–274.

[3] McEwen, B. S. Hormones as regulators of brain development. *Acta Paediatrica* 1997; 422:41–44.

[4] Taira, D. A., et al. The relationship between patient income and physician discussion of health risk behaviors. *Journal of the American Medical Association* 1997; 278:1412–1417.

[5] Adler, N., et al. Socioeconomic inequalities in health. *Journal of the American Medical Association* 1993; 269:3140–3145; Wilkinson, R. G. Income distribution and life expectancy. *British Medical Journal* 1992; 304:165–168.

[6] Gruman, J. Introduction for superhighways for disease. *Psychosomatic Medicine* 1995; 57:207.

[7] Pratt, L.A., et al. Depression, psychotropic medication, and risk of myocardial infarction. *Circulation* 1996; 94:3123–3129.

[8] Maunsell, E., Brisson, J., and Deschenes, L. Social support and survival among women with breast cancer. *Cancer* 1995; 76:631–637.

[9] Spiegel, D., et al. Effect of psychosocial treatment on survival of patients with metastatic breast cancer. *Lancet* 1989; 2:888–890.

[10] Cohen, S., et al. Social ties and susceptibility to the common cold. *Journal of the American Medical Association* 1996; 277:1940-1944.

[11] Oxman, T. E., Freeman, D. H., and Manheimer, E. D. Lack of social participation or religious strength and comfort as risk factors for death after cardiac surgery in the elderly. *Psychosomatic Medicine* 1996; 57:5–15.

[12] *The Global Burden of Disease.* Murray, C.J.L, and Lopez, A. D. (eds.). Cambridge, MA: Harvard University Press, 1996.

[13] Kuhn, T. *The Structure of Scientific Revolutions*, 3rd ed. Chicago: University of Chicago Press, 1996.

Chapter 18: Expanded Perspective on Health

APPENDIX

The Reactions

As an appendix to the forecast, the Foundation and the Institute asked eleven national experts to comment on different aspects of the forecast, focusing on their areas of expertise. Dr. Francis Collins, Ms. Laurie Flynn, Ms. Irma Godoy, Dr. Alan Guttmacher, Mr. Charles Kahn, Mr. David Lansky, Ms. Molly Mettler, Mr. Kevin B. Piper, Dr. H. Denman Scott, Dr. Kenneth Shine, and Mr. Gail Warden all contributed their ideas to this Appendix. These experts wrote essays that reflect their opinions of the Institute's portrait of the future. Collectively, they constitute an original, thoughtful, and realistic counterpoint to the forecast, offering both support for and disagreement with the scenarios of the future.

Both the Foundation and Institute staffs are grateful to these authors for the time and care that went into creating these essays. The utility of any forecast lies in its ability to help people understand the landscape of the future and either prepare for it or attempt to change it. These eleven experts have added the wisdom gained from their years of experience in the field to our portrait of the landscape, enriching our description of what lies ahead.

In addition, Tina Grande, Julie Koyano, and Danielle Gasper, of the Institute for the Future, and Maureen Cozine and Ann Searight, of The Robert Wood Johnson Foundation, all assisted with the compilation and production of these essays.

With thanks,

Wendy Everett

Director
Institute for the Future

Author Biographies

FRANCIS S. COLLINS, M.D., PH.D., is a physician-geneticist and the director of the National Human Genome Research Institute, of the National Institutes of Health (NIH). In that role, he oversees a complex multidisciplinary project aimed at mapping and sequencing all of the human DNA, and determining aspects of its function. Prior to joining the NIH, he was a member of the faculty at the University of Michigan. Dr. Collins obtained his undergraduate degree in chemistry at the University of Virginia, and a Ph.D. in physical chemistry at Yale University. Recognizing that a revolution was beginning in molecular biology and genetics, he changed fields and enrolled in medical school at the University of North Carolina. After a residency and chief residency in internal medicine in Chapel Hill, he returned to Yale for a fellowship in human genetics. His accomplishments have been recognized by election to the Institute of Medicine and the National Academy of Sciences, and numerous national and international awards.

LAURIE M. FLYNN has served as the executive director of the National Alliance for the Mentally Ill (NAMI) since 1984. NAMI is the nation's leading grassroots advocacy organization dedi-cated solely to improving the quality of life for people with severe mental illnesses and their families. Ms. Flynn is a member of many national advisory boards and professional association com-mittees concerned with the care of the severely mentally ill, the quality of mental health care and family support, as well as research and ethical aspects of the treatment of mental illness. She is also the recipient of many service awards and commendations from national foundations and associations, including three from the American Psychiatric Association. Ms. Flynn is the author of several articles, books, and book chapters on health services for the mentally ill and family support. She has a daughter with a serious mental illness.

IRMA GODOY is a young, Spanish-speaking mother living in Florida. She has cancer of the thyroid and is uninsured.

ALAN E. GUTTMACHER, M.D., is currently senior clinical advisor to the director at the National Human Genome Research Institute, of the National Institutes of Health. His major responsibilities are educating health professionals and the public about the use of genetics in clinical medicine and working toward incorpo-rating genetic medicine into the nation's health care. Previously, Dr. Guttmacher was associate professor of pediatrics and medicine at the University of Vermont College of Medicine, where he directed the Vermont Regional Genetics Center and Pregnancy Risk Information Service. Dr. Guttmacher is a graduate of Harvard College and Harvard Medical School. He com-pleted a residency in pediatrics and a fellowship in medical genetics at Children's Hospital of Boston and Harvard. He is a fellow of the American Academy of Pediatrics and of the American College of Medical Genetics.

CHARLES N. KAHN III, M.P.H., president of the Health Insurance Association of America (HIAA), is a nationally known health policy expert specializing in health care finance. Prior to his current position, he was vice president of HIAA and directed the Office of Financial Management Education at the Association of University Programs in Health Administration. He has taught health policy at Johns Hopkins, George Washington, and Tulane universities. Mr. Kahn serves on the board of visitors of Indiana University's School of Public and Environmental Affairs and is on the Medicare Competitive Pricing Advisory Committee. He holds a B.A. degree from Johns Hopkins University and an M.P.H. degree from the Tulane School of Public Health and Tropical Medicine.

MOLLY METTLER, M.S.W., is senior vice president of Healthwise, Inc., a not-for-profit research and development group located in Boise, Idaho. Healthwise is best known for the *Healthwise Handbook*, now in its 14th edition. Ms. Mettler is known nationally as an expert in medical self-care program design, medical consumer issues, and patient empowerment. She devotes her time speaking to national audiences and writing about how to empower patients and improve doctor-patient partnerships, and on the concept of shared medical

decision making. In 1995, Ms. Mettler began directing the Healthwise Communities Project, a community-based health education project. Its vision is to make the 278,000 residents of four southwestern Idaho counties the most empowered, best informed medical consumers in the world. The project won the 1996 Spirit of Innovation Award, co-sponsored by InterHealth and 3M Health Care. Ms. Mettler holds a master's degree in social work from the University of Washington.

H. DENMAN SCOTT, MD, MPH, is director of the Brown Center for Primary Care and Prevention, serves as physician-in-chief, Department of Medicine, Memorial Hospital of Rhode Island. Dr. Scott's extensive experience in public health and health policy combined with his roles as an educator and practicing physician make him uniquely qualified to lead this collaborative research center. He also heads up two of the Center's grants-Reach Out and Volunteers in Health Care, which are funded by the Robert Wood Johnson Foundation. The grants support initiatives and provide technical assistance to organizations throughout the United States that provide health care for the uninsured and underserved. care for the uninsured and underserved. His previous administrative posts include serving as Director of Health for the State of Rhode Island, and Senior Vice President for Health and Public Policy at the American College of Physicians. A sought after speaker and lecturer, Dr. Scott has published extensively on public health and healthcare topics in peer-reviewed publications.

KENNETH I. SHINE, M.D., is president of the Institute of Medicine, of the National Academy of Sciences, and professor of medicine emeritus at the University of California, Los Angeles (UCLA) School of Medicine. He is UCLA School of Medicine's immediate past dean and provost for medical sciences. Dr. Shine's research interests include metabolic events in the heart muscle, the relation of behavior to heart disease, and emergency medicine. Currently he is clinical professor of medicine at the Georgetown University School of Medicine. A cardiologist and physiologist, Dr. Shine received his A.B. from Harvard College in 1957 and his M.D. from Harvard Medical School in 1961. His advanced training was at Massachusetts General Hospital (MGH), where he became chief resident in medicine in 1968. Following his postgraduate training at MGH, he held an appointment as assistant professor of medicine at Harvard Medical School.

GAIL L. WARDEN, M.H.A., is president and chief executive officer of Henry Ford Health System, in Detroit, one of the nation's leading vertically integrated health care systems. Mr. Warden is an elected member of the Institute of Medicine, of the National Academy of Sciences. He is a mem-ber of the board of trustees of The Robert Wood Johnson Foundation and director emeritus and past chairman of the board of the National Committee on Quality Assurance. He is chair-man of the Health Research and Educational Trust and serves on the board of the National Resource Center on Chronic Care Integration. He recently was named chairman of the National Forum on Health Care Quality Measurement and Reporting. Before joining Henry Ford Health System in April 1988, Mr. Warden was president and chief executive officer of Group Health Cooperative of Puget Sound, in Seattle. Prior to that position, he was executive vice president of the American Hospital Association and executive vice president and chief operations officer of Rush-Presbyterian-St. Luke's Medical Center. He is a graduate of Dartmouth College, with a master's degree in health care management from the University of Michigan. He holds an honorary doctorate in public administration from Central Michigan University.

FRANCIS S. COLLINS AND ALAN E. GUTTMACHER

The Human Genome Project and Our Future Health

Francis S. Collins is director of the National Human Genome Institute, National Institutes of Health.

Alan E. Guttmacher is senior advisor to the director for clinical affairs, National Human Genome Institute, National Institutes of Health.

As the forecast appropriately highlights, both genetic mapping and testing should have real and important impacts on health and health care in the coming decade. These are not, however, the only means by which the products of the Human Genome Project (which is now slated to completely sequence the human genome by 2003) will significantly affect health care between now and 2010. The area of pharmacogenomics, for instance, should not only grow considerably in the next ten years, but during that time will likely start to have a demonstrable effect on health and health care.

New genetic knowledge and techniques will allow both more rational drug design and more rational drug use. In terms of drug design, genetics will provide new insights into the basic molecular pathophysiology of many disorders, thus allowing development of drugs that attack many disorders at an earlier and more vulnerable stage of their path toward the disease state. This will amount to treating the cause instead of a downstream consequence. In terms of drug use, the next decade should also witness the start of what promises to be a major change in how drugs are prescribed, using information from genes to individualize the use, and also, when needed, the avoidance, of specific drugs. It has long been obvious that many drugs have desired effects in only a portion of people who use them. Similarly, many drugs have undesired effects, sometimes even lethal ones, in only a portion of those who use them. While many factors contribute to both drug efficacy and toxicity, genetically determined drug metabolism is often the key influence. At present, clinicians are rarely able to individualize drug use through knowledge of a specific patient's genetic makeup, and instead usually must rely on a "trial-and-error" approach that may delay effective therapy for some time. Within the coming decade, however, the computer chip-based technology the forecast cites should enable clinicians to make informed decisions about which of several potentially useful drugs will be most efficacious for a given patient before prescribing, rather than much later. Furthermore, the ability to predict which individuals will suffer significant toxicity from a specific agent will broaden the clinician's armamentarium, by allowing use of pharmaceuticals now usually avoided because of serious side effects that may occur in only a small proportion of patients using them.

In considering key barriers, the forecast correctly draws attention to the need to educate health professionals if genetics is to have an optimal effect on health. However, it is not only the provider but also the patient who must be more knowledgeable for such success to occur. Moreover, since the "new genetics" spawned by the Human Genome Project will be of use in the care of virtually all individuals, rather than the relative few for whom genetics has thus far been clinically germane, there is a need to educate the entire population about genetics. This is especially true if this "cutting-edge" area of medicine is to benefit the entire population, rather than only those of certain socioeconomic and educational backgrounds.

The forecast properly emphasizes the promising area of gene therapy, but in doing so may suggest too strongly that it is through gene therapy that genetics will have its greatest effect on health. Especially in the coming decade, the greatest impact of genetics will come from DNA-based diagnostics and the opportunity it will begin to offer to indi-vidualize patient care, in terms of diagnosis, treatment, and prevention. This will allow each of us, in consultation with our health care providers, to use knowledge of our personal genetic disease predispositions to construct an individualized dietary, behavioral, and medication strategy to preserve health.

Indeed, as this application of genetics becomes real, it will help move medicine away from its present emphasis on treatment of morbid illness toward one of health preservation.

It is in the area of cancer that the Human Genome Project and the resultant "new genetics" will have their earliest large impact. However, in the coming decade, genetic medicine will also start to be a significant influence in many other areas, including cardiovascular and neuropsychiatric medicine. Indeed, genetics' impact will start to be so widespread as to become the proper, in fact necessary, purview not only of the specialist but also of the primary care provider.

LAURIE M. FLYNN

A New Image of Mental Health

Laurie M. Flynn is executive director of the National Alliance for the Mentally Ill.

No area of health care will see more change in the next decade than mental health. There are many reasons for this, as outlined in the forecast. Several of the factors driving health care broadly will have a special impact in mental health. The three biggest drivers of change are science and research, the information revolution, and consumerism.

SCIENCE AND RESEARCH

During the 1990s, the congressionally designated "Decade of the Brain," we saw a revolution in our understanding of mental disorders. Rapid advances in neuroscience have provided evidence that serious mental illnesses are brain disorders. Sophisticated electronic imaging techniques allow researchers to see into the living brain. Scientists are able to discern which areas of the brain are malfunctioning in specific illnesses, and we may soon be able to target treatments more effectively. More than a dozen new medications for serious mental illness were introduced in the 1990s and more are expected in the next decade. These new drugs are both more effective at treating symptoms and have fewer side effects.

Given that severe mental illness affects 5 percent of the population, this new understanding of the workings of the human brain—and medicine's improved ability to control the symptoms of mental illness—have profound implications. In the near term we will be able to treat severe depression, the most deadly mental disorder, more effectively, and perhaps reduce the rising suicide rate. More than 30,000 lives are lost each year to suicide, with the fastest rates of increase in the elderly. Better-targeted treatments and new medications will also help people who have schizophrenia—the most disabling and devastating mental illness. A new generation of antipsychotic drugs now offers real hope for improved outcomes for people with this illness, which is also the most frequent diagnosis among the homeless population.

With limited dollars in the health care system, the new science will help policymakers understand the difference between common mental health problems, such as stress, and serious brain disorders. Health insurance parity legislation in many states makes this distinction now, with equal insurance coverage mandated for schizophrenia, bipolar disorder, depression, and other severe illnesses for which ongoing medical treatment is vital. It is likely that there will be a move to recognize these and other chronic mental illnesses as part of physical medicine—and to include these diagnoses in "medical listings" in insurance policies.

As with all of health, treatment for mental disorders will be increasingly evidence based. Over the next few years, state and county mental health authorities will not reimburse treatment that cannot meet this important criterion. Thus, specific proven interventions, especially newer medications and research-based Assertive Community Treatment programs, will become the dominant modes of therapy. For many patients, a combination of medication and intensive community care will offer long-term stability for their conditions.

THE INFORMATION REVOLUTION

The information revolution, especially the rise of the Internet, will have a startling effect on the recognition and treatment of mental health problems. The Internet affords anonymity, which is still important given the stigma attached to mental disorders. Today consumers can access a wide range of information sites, with all manner of guidance on treatment options. Research results will become accessible as consumers go online to evaluate whether and where to get therapy. Confidential screening for possible symptoms of illness, online question-and-answer sessions with practitioners, and even psychotherapy online all are part of the future. Highly popular chat rooms already dominate mental health sites, which are among the most popular destinations on the Internet. Virtual support groups are forming as people with a wide array of issues and experiences help each other cope with mental illness. In the next decade, self-help will take a larger role in mental health services. Many of the functions of a traditional Employee Assistance Program will soon be offered more effectively and inexpensively via Web-based services. A major benefit of the openness and availability of this information will be a dramatic reduction in stigma. It will cost employers a little more to provide mental health treatment, but savings will accrue in the long run as productivity remains strong and disability associated with more severe illness is reduced.

CONSUMERISM

New psychiatric medications will be advertised directly to millions of potential customers, further changing the balance of power in the doctor-patient relationship. Pharmaceutical companies have demonstrated the strength of customer demand as a market force, and we can expect more and more aggressive advertising as new products come into a highly competitive market.

The increased focus on severe mental illness, driven by new treatments and insurance parity legislation, will push policymakers to deal with some tough issues. Concerns about protection of human subjects in research has already made headlines, as some ethical lapses become known. The National Bioethics Advisory Commission report will lead to attempts at more stringent regulations, and the resulting debate may slow the pace of clinical trials that lead to introduction of new medications. In the end, society should be able to accommo-date the need for stronger protections for vulnerable subjects and keep the pace of new research on track.

There are even thornier concerns about the persistence of homelessness and the random violence that are signs of a frag-mented and inadequate public mental health system. Spurred by a landmark Surgeon General's report on mental health, legislators will seek more accountability for the hundreds of mil-lions of dollars now supporting a failed public mental health system. Sustained pressure for improved and innovative community services and, in some cases, mandated treatment will help ease this public health crisis. The huge gap between what we *know* about mental ill-ness and what we *do* to help those with severe disorders will narrow. By the end of the decade, a new image of mental health will take hold, with a focus on early recognition, effective treatment, rehabilitation, and recovery for most patients. Mental health will be under-stood as an integral part of general health and essential to optimal function-ing and total well-being.

IRMA GODOY

My Story: One of 44 Million

Irma Godoy is an uninsured patient.

This is her legislative testimony.

I don't know anyone who has health insurance. At least, no adults in my family, nor any of my neighbors, have insurance. It's not that they don't work. All of my brothers, my father, and my husband work in construction, but they don't get health benefits. They wouldn't go to a doctor, anyway. If they ever miss a day of work, they'd risk not having a job to come back to.

I, on the other hand, have visited so many clinics that I've lost count. I sought prenatal care at a medical mobile unit that I saw parked in front of the local school. I climbed in and it felt like a boat. The nurse practitioner was very concerned about me, not because of the pregnancy but because of my thyroid. She referred me to the public hospital. That's when I got caught up in a tangle of clinics. They did so many tests, but I could never get a definitive answer. After the delivery, the baby had to stay in the hospital for a week. I would go every day and spend the day there. After a week, they released him. Then I had to have gallbladder surgery, which I didn't want.

But that wasn't the real problem. Apparently, there was something wrong with my thyroid. Scans, biopsies, and blood tests didn't show anything definite. We got so worried. You know it was bad, because I won't tell you what a sacrifice it was to scrape up the money for a private doctor. Every time that he could, my husband would give me money to put away. I used a coffee can on a shelf, in the closet, which coincidentally was next to a figurine of La Virgen de la Guadalupe. Once, my mother saw the coffee can and asked me about it. I told her it was for the medical tests. During the hurricane, I needed to borrow money out of the pot. When I put my hand in, there was a clove of garlic and a twig of *yerba buena* (peppermint). I laughed and cried at the same time. My mother had thought the can was an offering to the Virgin for a cure!

Not to say I didn't pray. I did. I desperately needed to know what was going on in my body. No doctor or nurse would ever explain what it was all about. I was embarrassed to take too much time, they seemed so busy. I don't know what was worse: the sickness in my body or the worrying about it. I was so upset that I became strange, not myself, arguing and crying without reason. I think it was the feeling of impotence and powerlessness. I would be so worried about dying and leaving my two children. This made my head pound, my heart ache, and my stomach feel like I had swallowed lead marbles. Thank God for my family. I don't know what would have happened if I were alone. I feel for those old people who are so lonely.

When we finally saved enough to go to a private doctor, he told me that I needed an operation, but, of course, we couldn't afford it. We tried an indigent care fund, but I didn't meet the requirements. I fell through the cracks. I went back to the mobile van not knowing where else to go. They then referred me to a free clinic, a trailer on the grounds of a church. I needed to bring the necessary paperwork to be accepted. I knew it would take a long time for an appointment there. But, really, I didn't have a choice, and I am so glad I found them. The doctor and her staff were angels. She said that we would start again and redo the studies and the blood work. They had a volunteer doctor who was a specialist, who cared for me for free. The whole ordeal took about two years. It was a sinister web and I felt like I was walking a tightrope. At 23 years old, uninsured, and with two babies, I finally got a diagnosis: thyroid cancer.

It's almost as if I had two lives, the one in Mexico and the one here. The one before being a mother. The one before being sick. I feel so young and the burden so heavy. But, even though I have a life-threatening illness, I feel lucky. Somehow I've been able to hold on to the life strings of a safety net, though sometimes if feels like a delicate thread. I know of others who haven't been blessed with the generous hearts of volunteer doctors and nurses. Those who haven't been able to access care, who postpone it, deny the pain, or cover the symptoms.

A neighborhood boy recently died of a burst appendix. I don't blame his parents. They had taken him to the hospital before and he had been released. They just hesitated a bit too long, thinking of the interminable debt. I know another woman who is diabetic but can't pay for her insulin, so she injects half the amount. Others get vitamin shots, hoping that will tide them over until they can get to the doctor. All of this seems strange in a great country where everything is in such abundance, so orderly and neatly planned.

CHARLES N. KAHN III

Health Insurance in America: A Future of Wild Cards

Charles N. Kahn III is president of the Health Insurance Association of America.

One of the most interesting trends in the health insurance market over the past two years has been the decline in the growth of HMO enrollment. This recent decline is relatively small, just a few percentage points of covered Americans, but contrasts the trend envisioned in the forecast. The Institute for the Future (IFTF) staff predicts a three-tier health insurance system with HMOs as the predominant form of coverage used by Americans. The forecasting business is tough in regard to health care coverage in this nation. However, the strength of the HMO model as the coverage product of preference appears to be waning, due to consumer demand for coverage with fewer restrictions on choice of providers and a growing regulatory aversion to aspects of managed care.

Further, key players in the health insurance market are now reluctant to associate their products with the HMO label. And, one company, United Healthcare Group, recently decided to cease precertification for most procedures or treatments, a move away from controls commonly used in HMOs as well as other managed care products. Part of the reason United Healthcare was able to make this change was that much of its business is already PPOs or indemnity.

In this case, the change in approach should lead to minor savings from spending and, more important, to a new challenge in the marketplace for others fielding more deeply managed coverage.

Besides the forecast concerning the nature of health insurance coverage in the United States, IFTF also examines the factors behind the growth in the number of uninsured Americans; the potential changing role of employers in financing insurance, particularly small businesses; and wild-card factors that could alter the future of health insurance.

THE UNINSURED

The number of uninsured is increasing faster than even projected in this forecast. The forecast assumes that 44 million Americans will be uninsured by 2002, yet current projections put the number of uninsured at that number today, in 2000. Two factors appear to be driving that number. First, welfare reform is reducing the Medicaid rolls. Second, coverage by small employers has been relatively static since 1996—although on the one hand, other employers have added to the number of insured Americans, while on the other, corporate restructuring is leaving many to fend for their own benefits as they become contractors rather than employees. These trends in insurance can be sustained by the system for some time, but eventually may be politically destabilizing, particularly if there is an economic downturn and insured middle-class citizens becomes anxious about their coverage.

ROLE OF EMPLOYERS

A case can be made that the models for insurance coverage may look different from those predicted, that the employer-based system is doing a better job of covering Americans than is described. Between 1993 and 1997, the number of Americans with employer coverage increased from *145* million to *152* million, and there is every reason to believe that trend will continue.

As IFTF points out, besides the elderly, disabled, and categorically indigent, most Americans receive their health coverage through employment. In the late 1980s and early 1990s, employers, in response to growing health care costs and a weak economy, demanded that insurers contain the growth of health insurance premiums paid for employees and their dependents. In response, many traditional health insurers, as well as a number of new players in the market, turned to managed care in the form of the HMO product as the coverage model of choice.

This generation of managed care products tended to limit choices of doctors and hospitals. And, despite the fact that HMOs turned out to have a good record on quality care, consumer anxiety and preferences have resulted in less restric-

tive forms of coverage becoming more popular and pervasive. Further, many physicians have become alienated from insurers in this new era of managed care, and they have fueled this consumer anxiety. Many HMO-centered companies have been compelled to offer products with out-of-network options, and the PPO is now the product of choice for many Americans and their premium-paying employers. This last point flies in the face of predictions that the PPO was a transitional product that would ultimately be replaced by closed-network HMOs.

WILD CARDS

The general future of the employer-based system of coverage and the private voluntary system in the United States could be significantly affected by certain wild cards described in the forecast. IFTF's wild cards illustrate the challenge to the current system from the political right, where an individualized system for purchasing insurance, based on some type of voucher for all or part of the premium payment, is espoused by key policymakers. On the left side of the political spectrum, there is not much talk of a single payer, government-run system, but there are potential factors that could undermine the current system and lead to a government takeover. On the other side, certain policymakers on the political right would like to see the United States move away from the employer-based system to one with individualized choice and taxpayer subsidy for coverage through income-related tax credits, rather than the current tax exclusion for employer-purchased premiums.

The single-payer alternative increases in likelihood if certain additional wild cards turn events in a problematic direction for the current private system, or turn to this idealized individual system. These wild cards are health care costs, which are driving premiums to double-digit increases this year; legislation at the federal level enabling health insurers and employers to be sued for punitive damages by consumers; and the class-action suits that challenge basic health plan management and payment policies. Continuous double-digit inflation in health care costs could make premiums unaffordable for many employers, and the class-action suits, if they are not thrown out by the courts, could threaten the viability of major companies in the health insurance market. The attorneys who have brought these class-action suits clearly intend to change the nature of the way insurance is provided in America.

The combination of these new wild cards and those in the forecast may determine the future of the nation's private health care system. However, at the end of the day, the major factors may be the insurance industry's ability to mold and refine managed care to build bridges to the physician community, which has become alienated from the carriers, and to reduce consumer anxiety about coverage—all while keeping cost growth within acceptable bounds for employers. The industry does not have an easy task in the decade to come.

MOLLY METTLER

That Patient Is Not Diabetes Case #115491 —She's Me

Molly Mettler is senior vice president of Healthwise, Inc.

"May you live in interesting times," was intoned by the ancient Chinese as a curse. According to the cultural dictates of the time, fortune smiled on those who lived and prospered in periods of stability, predictability, and calm. "Interesting times" implied just the opposite. Alas, the Institute for the Future forecasts "interesting times" in health and health care over the next decade. Perhaps, though, within the curse lies the seed of a blessing. However wild and bumpy the health care ride will be over the next ten years, we might see the emergence of a sane, centered, and effective system that will balance cost and quality by shifting power to the consumer.

Welcome to the world of consumer-centered care and to the most dramatic and fundamental shift of all: the consumer management of chronic disease. The blossoming of new consumer attitudes, the codification of evidence-based medicine, and the reach of the Internet are combining to turn the current-day practice of disease management upside down. These trends, all documented by the forecast, point to a future in which the majority of chronic illness care will be custom designed for and by each individual patient.

THE JUGGERNAUT OF CHRONIC ILLNESS

Why pick on disease management and chronic illness as ground zero for change? Because it's huge, it's costly, and it's accelerating. Consider this—by the year 2010:

- Some 120 million Americans, about 40 percent of the total population, will be living with a chronic illness. Of those, 40 percent will have at least two such conditions.

- The direct medical costs of chronic conditions in the United States will total $600 billion per year.

- The leading edge of the baby boomers will be hitting age 65, heralding a relentless influx of new chronic-care patients with each passing year.

This has all the makings of a crisis in care of enormous proportions. If we try to extend today's approach to chronic care, which is fragmented, system-centric, and non-empowering, the system simply will collapse. We can't train enough providers to meet the need. There is a widening gap, made even more apparent with the aging of the population, between the health care needs of the people and the medical remedies of the health care system.

SHORTCOMINGS OF THE CURRENT SYSTEM

The trend toward population management is helpful, but mass interventions for chronic disease will miss the mark. While myriad disease management programs are being introduced into the health arena, and providers and payers are jousting over who gets to develop the protocols and guidelines, the daily burden of the illness is borne by the patients and their families.

Current disease management materials and programs do not always meet the needs of the individual patients. Long on "shoulds" and short on acceptance of personal values and preferences, typical disease management becomes an issue of "managing patient compliance" rather than encouraging patient choice, involvement, and adherence. Simply preaching to a person with diabetes that he must lose weight, exercise, change his diet, take his medicine, and prick his finger once a day will most likely bring on nothing but depression and *ennui*. For payers and providers, it is an illness to be managed; for patients, it is part of the fabric of everyday life. Health care provider time for patient education and support is constrained in the office, and, for the most part, does not extend to the home, which is the 24/7 frontline of illness management. Finding a way to actively involve the patient as a member of the provider team will produce far more positive results.

WHAT'S A HEALTH CARE SYSTEM TO DO?

The consistent application of best practices for disease management is not a matter to be left to systems-thinkers,

statisticians, and clinical teams alone. Effective disease management will require full patient involvement and a strong, vital doctor-patient partnership.

Patient involvement is a given, as the forecast points out. More and more of us will expect and demand a formative role in so personal an issue. We'll want and expect highly personalized treatment interventions and support. We'll demand to see not the XYZ Guidelines for Asthma Management, but the Liz Jones Program for Asthma Management, the Bob Smith Plan for Living with Diabetes, and more. Luckily, the tools are there to support mass personalization. Evidence-based medicine, personal health assessments, information therapy, support groups, and much more are as close as a modem and a mouse. Voice recognition, virtual reality, videoconferencing, and interactive multimedia technologies will provide self-management tools never before imagined.

Diagnosis of chronic illness is a life-changing event for patients and their loved ones. Serious illness provides patients with an opportunity to move to a new level of health care empowerment, self-determination, and perhaps even a higher level of wellness and personal growth.

Health is such a profoundly personal thing: we, the consumers of health care, do not think of Diabetes Case #115491, we think of Mom, Dad, spouse, us. It makes sense for us to think through how we ourselves can become the ultimate managers of our own health. In order for all of us to survive and flourish, the health system needs to help us do that.

KENNETH I. SHINE

The Future Practice of Medicine

Kenneth I. Shine is president of the Institute of Medicine.

For an enterprise to account for one-seventh of the gross domestic product of the United States, while functioning in many ways as a cottage industry, is remarkable. As noted in the forecast, 40 percent of all office-based physicians still deliver care in individual or two-physician practices. It is only recently that any serious effort has been made to collect information about what works and what does not work in the everyday practice of medicine. Information systems, computer and telecommunications technologies that have revolutionized other aspects of life in America, have only barely begun to be applied effectively in health care. The computerized patient record functions superbly in some isolated parts of the health care system, yet many hospitals' information systems cannot communicate within a hospital, much less with other institutions.

The trends toward group practice are compelling and the progressive increase in employed physicians is important. These developments are crucial if information systems are to be effectively used not only to monitor quality of care, but also to collect fiscal and demographic data that would allow physician groups to negotiate contracts and to manage their revenue and expenses.

The Institute for the Future forecasts a slow transition from a world of independent entities to one of more corporate systems. The crucial challenge remains to maintain patient-oriented professionalism in the health care system. While a diverse set of corporate structures will persist, the best hope for professionalism is an increasing role of physician managers and corporate structures controlled by providers. Accomplishing such a goal will take determination, leadership, and capital.

The forecast assumes some acceleration in the rate of decrease of hospital beds to 2 percent per year, suggesting that beds will decline to something more than 670,000 in 2010 and that "hospital services will stabilize at approximately 32 percent of health spending after 2002." I suspect that these projections have the right direction, but underestimate velocity. The continued explosive growth of procedures that can be carried out in the ambulatory arena, improved techniques for shortening lengths of stay, and the increased recognition that it will take substantial rather than minimal, incremental steps to decrease the inventory of unused beds will accentuate these processes. Moreover, the progressive growth of expenditures for pharmaceuticals and devices will increase their share of the health care dollar at the expense of hospital and physician expenditures. Indeed, today in the Boston and New York areas, hospital expenditures are now in the range of 25 to 27 percent of the health care dollar. In-patient hospital beds will continue to play a smaller and smaller role in the overall health care system.

The roles of multidisciplinary group practice and ambulatory technology have only slowly been recognized by academic health centers. Many hospitals have continued to have positive financial results from in-patient services financed through Medicare, while losing money on Medicare services in the ambulatory arena. It does not make sense for hospitals to run physician offices as more and more patients are enrolled in Medicaid and Medicare managed care plans, the children's health insurance plan, and other strategies for covering the uninsured. Hospitals that do not have convenient, efficient, cost-effective ambulatory services will lose these patients to sites and physicians who can meet patient needs and demands. The separation of outpatient services so that they are managed by faculty practice plans, which are responsible for revenue and expenses, and are equally responsible for quality of care and patient satisfaction, will increase the effectiveness of these services. Moreover, any rational use of government monies for graduate medical education will require that the significant portion of these funds be put in the care of the faculty who are educating students and residents in the ambulatory arena.

Although local politics, particularly as related to employment, will continue to make true consolidation of hospitals difficult, these changes are inevitable. Cost-containment efforts place great strain on the cross-subsidy for education and research in academic health centers, but medical faculties have been extremely slow to accept that academic health centers must be operated efficiently and cost effectively. The lack of accurate cost accounting, which has only recently been introduced in some academic medical centers, has made discussion of cross-subsidies abstract and unreliable.

A number of funding options are discussed in the forecast analysis. The progressive decline in the proportion of care provided through the fee-for-service mechanism is inevitable. Not only are the incentives wrong in the fee-for-service system, but the system encourages an increase in volume in order to make up for any decrease in price—well exemplified by experiences in the Canadian province of Ontario. It is likely that a blended reimbursement system, which includes both capitation and a variety of reinsured risk reimbursements, is likely to emerge for the health care system in general, including Medicare. Through capitation, physicians and other providers have incentives to provide preventive services and cost-effective primary care. Through some form of risk-based reimbursement, providers can be insured against catastrophic illnesses and reduce the impact of high-cost diagnoses. Due to a growing surplus of physicians, especially specialists, physician incomes increasingly will decline; this is well documented now in California and Minnesota. But if groups of providers can learn to manage their practices, capitation can dramatically reduce the amount of nonmedical administrative interference and oversight.

Three additional wild-card items should be emphasized. First, serious increases in insurance coverage for the uninsured would have a major impact on the health care system. This will have a salutary effect in reducing uncompensated care and could decrease many of the problems associated with adverse selection, privacy, and related system problems. It will not necessarily help academic health centers, which are likely to lose significant numbers of individuals covered by Medicaid managed care, and by other insurance plans if patients have an option to go to more user-friendly environments. This is an important reason for improving accessibility and convenience, as well as quality of care, for all patients seeking ambulatory services at academic health centers. Second, a serious financial recession, prolonged for more than a year or two, could dramatically accelerate change in all aspects of the health care system, as the number of uninsured rise, corporate profits fall, and unemployment increases. Individual practice associations have

emerged as the most rapidly growing organizational strategy over the past several years. They reflect physicians' desires for autonomy and patients' desires for choice. But they remain inefficient and ultimately will have to be modified. The notion that an individual physician accepts patients from multiple managed care organizations restricts the interests of any one organization to invest in information systems or to develop systems for quality of care.

This forecast states that "although patients will be involved in all stages . . . most of the action will be driven externally by employers, governments, and health insurers." This may underestimate the growing importance of consumerism in the United States and the potential for real partnerships to emerge between providers and patients. Physicians should welcome such partnerships as a way to enlist the public's help in dealing with the monoliths in the insurance and managed care industry. This would require some real sharing of information and responsibility, but it is another important wild card in forecasting the future.

GAIL L. WARDEN

Challenges and Opportunities in Seeking a Balanced Health System

Gail L. Warden is president and CEO of Henry Ford Health System.

When the Institute for the Future made its ten-year forecast for health care providers, it was correct in its prediction that continued organizational change, a changing role of intermediaries, a potential oversupply of hospital beds and physicians, and a struggle over control of medical management will be major issues facing all provider organizations. The major factor that the ten-year forecast did not anticipate was the impact of the Balanced Budget Act on the health care delivery system. The Balanced Budget Act severely limited resources. It forced important choices by health care organizations about the services they could afford. It brought about a rationalization of services, more consolidation of organizations, and an increased emphasis on productivity. Consequently, the landscape began to change. As it changes, challenges and opportunities present themselves in the following areas.

UPWARD COST PRESSURES

It is clear that upward cost pressures in health care are here to stay. Overall spending will increase as the population ages, as the demand for leading-edge technology and pharmaceutical innovations continues, and as we book the cost

of the transition to Year 2000 information technology standardization.

DEMAND FOR EFFICIENCY AND PRODUCTIVITY

The demand for efficiency and productivity is also increasing as providers are forced to do more with fewer resources, and as they realize that some of the mergers and joint ventures of the early and mid 1990s have not achieved the savings that were expected or intended. Further, providers' market share of patients has not grown as expected, and the leverage for improvement of services has been difficult.

MANAGED CARE

Managed care has continued to grow and in doing so has had an effect on cost and quality. Despite the HMO backlash, most consumers and employers like managed care, and as was predicted, the government purchasers are moving Medicaid and Medicare beneficiaries into managed care programs. Care management continues to be a challenge, but the goals are sound: to ensure quality and appropriateness of care, to address utilization opportunities, to provide accountability, and to enhance the opportunities for managing risk. Most organizations are giving priority to preadmission screening, consolidated pharmacy cost-management strategies, disease-specific utilization management, coordination of benefits, and health plan contract reviews.

THE VOICE OF CONSUMERS

The voice of consumers has put them in charge, as we see increased demand for provider and insurer responsiveness and a greater focus on patient satisfaction, especially in an encounter with the health care system. The demand for alternative or complementary medicine and a strong emphasis on choice also seem to be recurring themes.

INFORMATION TECHNOLOGY

Information technology is driving the future of provider organizations, and in the long run, the use of information technology through automated medical records and the Internet may be as important as the introduction of antibiotics in the 1940s.

COMPETITION BASED ON QUALITY

Health care providers and insurers are competing on quality, and quality has become a differentiating factor for purchasers. A greater emphasis and investment is being placed on quality measurement and reporting through the establishment of the National Forum on Quality Measurement and Reporting. Further, evidence-based medicine is becoming the gold standard for patient care.

HEALTH CARE AS A COMMODITY

Health care has become a commodity, and as such, we see spot buying of expensive procedures, carve-out companies specializing in highly profitable product lines and disease management, and virtual systems built by linking carved-out services.

PERSONNEL SHORTAGE

The greatest resource constraint in the future will be the shortage of personnel. There is a serious nurse shortage across the country, particularly in bachelor of science graduates and nurse practitioners. More physicians, particularly young physicians, are migrating to group practices. Within those group practices there continues to be unrest about the fact that physicians feel they've lost their autonomy, their income-earning potential is flat, and they suffer the burdens of managed care. In some cases this physician unrest is leading to threats of unionization, and even the American Medical Association is supporting such a movement.

THE PURCHASERS PREVAIL

While the power of the private and governmental purchaser continues to prevail, we see a number of changes. Group health care purchases are expanding. Purchasers are leading the way and creating a more informed consumer. Performance measures are more specific and publicly reported. Value-based health care is coming into its own as the emphasis changes from providing sick care toward maintaining health status, disease prevention, and productivity of the workforce.

THE FUTURE

The future, as of the beginning of the millennium, appears to be one in which we will have collaborative networks of providers, payers, and purchasers; well-informed consumers making decisions based upon empirical data; and an organized continuum of care that is virtually linked with high quality and efficiency across episodes of illness and pathways to wellness.

Provider organizations of the future will become financially and organizationally lean, customer driven, and community focused. They will use a series of relationship-building and model-redesign strategies that enhance horizontal and vertical integration. They will focus on product differentiation and improving core processes, and will continue to recognize the importance of community benefit by partnering with community organizations to meet local health care needs.

H. DENMAN SCOTT

Public Health Services: A Challenging Future

H. Denman Scott is director of the Brown Center for Primary Care and Prevention and is Physician-in-Chief of the Department of Medicine, Memorial Hospital of Rhode Island

The report gives a gloomy assessment of public health over the past thirty years and predicts that "public health will continue to be under funded and marginalized." Many public health departments have been overwhelmed by demand for personal health services from the growing millions of uninsured. It is highly probable that this stress on public health will continue over the next decade. As difficult as this problem is, there is a more rosy perspective in the domain of disease prevention and health promotion. Consider these five examples.

■ Over the past thirty years morbidity and mortality from heart disease has steadily declined by almost fifty percent as a result of healthier life styles, treatment of hypertension and elevated cholesterol, and effective treatment of disease once expressed. Much remains to be done and the next decade should see further improvements.

■ Vaccine preventable diseases have virtually disappeared. Newer vaccines such as H. influenzae B have been widely deployed to all population groups because of federal support for vaccine purchase and the diligent efforts of local health departments to reach all vulnerable children. There are still opportunities for improve-

ment, but public health at all levels should be proud of accomplishments in this area.

■ Unintentional injuries and gun violence have been redefined as public health issues thanks to the leadership of many public health professionals. These leaders have influenced policy and designed programs that have and are reducing morbidity and mortality. The next decade should see much more progress.

■ Since the publication in the mid-1960s of the first Surgeon General's report on smoking and health when almost half of Americans smoked cigarettes, millions of Americans have quit and millions more have chosen never to take up the habit. We still have much to do with a national smoking rate of 25 percent. In the next decade other states would do well to emulate programs California, Minnesota, and Utah where the smoking rates have fallen to about 18 percent in the California and Minnesota, and to just over 13 percent in Utah.

■ HIV/AIDS has evoked a massive national effort over the past eighteen years. Remarkable advances in prevention and treatment have occurred.

Persistent, painstaking work over the next decade may give us the ultimate solution to this scourge-a safe, effective vaccine.

The U.S. Surgeon General recently released Healthy People 2010, a document that outlines goals for several hundred public health problems. As its predecessors have, this new compilation will focus the attention of Congress, state legislatures, and local elected officials on an array of possibilities. The document is a superb example of public health assessment and will play a key role in policy development at all levels of government. What actually occurs over the next ten years will reflect the politics and priorities of our communities and our nation. Public health professionals in large numbers will have essential roles in bringing expertise and evidence to these debates.

THE IDENTITY OF PUBLIC HEALTH

The report correctly notes the confusion among the public about the definition of public health. On the one hand, the definition embraces myriad dimensions, many risk factors, and involves numerous interest groups. On the other hand, many people construe public health as narrowly focused on the poor. However, individuals do relate and react to an outbreak of meningitis in their schools or pesticide contamination of their drinking water. Moreover, they are impressed when a health department manages these threats with skill and dispatch. Once concluded, these episodes recede from the public's mind and are replaced by other concerns. The challenge is how to

keep the mission and goals of public health before the people on a regular basis. Over the next ten years those responsible for enunciating the mission of public health would be well advised to employ frequently the tools of social marketing to define in concrete terms the goals of public health. The future image of public health may remain a bit fuzzy, but social marketing can make it much sharper than it is today.

PUBLIC HEALTH AND PRIVATE MEDICINE

In many communities the local health department has become the provider of medical services for those who cannot afford a private physician or for those whom a private physician will not see. The typical scenario depicts a wide gulf between the public health clinic and the private practitioners office.

There is another important scenario emerging in many communities, one of remarkable collaboration between public health and the private sector. In one version public health nurses, employed by the local health department, are working with private physicians. The nurses perform medical screening and case management services which permit the doctors to see patients in their offices-patients whose social and economic problems would ordinarily overwhelm the office staff's capacity to deal with them. In another version public health clinics are working with groups of medical and surgical specialists, and dentists to provide services either in their clinics or in the doctor's office. The participating physicians and dentists either volunteer their services or accept reduced fees. These arrangements are helping to solve the long-standing problem of obtaining specialty services for the patients of the public health clinics.

Local leadership inspires and sustains these programs. Leaders in medicine, public health, dentistry, hospitals, health insurance companies, and local elected officials have in various combinations come together to create thriving programs that benefit the health of several hundred to several thousand individuals. They do not solve the massive problem of access to care for the underserved and uninsured, but they make important contributions in community after community.

As this decade proceeds, it is unlikely that some form of universal insurance will come about. The health needs of the uninsured are with us this year, and will

continue each year for the foreseeable future. It is, therefore, necessary that local communities without functional public private coalitions be encouraged to learn about and emulate the communities with well-developed programs.

OTHER THEMES

World population mobility, environmental hazards in food, water, and air, the definition of the human genome, and information technology are complex themes discussed in the report. They will surely impact public health, but to what extent is difficult to predict. Not mentioned in the report but worthy of note is the threat of bioterrorism. These areas all require regular scrutiny and periodic assessment to take advantage of opportunities to improve public health and to avoid policies deleterious to our health or our our liberties

KEVIN B. PIPER

Health Care Purchasing in 2010

*Kevin B. Piper is director of
the National Health Care
Purchasing Institute and vice
president of the Academy for
Health Services Research and
Health Policy.*

The Institute for the Future performed
an outstanding service by laying out a
road map for the future of health and
health care in America. By anticipating
the future transformations of health and
health care, we are better positioned to
influence the nature and consequences of
change.

However, there was a notable omission
from the Institute's forecasts: the future
of health care purchasing by public and
private employers and public programs
like Medicare and Medicaid. Purchasers,
particularly leading Fortune 500 companies like General Motors and General
Electric, are actively leveraging their
market power to improve quality of care.
They are leading the way for what will
be a dramatic transformation of health
care purchasing over the coming decade.

FORECAST

To help address the lack of a forecast for
health care purchasing in the Institute's
excellent report, the following describes
two major forecasts for the increasingly
influential world of purchasing:

HEALTH CARE PURCHASING AS A
MANAGEMENT DISCIPLINE

At its core, health care purchasing is
about an economic exchange of value,
denominated in cost and quality. Health

care purchasing—as a strategy, policy
set, and management discipline—is the
cornerstone of major public and private
sector efforts to improve the performance
of America's health care system.

As a strategy, health care purchasing is
about leveraging the economic power of
purchasers to generate greater value for
the dollar invested in care. The purchaser's policy set of contract specifications, performance measures and
standards, and beneficiary education
reflects a new performance-oriented paradigm. As a management discipline,
health care purchasing is all about the
effective deployment of incentives, systems, and techniques to achieve direct
accountability of health plans and
providers for their substantive results,
clinical and financial.

Most purchasers instinctively understand
the strategic intent of the results-driven
approach, despite lingering challenges in
conceptualization and execution for some
traditional, regulatory-oriented purchasers. Further, many organizations are
actively embracing the basic policy set of
results or value-based purchasing in their
managed care contracting. However,
health care purchasing's greatest promise
resides in its development as a unique
management discipline, an equal in rigor
to the traditional corporate disciplines of
finance, human resources, and marketing.

For a number of reasons, health care purchasing is steadily evolving as a management discipline. First, the participants, whether in the public or private sector, share a common set of core values centered on maximizing the clinical and financial performance of the health care system for the joint benefit of beneficiaries and stockholders or taxpayers. Second, purchasing executives perform a separate, distinct, and increasingly complex managerial function requiring planning, direction, organization, control, execution, and evaluation—the hallmarks of any management discipline. Finally, health care purchasing is further defined by its reliance on a unique knowledge base and skill set. This knowledge base and skill set—distinct from health care purchasing's sister disciplines of finance and human resources— is built upon a number of other areas, including business and public administration, economics, human resources, business law, decision theory, actuarial science, and information technology.

By 2010, health care purchasing will be readily accepted as a management discipline in its own right, with a significant impact on the provision of health care to employees and public program beneficiaries. The impact of this professionalization process will be felt through greater acceptance and wider use of value-based purchasing tools to drive quality improvements at the health plan and provider levels. These tools will include:

- Incentives—financial and non-financial—to reward the higher performing plans and providers, including targeted results-based payments, increased patient volume, and marketplace recognition.

- Patient safety standards to save the lives of employees and beneficiaries.

- Practices to empower and directly incentivize consumers to choose higher quality health plans and providers.

THREE TIERS OF HEALTH CARE PURCHASING

By 2010, the world of health care purchasing will be roughly divided in three parts:

- Active purchasers of health care

- Passive purchasers of health care

- Defined contributors

The active purchasers of health care, which will include many Fortune 500 companies and some state Medicaid programs, will engage in value-based purchasing using the tools described above. While they will represent only a segment of the total marketplace, each is a multi-billion dollar purchaser and will greatly determine the baseline of contracts, tools, and practices used by other employers and government agencies. They will serve as the knowledge leaders and standard barriers for the buying of health care in America.

The passive purchasers will still function largely as payors of health care, albeit through premium-based health plans. Most employers, particularly small and mid-sized companies, will not try to actively leverage their buying power to affect outcomes. However, as health care purchasing advances as a management discipline with a refined toolset, these passive purchasers will increasingly follow the lead of their active colleagues in such areas as performance standards and patient safety protections. The real unknown here is whether the federal Medicare program, the nation's largest buyer of health services, will continue to be a passive payor or ultimately evolve into an active purchaser. Necessity would say yes, while history and politics would say no.

The final tier—and potentially the largest segment—will be employers using the defined contribution approach to paying for employee health care. If patient rights legislation creates liability for purchasers, defined contribution will become commonplace. While fraught with complications, the defined contribution approach still affords some opportunity for leveraged buying. For example, employers could still use performance standards to pre-qualify available plans. In addition, it has the potential of bringing consumers back into the purchasing process. However, the positive impact of defined contributions, if any, will be highly dependent on the continued engagement of employers as purchasers and the underlying decision support systems made available to consumers.

DAVID LANSKY

Health & Health Care 2010 Commentary—Consumer Power as a "Wild Card"

The forecast at once excites us about the possibilities for biomedical breakthroughs and reminds us of our historic failure to use medical technology appropriately, equitably, and humanistically. While today's consumers are seeking new health care arrangements consistent with an "expanded view of health"—alternative providers, self-care resources, support groups, web sites, and health media, and today's experts are noting an array of demographic, cultural, and environmental shifts that seem to cry out for new forms of health care delivery, the dominant health care systems respond with only trivial changes.

As we look at the decade ahead, is there any reason to think that the professions and managers who control our $1.2 trillion health system will undertake fundamental redesign of that system? Will sudden insights, or the maturing of a newer generation of physician leaders, or the oscillations in Federal health financing create an environment that facilitates reallocation of health care resources to optimize health? We can appreciate the richness and subtlety of the forecast, but ultimately wonder: what will it take to materially change our health system?

In the 1990s, it was widely thought that a market-based health system would focus on quality care when group purchasers used their clout to demand population health improvements. But the experience has been disappointing. It turns out that public sector purchasers are constrained by intensely political factors and private sector purchasers lack market mass, are fearful of interfering in employee-provider relationships, and have not resolved the tension between their roles as population health managers and as agents of individual needs.

In the past decade, it has become commonplace to observe that medical care has a small influence on human health. Why, then, do we spend 15% of our national wealth on it? As the number of uninsured climb and the quality deficiencies of our system become more evident, it may be time for a more probing re-thinking of the role of the institutional health care system in our society.

The next decade may witness many interesting experiments and improvement initiatives, but it is not primarily about improving systems of care or introducing breakthrough medical technology. It will be primarily about shifting the power to decide *what's important* from our historic medical leadership to the public itself. Alas, there is only one unequivocal stakeholder for the quality of health care—and it's the one you see when you look at a frail parent, a sick child, or in the mirror. A meaningful transfer of power to consumers will be difficult and complex, but it's essential to the proper organization of health care in a democratic society.

In one wave of health care "reform" after another, various large institutions have wrestled for control over the allocation of health care resources—dueling each other for the right to extend their particular paternalism over the judgment of the patient and family. Should the doctor decide what's right for the patient? No, the health plan should decide. No, the employer should decide. No, the government should decide. In what other area of life would we cede our personal ability to make vital decisions to our employer or an expert—our housing, our children's education, our food?

In hundreds of focus groups, surveys, and interviews we have found that ordinary Americans—particularly those who need vital health care services—are able to articulate their needs in a complex and balanced way. But in equal measure, we hear that they cynically question the health system's interest in meeting those needs and feel powerless to alter the behavior of this vast, impenetrable array of institutions. Nothing in the behavior of the medical professions, the government, the insurance industry, or the private employers gives American consumers confidence that their health needs will be met. Where, then, should we look for the energy and focus that could allow the health system to become

centered on the patient and embrace a more complete picture of health?

Consumer action—both organized and personal—is the necessary prerequisite to the reengineering of our health care system. For group and individual consumer action to succeed, several transitions must occur.

- Increasing numbers of Americans must see their doctor as a partner and advocate, rather than an omniscient and unbiased healer.

- Consumers must amplify their personal decisions, by telling their stories to each other, to the media, to their children, and to their health care providers.

- Consumers must have the ability to direct their health care dollars to the services and service providers that they value.

- Consumers must learn about and embrace the moral implications of their own health care decisions, and understand the interdependency of all of us in managing financial and health risks.

- Consumers must develop a policy agenda that facilitates system reengineering. They must ask their political parties and representatives to permit innovators to reallocate health dollars where they do the most good.

- Physicians and other health professionals must support their patients' interest in taking more responsibility for health and health care decisions.

Some of these trends will occur without the say-so of any politician, doctor, or employer—just because they are intrinsic to modern society. But others won't happen until there is sufficient, focused public pressure to permit the millions of well-intentioned health care providers and policy leaders to "do the right thing". Existing consumer organizations—unions, advocates, service agencies—will need to add support of this movement to their portfolio of activities, or perhaps a new organization will emerge to channel the public's anxiety about healthcare. The "wild card" of the next decade may be the massed demand of consumers to take back their health care from the system that has been so unresponsive.

Glossary

Listed below are brief explanations of common health care terms used in this forecast. Many of these glossary terms and resource citations are taken from the Public Health and Health Care Administration Glossary of Terms Web page of the University of Washington (http://weber.u.washington.edu/~hserv/hsic/resource/glossary.html).

ACADEMIC MEDICAL CENTER (AMC)

A group of related institutions including a teaching hospital or hospitals, a medical school and its affiliated faculty practice plan, and other health professional schools.

ADJUSTED AVERAGE PER CAPITA COST (AAPCC)

A county-level estimate of the average cost incurred by Medicare for each beneficiary in the FFS system. Adjustments are made so that the AAPCC represents the level of spending that would occur if each county contained the same mix of beneficiaries. Medicare pays health plans 95 percent of the AAPCC, adjusted for the characteristics of the enrollees in each plan. See also Medicare Risk Contract.

AID TO FAMILIES WITH DEPENDENT CHILDREN (AFDC) PROGRAM

A federally financed program for single-parent families, designed to provide welfare for single parents who cannot, without assistance, take proper care of their children.

AMBULATORY CARE

Medical services provided on an outpatient (nonhospital) basis. Services may include diagnosis, treatment, surgery, and rehabilitation.

BENEFIT PACKAGE

Services covered by a health insurance plan and the financial terms of such coverage, including cost sharing and limitations on amounts of services.

CAPITATION

A method of paying health care providers or insurers in which a fixed amount is paid per enrollee to cover a defined set of services over a specified period, regardless of actual services provided.

CASE MANAGEMENT

Monitoring and coordinating the delivery of health services for individual patients to enhance care and manage costs; often used for patients with specific diagnoses or who require high-cost or extensive health care services.

CASE MIX

The mix of patients treated within a particular institutional setting, such as the hospital. Patient classification systems like DRGs can be used to measure the hospital case mix.

COPAYMENT

A fixed amount of money paid by a health care plan enrollee (beneficiary) at the time of service. The health plan pays the remainder of the charge directly to the provider. This is a method of cost sharing between the enrollee and the plan and serves as an incentive for the enrollee to use health care resources wisely.

DEDUCTIBLE

The amount of money an insured person must pay "at the front end" before the insurer will pay. The reason for introducing this concept into health care coverage is primarily to discourage unnecessary use of services, and also to reduce insurance premiums, as all claims have a minimum amount that the insurer will be spared on every claim.

DIAGNOSIS-RELATED GROUP (DRG)

A hospital patient classification system developed at Yale University. The current payment system for Medicare is based on the federal government's setting a predetermined price for the "package of care" in the hospital (exclusive of physician's fees) required for each DRG. If the hospital can provide the care for less than the DRG price, it can keep the difference; if the care costs the hospital more than the price, the hospital has to absorb the difference. Originally each DRG was intended to contain patients who were roughly the same kind of patient in a medical sense and who spent about the same amount of time in the hospital. The groupings were subsequently redefined so that, in addition to medical similarity, resource consumption was approximately the same within a given group.

DIRECT CONTRACTING

Direct contracting usually refers to a service (e.g., substance abuse treatment) that an employer contracts directly to save money on its employees' health plan, leaving employees free to choose among other eligible providers for their primary, obstetric, pediatric, and other medical care needs.

DISPROPORTIONATE SHARE HOSPITAL (DSH)

A Medicare term for a hospital serving a higher than average proportion of low-income patients.

ENROLLEE

A person who is covered by health insurance.

ERISA

The Employee Retirement Income Security Act. ERISA exempts self-insured health plans from state laws governing health insurance, including contribution to risk pools, prohibitions against disease discrimination, and other state health reforms.

FEE-FOR-SERVICE (FFS)

A method of paying the provider whatever fee he or she charges on completion of a specific service.

GATEKEEPER

The person responsible for determining the services to be provided to a patient and coordinating the provision of the appropriate care. The purposes of the gatekeeper's function are (1) to improve the quality of care by considering the whole patient, that is, all the patient's problems and other relevant factors; (2) to ensure that all necessary care is obtained; and (3) to reduce unnecessary care and cost. When, as is often the case, the gatekeeper is a physician, she or he is a primary care physician and usually must, except in an emergency, give the first level of care to the patient before the patient is permitted to be seen by a specialist

GRADUATE MEDICAL EDUCATION (GME)

The period of medical training that follows graduation from medical school, commonly referred to as internship, residency, and fellowship training.

GROSS DOMESTIC PRODUCT (GDP)

The total current market value of all goods and services produced domestically during a given period; differs from the gross national product by excluding net income that residents earn abroad.

GROUP-MODEL HMO

An HMO that pays a medical group a negotiated, per capita rate, which the group distributes among its physicians, often under a salaried arrangement.

HEALTH CARE PROVIDER

An individual or institution that provides direct medical services (e.g., physician, hospital, laboratory). This term should not be confused with an insurance company, which "provides" insurance.

HEALTH PLAN EMPLOYER DATA AND INFORMATION SET (HEDIS)

A set of standardized measures of health plan performance. HEDIS permits comparisons between plans on quality, access and patient satisfaction, membership and utilization, financial information, and health plan management.

HEALTH INSURANCE

Insurance that covers the patient for health care, including physician and hospital services.

HEALTH INSURANCE PURCHASING COOPERATIVE (HIPC)

A local board created under managed competition to enroll individuals, collect and distribute premiums, and enforce the rules that manage the competition.

HEALTH MAINTENANCE ORGANIZATION (HMO)

A managed care plan that integrates financing and delivery of a comprehensive set of health care services to an enrolled population. HMOs may contract with, directly employ, or own participating health care providers. Enrollees are usually required to choose from among these providers and, in return, have limited copayments. Providers may be paid through capitation, salary, per diem, or prenegotiated FFS rates.

HEALTH PLAN

An organization that acts as an insurer for an enrolled population.

INDEPENDENT PRACTICE ASSOCIATION (IPA)

An HMO that contracts with individual physicians or small physician groups to provide services to HMO enrollees at a negotiated per capita or FFS rate. Physicians maintain their own offices and can contract with other HMOs and see other FFS patients.

MANAGED CARE

Any system of health payment or delivery arrangements where the plan attempts to control or coordinate use of health services by its enrolled members in order to contain health expenditures, improve quality, or both. Arrangements often involve a defined delivery system of providers with some form of contractual arrangement with the plan.

MEDICAID

A state/federal health benefit program for the poor who are aged, blind, disabled, or members of families with dependent children. Each state sets its own eligibility standards.

MEDICAL LOSS RATIO

The ratio of benefits paid out to premiums collected for a particular type of insurance policy. Low loss ratios indicate that a small proportion of premium dollars were paid out in benefits, while high loss ratios indicate that a high percentage of the premium dollars were paid out as benefits.

MEDICAL SAVINGS ACCOUNT (MSA)

A health insurance option consisting of a high-deductible insurance policy and a tax-advantaged savings account. Individuals would pay for their own health care up to the annual deductible by withdrawing from the savings account or paying out of pocket. The insurance policy would pay for most or all costs of covered services once the deductible is met.

MEDICARE

The federal health benefit program for the elderly and disabled that covers 35 million Americans or about 14 percent of the population for an annual cost of over $120 billion.

MEDICARE RISK CONTRACT

A contract between Medicare and a health plan under which the plan receives monthly capitated payments to provide Medicare-covered services for enrollees and thereby assumes insurance risk for those enrollees. A plan is eligible for a risk contract if it is a federally qualified HMO or a competitive medical plan.

MEDIGAP INSURANCE

Privately purchased individual or group health insurance policies designed to supplement Medicare coverage. Benefits may include payment of Medicare deductibles and coinsurance and balance bills, as well as payment for services not covered by Medicare. Medigap insurance must conform to one of ten federally standardized benefit packages.

MORBIDITY

A measure of disease incidence or prevalence in a given population, location, or other grouping of interest.

MORTALITY

A measure of deaths in a given population, location, or other grouping of interest.

NATIONAL HEALTH EXPENDITURES (NHE)

Total spending on health services, prescription and over-the-counter drugs and products, nursing home care, insurance costs, public health spending, and health research and construction.

NETWORK-MODEL HMO

An HMO that contracts with several different medical groups, often at a capitated rate. Groups may use different methods to pay their physicians.

OUT-OF-POCKET EXPENSE

Payments made by an individual for medical services. These may include direct payments to providers as well as payments for deductibles and coinsurance for covered services, for services not covered by the plan, for provider charges in excess of the plan's limits, and for enrollee premium payments.

OUTCOME

The result of a medical intervention on a patient.

PART A MEDICARE

Medical Hospital Insurance (HI) under Part A of Title XVIII of the Social Security Act, which covers beneficiaries for inpatient hospital, home health, hospice, and limited SNF services. Beneficiaries are responsible for deductibles and copayments.

PART B MEDICARE

Medicare Supplementary Medical Insurance (SMI) under Part B of Title XVII of the Social Security Act, which covers Medicare beneficiaries for physician services, medical supplies, and other outpatient treatment. Beneficiaries are responsible for monthly premiums, copayments, deductibles, and balance billing.

PARTIAL CAPITATION

An insurance arrangement where the payment made to a health plan is a combination of a capitated premium and payment based on actual use of services; the proportions specified for these components determine the insurance risk faced by the plan.

PER DIEM PAYMENTS

Fixed daily payments that do not vary with the level of services used by the patient. This method generally is used to pay institutional providers, such as hospitals and nursing facilities.

PERSONAL HEALTH CARE EXPENDITURES

These are outlays for goods and services related directly to patient care.

POINT-OF-SERVICE (POS) PLAN

A health plan with a network of providers whose services are available to enrollees at a lower cost than the services of nonnetwork providers. POS enrollees must receive authorization from a primary care physician in order to use network services. POS plans typically do not pay for out-of-network referrals for primary care services.

PRACTICE GUIDELINE

An explicit statement of what is known and believed about the benefits, risks, and costs of particular courses of medical action, intended to assist decisions by practitioners, patients, and others about appropriate health care for specific clinical conditions.

PREFERRED PROVIDER ORGANIZATION (PPO)

A health plan with a network of providers whose services are available to enrollees at lower cost than the services of nonnetwork providers. PPO enrollees may self-refer to any network provider at any time.

PREPAID GROUP PRACTICE PLAN

A plan in which specified health services are rendered by participating physicians to an enrolled group of persons, with a fixed periodic payment made in advance by or on behalf of each person or family. An HMO is an example of a prepaid group practice plan.

PRIMARY CARE

Primary care is the provision of integrated, accessible health care services by clinicians who are accountable for addressing a large majority of personal health care needs, developing a sustained partnership with patients, and practicing in the context of family and community.

PRIMARY CARE CASE MANAGEMENT (PCCM)

A Medicaid managed care program in which an eligible individual may use services only with authorization from his or her assigned primary care provider. That provider is responsible for locating, coordinating, and monitoring all primary and other medical services for enrollees.

PROSPECTIVE PAYMENT

A method of paying health care providers in which rates are established in advance. Providers are paid these rates regardless of the costs they actually incur.

PUBLIC HEALTH

Activities that society does collectively to ensure conditions in which people can be healthy. This includes organized community efforts to prevent, identify, preempt, and counter threats to the public's health.

RELATIVE VALUE SCALE (RVS)

An index that assigns weights to each medical service. The weights represent the relative amount to be paid for each service. The RVS used in the development of the Medicare Fee Schedule consists of three cost components: physician work, practice expense, and malpractice expense.

RESOURCE-BASED RELATIVE VALUE SCALE (RBRVS)

A relative value scale that is based on the resources involved in providing a service.

RISK ADJUSTMENT

Increases or reductions in the amount of payment made to a health plan on behalf of a group of enrollees to compensate for health care expenditures that are expected to be higher or lower than average.

RISK SELECTION

Enrollment choices made by health plans or enrollees on the basis of perceived risk relative to the premium to be paid.

SINGLE-SPECIALTY GROUP PRACTICE

Physicians in the same specialty pool their expenses, income, and offices.

SKILLED NURSING FACILITY (SNF)

An institution that has a transfer agreement with one or more hospitals, provides primarily inpatient skilled nursing care and rehabilitative services, and meets other specific certification requirements.

SOLO PRACTICE

A physician who practices alone or with others but does not pool income or expenses.

STAFF-MODEL HMO

An HMO in which physicians practice solely as employees of the HMO and usually are paid a salary.

SUPPLEMENTAL INSURANCE

Any private health insurance plan held by a Medicare beneficiary, including Medigap policies and postretirement health benefits.

SUPPLEMENTAL MEDICAL INSURANCE (SMI)

The part of Medicare through which persons entitled to Part A Medicare, the Hospital Insurance Program, may obtain assistance with payment for physician's services, diagnostic tests, and other outpatient services. Individuals participate voluntarily through enrollment and the payment of a monthly fee.

TERTIARY CARE

Care of a highly technical and specialized nature, provided in a medical center—usually one affiliated with a university—for patients with unusually severe, complex, or unusual disorders. Tertiary care is the highest level of care.

TERTIARY CARE CENTER

A large medical institution, usually a teaching hospital, that provides highly specialized care.

THIRD-PARTY PAYER

An organization, private or public, that pays for or insures at least some of the health care expenses of its beneficiaries. Third-party payers include commercial health insurers, Medicare, and Medicaid.

UNDERWRITING

The process by which an insurer determines whether and on what basis it will accept an application for insurance. Some insurers use medical underwriting to exclude individuals, groups, or coverage for certain health conditions that are expected to incur high costs.

UTILIZATION REVIEW (UR)

The review of services delivered by a health care provider to evaluate the appropriateness, necessity, and quality of the prescribed services. The review can be performed on a prospective, concurrent, or retrospective basis.

Index

International medical students (IMGs), 95, 96, 226

International Recording Media Association, 136

Internet, 8, 50, 52, 55, 58, 137, 140, 143, 144, 196, 199, 205–206, 306

Interstudy, 5

J

Johns Hopkins University, 80, 241

Johnson, L. B., 166

Journal of the American Medical Association, 225, 281, 312

K

Kaiser Family Foundation/Health Research and Educational Trust, 39, 48, 57, 240

Kaiser Permanente, 38, 69, 309

Kennedy-Kassebaum Act, 71, 139

Knickman, J. R., 280

Kuhn, T., 345

L

Labor markets, 38

Laparoscopy, 118–119

Lasker, R., 166

Leapfrog Group, 54, 57

Legislation, 1–2

Leung, A., 232

Licensed practical nurses (LPNs), 103, 266, 267

Licensed vocational nurses (LVNs), 266, 267

Little, J. S., 37

Long-term care (LTC), 221, 254, 266, 267–270

Los Angeles, 20, 39, 171, 176, 236

Louis Harris & Associates, 98, 136

Lovelace Health System (New Mexico), 79, 309

M

Magnetic resonance imaging (MRI) technology, 115, 117, 119, 193

Magnetic resonance technology (MRN), 115

Managed behavioral health organizations (MBHOs), 213, 214

Managed care: and cost consequences of regulation, 51–52; drivers, 49–51; as experiments in reinvention, 47–64; forecast, 54–60; issues, 47–49; and patterns of power, 60–63; and potential

barriers to information technology implementation, 52–54; and public health, 183–184

Management services organization (MSO), 80

Mannino, D. M., 172

Manton, K., 262

Marijuana, 313, 314

Market dynamics, 28–29

Massachusetts, 74–75, 342

McEwen, B., 341

McGinnis, J. M., 312

M.D. Anderson Cancer Center, 79

Measles, 113, 170

Med Partners, 59

MedCath, 79

Medicaid, 4, 12, 25–33, 41, 68, 71, 151–153, 166, 178, 221–225, 243

Medical management, 8; background to, 82; battle over control of, 68; for the chronically sick, 83–84; issues in, 82–83; and medical managers, 102

Medical technologies, 6–7; and advances in imaging, 114–117; and artificial blood, 128–129; and disease management, 306–307; and gene therapy, 123–126; and genetic mapping and testing, 120–123; and minimally invasive surgery, 117–120; and rational drug design, 112–113; and stem cell technologies, 131–133; and vaccines, 126–128; and xenotransplantation, 129–131

Medicare, 2, 4, 11–13, 25–33, 40–41, 67, 68, 71, 84, 153, 155, 166, 178; Catastrophic Coverage Act (1988), 223; drug benefit, 272–273; GME, 86, 88, 91, 101; PSN legislation, 88; Trust Fund, 271

Medicine and Public Health: The Power of Collaboration (Lasker), 166

Medscape, 52

Mental disease, 113

Mental health: challenges in, 187–189; economic and social costs of, 193; and incarceration, 193; most common disorders in, 191; parity for, 187; and prevalence and impact of mental illness, 190; priorities for public spending in, 190–193; public versus private spending in, 192; social implications of, 200

Scenario 1: Stormy Weather

★ Spending growth 2.5% above nominal GDP

★ Managed care fails to contain costs or improve quality

★ MD/consumer backlash

★ Gaming and adverse selection in Medicare choice

★ Hospital oligopolies sustain high prices

★ Large employers pay up; small ones drop insurance benefits

★ New medical technologies are costly and in high demand

★ IT systems costly and ineffective

★ No social consensus on limiting end-of-life spending

★ Safety net in tatters

➡ NHE 19% of GDP $10,200 per capita

➡ 65 million uninsured; 22% of Americans

➡ 60% of Americans worried about security of benefits

➡ Radical tiering of access and care

➡ Several major public hospitals go under

➡ Spending on Medicaid overwhelms state budget

➡ Baby boomers hit Medicare unprepared— meltdown

Scenario 2: The Long and Winding Road

★ Spending growth 1% above nominal GDP

★ Benefit cuts drive out-of-pocket costs up; utilization down

★ Employees keep pressure on plans

★ Continued "hassling" and rate pressure by plans

★ Limited adoption of organizational innovation

★ Government limits Medicare and Medicaid expenditures

★ Turbulent unorganized change

★ Open competition

➡ NHE 16% of GDP $8,600 per capita

➡ 47 million uninsured; 16% of Americans

➡ Continued 3 tiers of health care

➡ Safety net muddles through as usual

➡ Fragmented delivery of individual care

➡ No major policy reform in health care

Scenario 3: The Sunny Side of the Street

★ Spending growth 1% above nominal GDP

★ Competition among providers drives prices down

★ Efficient health care organizations emerge from wave of consolidation

★ Steady cost pressure closes hospital beds

★ Public/private partnerships

★ Effective risk adjustment for Medicare risk

★ Prospective payment works for ambulatory care

★ Willing and able PSNs

★ Clinical information technology improves care processes and outcomes

★ Cost-effective medical technologies adopted

➡ NHE 15% of GDP $8,100 per capita

➡ 30 million uninsured; 10% of Americans

➡ System well-equipped to absorb baby boomers after 2010

➡ Population and alternative preventive services prevail

➡ Best practices minimize practice variation

➡ Tiers of care by amenities, access, quality

➡ Medicare and private plans reward population management

2010

HEALTH AND HEALTH CARE THROUGH 20

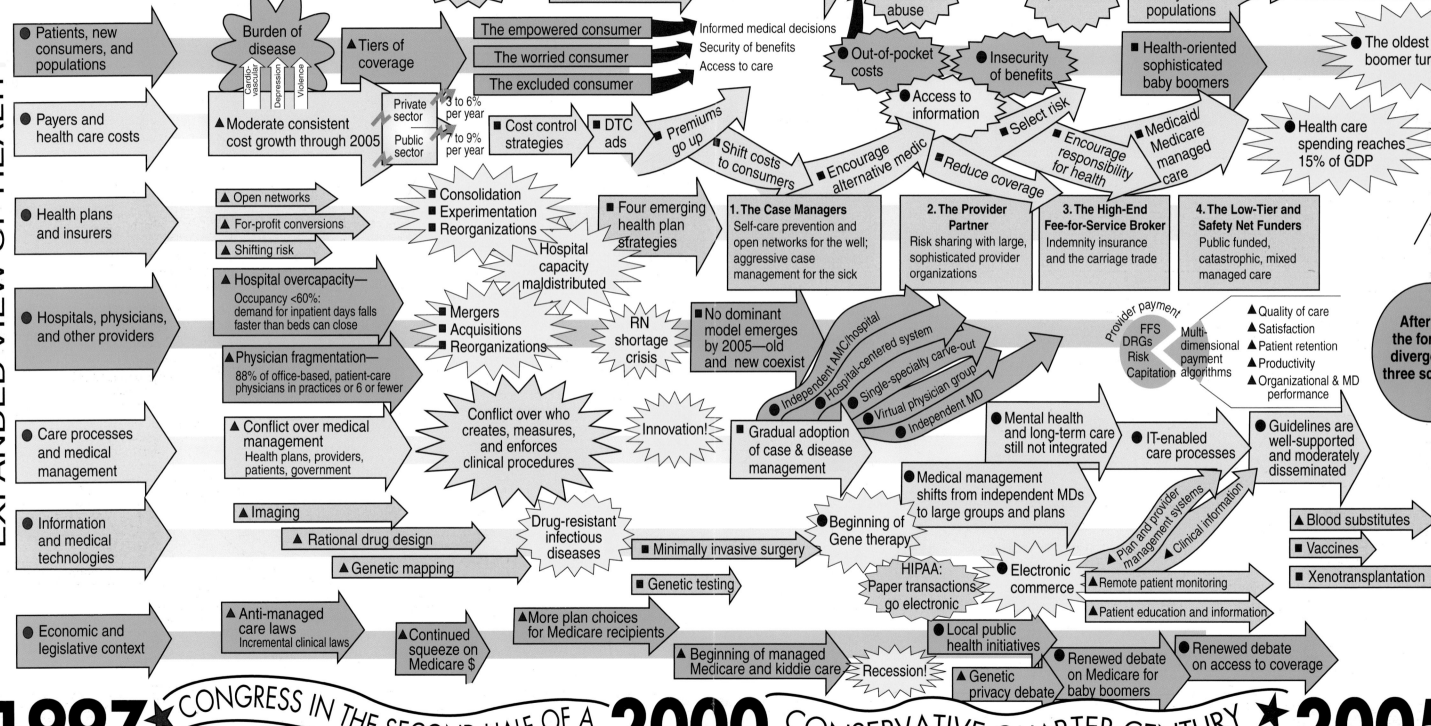